Linguistics in Clinical Practice
Second Edition

Linguistics in Clinical Practice

Second Edition

Kim Grundy

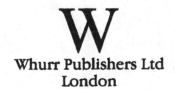

Whurr Publishers Ltd
London

© 1995 Whurr Publishers Ltd
First published 1989 by Taylor & Francis
Second edition published 1995 by
Whurr Publishers Ltd
19b Compton Terrace, London N1 2UN, England

Reprinted 1998, 2001, 2004 and 2005

British Library Cataloguing-in-Publication Data
A catalogue record for this book is available from the
British Library.

ISBN 1-897635-52-4

Contents

Chapter 14   329
Developmental Speech Disorders
Kim Grundy and Anne Harding

Chapter 15   358
Acquired Neurogenic Speech Disorders: Applying Linguistics to Treatment
Niklas Miller and Gerry Docherty

Index   385

Preface to First Edition

The introduction of linguistics to speech therapy courses has been relatively recent, and in this short time linguistics has come to have a profound influence on the approach to assessment, diagnosis and management of individuals with communication disorders. Although there are many excellent books available which introduce the subject of linguistics, these tend to have a theoretical rather than practical bias and newcomers to the subject may experience difficulty in linking theory with practice. This text has been written by practising clinicians and researchers actively involved with language disabled individuals and so offers a different perspective on the subject by specifically relating each of the relevant areas of linguistics to communication disorders likely to be encountered by clinicians. Further, although this is an edited volume, it is unusual in that the aim from the start has been to produce a textbook and not a series of related papers. Contributors have therefore collaborated with one another, often reading each other's drafts, in an endeavour to ensure that the chapters within the book form a cohesive whole.

The book is divided into three sections. Section I provides an introduction to the fields of linguistics and phonetics. Chapter 1 examines the nature of language, explains the fundamental distinction between speech and language and discusses issues surrounding the question 'How do children acquire language?' Chapter 2 defines many of the linguistic and phonetic terms likely to be encountered in clinical work and also serves as a glossary for the following chapters. The terms defined are specifically related to aspects of clinical work.

Each chapter in Section II takes one area of linguistics, discusses the purpose and value of assessing that aspect of an individual's linguistic ability and evaluates currently available assessment procedures. Several themes recur throughout this text and one of these is that although different aspects or 'levels' of language may be identified for the purposes of linguistic analysis, it is not always easy to separate these levels when evaluating an individual's linguistic capabilities. Thus, many of the chapters in Section II interrelate. Evershed Martin's and Grunwell's chapters consider the evaluation of disordered speech, the former from a phonetic perspective and the latter from a linguistic perspective. Both authors acknowledge the significant overlap between these two aspects of assessment. Garman examines the evaluation of syntactic aspects of expressive language and points out that such assessment cannot be satisfactorily under taken without considering the influence of phonological, semantic and pragmatic factors. Similarly, Dewart indicates that the influence of semantic and pragmatic variables cannot be ignored when evaluating an individual's understanding of syntactic structures. Landells suggests that one of the reasons why semantic assessment has been relatively neglected in speech pathology is the fact that all levels of language contribute to meaning and thus semantics is, perhaps, the most difficult aspect to isolate. McTear and Conti-Ramsden discuss the applications of recent developments in pragmatic theory and point to the many paralinguistic and non-linguistic variables which need to be considered when evaluating an individual's use of language. Brewster evaluates the role of prosodic aspects of speech production and indicates that while disrupted prosody may reduce an individual's ability to convey meaning, undisturbed prosodic features may actually be used to compensate for breakdown at other language levels. Section II closes with Myers' chapter which provides an overview of language assessment in the United States and she, too, suggests that current trends lead towards an evaluation of the interactions between different language levels.

The five chapters in Section III evaluate the role of linguistics and phonetics in the diagnosis and management of individuals with speech and language disorders. The issue of interactions between different levels of language is also taken up by these authors. Myers and Conti-Ramsden, for instance, both discuss the effects of 'over loading' the linguistic system; Myers in the context of children with dysfluent speech and Conti-Ramsden in the context of children with developmental language disorders. Both authors suggest that children with these types of language disorder may have difficulty in integrating all levels of language and that when linguistic demands upon them are too high, communication breakdown occurs. Ross provides a comprehensive overview of the linguistic description of acquired aphasia and relates this to the localizational model. Miller examines the relation between phonetic and linguistic aspects of speech production in the context of individuals with acquired speech disorders and Grundy points out that while it is important to separate these two levels in the diagnosis of developmental speech disorders, management often requires co-occurrent attention to both. All five chapters illustrate the value of linguistic and/or phonetic knowledge in the preparation of therapy programmes and offer practical guidelines for treatment.

A consensus of opinion has also emerged with regard to the classification of speech and language disorders. It becomes clear when reading these chapters that the current trend is turning away from group classification and towards individual assessment and diagnosis. That is, blanket labels such as 'expressive language disorder' are not particularly useful to clinicians who need to identify the precise features of each individual's speech/language disabilities in order that they may plan appropriate and effective, individually-tailored therapeutic programmes. All authors point out that linguistic/phonetic data alone do not provide a sufficient basis for such programmes and that clinicians draw on many sources of information during the management process. Linguistic skill is just one part of the individual's ability to communicate effectively and cannot be viewed in isolation from, for example, social, motor and cognitive skills. Conti Ramsden suggests that clinicians are, perhaps, in the unique situation of being the one person with access to *all* the different threads of information and that their role in bringing these together to form a complete picture is highly important and one that should be developed. Several of the chapters further suggest that it is inappropriate to approach language assessment and remediation by considering the individual with the language disorder only. Communication involves, at least, two people, and evaluation and therapy should, therefore, avoid focusing purely on the speech/language behaviour of the individual with the disorder, and should consider the effects of the communicative situation, listener response and so on. Another point raised is that, to date, the majority of research has concentrated on establishing profiles of development for the linguistically 'normal' population and that language-handicapped individuals may acquire language in a significantly different manner. This is not to undermine the value of such profiles, but to suggest that a useful direction of future research might be to investigate language acquisition in the language-handicapped population.

By providing an introduction to the fields of linguistics and phonetics with specific reference to speech/language disorders and with little assumption of pre-knowledge on the part of the reader, this text will be of particular value to student speech therapists. It also provides a useful focus of reference for those clinicians, who trained prior to the introduction of linguistics on speech therapy courses, and for other professionals working with language-disordered individuals, whose training included little in the way of linguistic study. Further, clinicians who have decided to specialize, or change their area of specialism, will find the chapters in Sections II and III particularly useful.

Kim Grundy
July, 1988

Preface to Second Edition

When I accepted Colin Whurr's invitation to produce a second edition of this volume, my view of my assignment was to ensure that each chapter was updated in the light of recent research and current clinical practice. Having now completed the task, I feel that something more has been achieved. What we have here is a collection of 'state-of-the-art' papers which manages to maintain cohesion within the overall framework of the book. Many more changes have been made than I anticipated at the outset.

Section I has been retitled *Fundamentals of Linguistics for Clinicians* to indicate its intention to provide a limited introduction to the field of linguistics as it applies to clinical work. Chapter 1 offers a historical overview of the development of the linguistic study of language and draws attention to those aspects of linguistic theory that have particular relevance for clinical work. In the light of many recently published texts in the field of language acquisition it seemed appropriate to reduce the section on language acquisition and direct the reader to this comprehensive coverage of the area. The second half of Chapter 1 now focuses on the contributions of linguistics to clinical work and sets the scene for the rest of the book. The presentation of chapter 2 has been modified for clarity and a list of suggested additional reading is offered at the end.

Section II has also been retitled. *Linguistics and Assessment of Speech and Language Impairment* gives a clearer indication that speech as well as language impairments are addressed in this section. In the first edition, an aspect of speech and language assessment was not included. This omission has been rectified by the addition of a chapter on *Assessment of Speech Perception*. Each chapter in this section addresses current issues relating to assessment of a specific area of speech/language production and/or reception. Section III has a new title *The Role of Linguistics in the Management of Clients with Speech and Language Impairments* which reflects the aim of each chapter in this section to exemplify the role of linguistics in the broad context of client management.

As in the first edition, there are several clear themes which recur.

Interestingly, in this edition there is no clear dividing line between themes which recur in Section II chapters and those which emerge in Section III chapters. All chapters reflect a more holistic approach to clients with speech and language impairments which is prevalent in current clinical practice. The significance of interactions between linguistic levels and the difficulties and potential dangers in attempting to maintain a separation of linguistic levels is evident throughout. The increasing influence of pragmatics in all aspects of clinical work is clearly indicated in all chapters. The emerging influence of psycholinguistics and cognitive neuropsychology is evident in Chapters 6, 7, 8 11 and 15.

It was important to me that contributors felt able to reflect what they consider to be the most significant advances and important issues in their particular linguistic or clinical area. Thus, some chapters focus mainly on discussion of selected pertinent issues while others have a greater emphasis on evaluation of specific assessments or treatment approaches.

I hope that this text will be helpful to the student speech and language therapist trying to understand the complexities of speech and language impairment. I anticipate that it will also be utilised by working clinicians and clinical researchers as an informative reference text.

Kim Grundy
May 1995

Acknowledgements to Second Edition

I would like to thank all contributors to the first edition for their willingness to revise their chapters, and the new contributors to this edition who have who have each added a fresh dimension to the book. Each chapter bears witness to the commitment of all contributors to present current, specialist knowledge within a cohesive and accessible framework.

Without the practical and moral support of my colleagues at De Montfort University, it feels unlikely that this edition would have been completed prior to the millenium! I would particularly like to thank Pamela Grunwell for her sage advice and generous help. Thanks to Colin Whurr for his patience and to the Whurr Publishing Team for their courtesy and efficiency.

To Terence and Elizabeth Davies, thank you for all your support and a quiet haven to work in; and to Ralph and Margaret Grundy, your understanding and consistent encouragement have helped me through some low points.

To Geoff, Maxine and Toby Campion, I couldn't have done what I did without you doing what you did. Thank you all.

Contributors

Catherine Adams
Centre for Audiology, Education of the Deaf and Speech Pathology
School of Education
The University of Manchester
Oxford Road
Manchester
M13 9PL

Kevin Baker
Department of Human Communication
De Montfort University
Scraptoft Campus
Scraptoft Leicester
LE7 9SU

Gina Conti-Ramsden
Centre for Educational Needs
School of Education
University of Manchester
Manchester
M13 9PL

Hazel Dewart
Division of Psychology
University of Westminster
309 Regent Street
London
W1R 8AL

Gerry Docherty
Department of Speech
University of Newcastle upon Tyne
Queen Victoria Road
Newcastle upon Tyne NE1 7RU

Susan Edwards
Department of Linguistic Science
University of Reading
Whiteknights
P O Box 218
Reading RG6 2AA

Susanna Evershed Martin
Department of Clinical Communication Studies
The City University
Northampton Square
London EC1V OHB

Michael Garman
Department of Linguistic Science
University of Reading
Whiteknights
P O Box 218
Reading RG6 2AA

Kim Grundy
Department of Human Communication
De Montfort University
Scraptoft Campus
Scraptoft
Leicester
LE7 9SU

Pamela Grunwell
Department of Human Communication
De Montfort University
Scraptoft Campus
Scraptoft
Leicester
LE7 9SU

Anne Harding
Department of Human Communication
De Montfort University
Scraptoft Campus
Scraptoft
Leicester
LE7 9SU

Allen Hirson
Department of Clinical Communication Studies
City University
Northampton Square
London EC1V OHB

Jenny Landells
Calderdale Healthcare (NHS Trust)
Speech and Language Unit
Clover Hill Annexe
Clover Hill Road
Halifax
HX1 2YP

Mike McTear
Department of Information Systems
University of Ulster
Newtownabbey
BT37 OQB
Northern Ireland

Nik Miller
Department of Speech
University of Newcastle upon Tyne
Queen Victoria Road
Newcastle upon Tyne NE1 7RU

Florence Myers
Department of Communicative Sciences and Disorders
Adelphi University
Garden City
Long Island
New York 11530
USA

Susan Peppé
Department of Human Communication Science
University College London
Chandler House
2 Wakefield Street
London WC1N 1PG

Alison Ross
Faculty of Health and Social Care
Leeds Metropolitan University
Calverley Street
Leeds
LS1 3HE

Maggie Vance
Department of Human Communication Science
University College London
Chandler House
2 Wakefield Street
London WC1N 1PG

Bill Wells
Department of Human Communication Science
University College London
Chandler House
2 Wakefield Street
London WC1N 1PG

Section I

Fundamentals of
linguistics for clinicians

Chapter 1
Introduction

KIM GRUNDY

What is Linguistics?

The above question may be answered by stating that linguistics is *the scientific study of language*. However, this definition begs two more questions: 'What is meant by scientific study?' and 'What is language?'. *Scientific study* can be taken to mean systematic and objective investigation of a clearly identified subject (for further discussion on linguistic science see Crystal, 1981). Thus, if linguistics is to be considered a scientific discipline its subject-matter – language – must be clearly delineated. The first part of this chapter is, therefore, mainly concerned with identifying language. Having identified the subject-matter of linguistics, discussion will then turn to identifying the contributions linguistics has made to clinical practice.

To people who have not undertaken any linguistic study, the question 'What is language?' may appear somewhat unnecessary because most people would consider that they know what language is. However, *knowing* that something exists and being able to use it is not the same as knowing its composition or how it works. We know what a telephone is and how to use one, but I doubt whether most people would consider that they know exactly how it works, or whether, if it stopped working, they could fix it. In some respects, language may be compared to a telephone. Each may be seen as a tool which is used for communication. We can readily accept that in order to correct a fault in the telecommunication system, telephone engineers must undergo extensive training; so too, must professionals concerned with remediating faults in the language system. Both must learn about the component parts of the communication system with which they are concerned, how each part interconnects with every other part and how the entire system works as an integrated whole. Training in anatomy, physiology and neurology provides the speech and language therapist with an understanding of the 'mechanics' of language; that is, how humans use their anatomical equipment to convey language to one another. Speech pathology combined with these

3

subjects provides knowledge of the ways in which anatomical, physiological and/or neurological impairment prevents humans from conveying language. Psychology and sociology contribute to our understanding of why human beings communicate and the different ways in which they do so. However, these subjects do not tell us *what* is being conveyed; what language is. Linguistics provides the final component to the system of human communication by addressing this fundamental question.

What is Language?

Ferdinand de Saussure (1857–1913) made the first major contribution to our current understanding of what language is and he is widely recognised as the founder of modern linguistics. He challenged the premises on which 'traditional' language study was based and created the framework within which twentieth-century linguistics has made its achievements.

In 1957, Noam Chomsky published a short volume entitled *Syntactic Structures* which is said by many to have revolutionised the linguistic study of language. The impact of Chomsky's theories was so great that some aspects of Saussure's theories were forgotten in the Chomskian revolution. The theories of Saussure and Chomsky are not entirely incompatible, however, and both concepts of language have profound implications for the remediation of language disabilities.

Saussure: His Theory of Language

Saussure insisted that to get at the true subject-matter of linguistics – language – it is necessary to adopt the point of view of the user and consider the act of spoken communication. This act will involve at least two people: speaker and listener. The speaker has an idea (or concept) which triggers in the brain a *sound pattern*. 'Sound pattern' is the term used by Saussure but it is important to appreciate that this term does not mean spoken sound. Spoken sound involves movement of speech organs (tongue, lips, larynx, etc.) and can be heard by a listener. Sound pattern can perhaps best be understood by considering what occurs when conducting a conversation or reciting some poetry 'in one's head'. When engaged in either of these activities, one *thinks* words but does not actually say them. Saussure uses the term 'sound pattern' to refer to words when they are in this 'think-state'. The association of concept and sound pattern can therefore be seen to occur within the brain and, as such, is a *psychological* phenomenon.

Concept having triggered sound pattern, the association centre in the brain then sends impulses to the speech organs and the speaker utters the appropriate word. This second stage, involving brain, nerves, chemicals and muscles, is *physiological*. Once the word has been uttered, a

speech sound-wave travels through the air, a purely *physical* occurrence, until it meets the ear of the listener. Then the same process occurs
in reverse. The speech sound-wave is received by the ear and transmitted, via nerves, to the brain (physiological). The sound pattern thus acti-
vated in the listener's brain then triggers the appropriate concept
(psychological). At this stage the listener may choose to respond to the
message, in which case the whole cycle is started again. This cycle Saussure termed the *speech circuit* (see Figure 1.1).

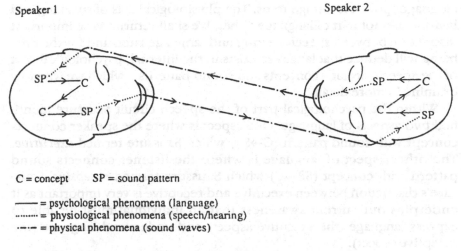

C = concept   SP = sound pattern

———— = psychological phenomena (language)
·········· = physiological phenomena (speech/hearing)
·—·— = physical phenomena (sound waves)

Figure 1.1 Diagrammatic representation of the speech circuit

Saussure did not claim this representation of spoken communication
to be complete. In speech pathology, for example, we are concerned
with the actual muscle movements involved in speaking, the way in
which the ear actually responds to sound and so on. (For a detailed
discussion of the phenomena and processes involved in the speech
circuit the reader is referred to Denes and Pinson, 1993). However, the
essence of this model is the clear distinction it makes between:

  (a) psychological phenomena: concepts and sound patterns;
  (b) physiological phenomena: speaking and hearing; and
  (c) physical phenomena: speech sound waves.

In addition, Saussure further divided the circuit into:

  (i)   an external part (sound waves travelling from mouth to ear) and
        an internal part (all the rest);
  (ii) a psychological part (a), and a non-psychological part (b) and (c);
  (iii) an active part – everything which goes from the association centre

of the speaker to the ear of the listener; and a passive part – everything which goes from the ear of the listener to his or her own association centre in the brain.

These initial distinctions provide the crucial basis for understanding what language is and, in turn, what linguistic study came to be concerned with. The physical phenomena, speech sound-waves, are not part of language. This may be easily appreciated when we think about listening to a language with which we are unfamiliar: we can hear the speech sound-waves but we cannot make any sense of them because the language spoken is foreign to us. The physiological acts of speaking and hearing are not part of language either. We shall return to the important distinction between speech/hearing and language later, and for the time being will deduce that language exists in the internal, psychological part of the speech circuit – concepts and sound patterns – which we will now examine in more detail.

Within the psychological part of the speech circuit Saussure identified two aspects of language. One aspect is where the speaker connects concept with sound pattern (C→SP) which Saussure termed *executive*. The other aspect of language is where the listener connects sound pattern with concept (SP→C) which Saussure termed *receptive*. Saussure's distinction between executive and receptive is very important as it underpins our current awareness that an individual must be able to express language (the executive aspect) and understand language (the receptive aspect).

The combination of *concept* and *sound pattern* Saussure called the 'linguistic sign'. He asserted that the notion of the linguistic sign, and the facts which surround it, are fundamental to understanding the true nature of language. These issues offer considerable insight for anyone concerned with language-impaired individuals, and their relevance will be discussed as they are explained.

1. The Two Parts of the Linguistic Sign Are Inseparable

Saussure uses the analogy of two sides of a piece of paper: 'we cannot cut one side without cutting the other also' (Saussure, 1916, translated by Harris, 1983, p. 157). In theoretical consideration it is, of course, possible to separate out concept and sound pattern. One can, for example, see a chair and be aware that *chair* is the sound pattern which matches this concept, but, for language to work, the two parts are inseparable. If we wish to convey the concept *movable, four-legged seat with a rest for the back* (OED) quickly and economically, in English, we must use the sound pattern *chair*. The inseparability of the two is evident in the fact that we do not consciously make the connection. For individuals with a language impairment, language does *not* work and the notion of the linguistic sign leads us to consider the possibility that some people may experience difficulty in learning or maintaining the *whole* sign. If such is the case we will want to ask: do they *know* the concepts of their language but have difficulty in matching sound patterns to them? Or do they not fully appreciate the concepts to which the sound patterns of their language are matched? Either case may be compared to attempting to clap with only one hand. In practice, clinicians will encounter people who have either or both of these difficulties.

2. Both Parts of the Linguistic Sign Are Totally Arbitrary

Arbitrariness of sound patterns is relatively easy to appreciate. There is no reason why, in English, an apple, for example, should not be known as an *apfel, pomme, mela* or even a *smugnot*, it just so happens that in English 'apple' is the sound pattern which matches the concept *round, firm, fleshy fruit of the Rosaceous tree* (OED). If we accept the fact that sound patterns are totally arbitrary, the nature of the problem for children who confuse opposite terms, for instance, is more easily appreciated. The concepts hot and cold, for example, exist as two ends of a heat continuum. The fact that, in English, *hot* is the sound pattern which matches the 'plus heat' end of the continuum and *cold* the sound pattern which matches 'minus heat' is a product of chance or accident. (In Italian, for example, *caldo* is the sound pattern for hot.) It is understandable therefore, that one of the difficulties which language-impaied individuals may experience is maintaining a spontaneous connection between each concept and its corresponding sound pattern.

Arbitrariness of concepts is more difficult to appreciate, though no less important. We have seen that there is no intrinsic link between a sound pattern and its corresponding concept (although it may be argued that onomatopoeic words, such as *slurp, plop, wuf*, might be seen as an exception to this). There is also no intrinsic reason for acknowledging the existence of a concept and for assigning a sound pattern to it in the first place. This fact becomes apparent when we consider translation from one language to another. If languages had a one-to-one correspondence of concepts, then translation would simply involve the exchange of one sound pattern for another and reorganisation of word order. The case is, however, that we often come across words of one language which have no direct translation in another. Comparison of English and Welsh colour systems provides an interesting illustration of this point. In English, part of the colour spectrum is divided and labelled *green, blue, grey, brown*. In Welsh, this same part of the spectrum is only divided into three sections labelled *gwyrdd, glas, llwyd*.

Another commonly used illustration of the arbitrariness of concepts is the fact that in English there is one linguistic sign *snow* whereas Eskimos have twelve different linguistic signs for snow. This may be because snow holds more significance for Eskimos than for English people and thus they are more attuned to noticing the fine variations of its substance which we do not necessarily notice. Each linguistic community divides 'reality' in its own unique way. English has two terms, *river* and *stream*. River and stream are differentiated on the basis of size: rivers are bigger than streams. French has the two terms *rivière* and *fleuve*. A *fleuve* is not necessarily bigger than a *rivière* but it flows into the sea whereas a *rivière* does not.

Conversing with someone who has a different native tongue to one's own results, on occasions, in one person saying 'oh, how do you say...'. Sometimes these uncertainties are resolved because the individual is searching for a sound pattern from the other language which can be readily provided by the listener. For example, 'what do you call those metal things attached to the wall with water in, which heat the room?' – 'radiators' – 'yes, that's it, well the radiator in my room is broken.' In other instances the uncertainty is not satisfactorily resolved and results in the foreign-language speaker saying 'well, that's sort of what it means but not quite' because there is not commonality of concepts. For example, in Afrikaans there is a phrase *skop skiet en donder* which literally translated means *kick, shoot and thunder*. The phrase is used to apply to a genre of films which are action-packed, fast-moving and violent. In English we can find words to attempt to identify the concept *skop skiet en donder* but we do not have a phrase which instantly conveys that concept to another person. In other words, the specific concept conveyed by the phrase *skop skiet en donder* does not exist in English.

This discussion of arbitrariness of concepts may seem somewhat laboured but it is considered to be extremely pertinent to the work of the speech and language therapist. For those of us who, by fortune, had no difficulty in acquiring our language, it takes a good deal of reflective thought to acknowledge that the conceptual divisions of our language are, indeed, arbitrary and socially created. It is suggested here that, if we are to appreciate fully the nature of the difficulties of language-impaired people, we must reflect on the possibility that they may not share the same conceptual perceptions as ourselves. The linguistic signs that we use may seem 'natural' or 'logical' to us, but how does the world look to a child, or to an adult with brain damage? What are their perceptions of time, space, touch, taste, colour, emotion, quantity, quality...? In some cases, individuals with a language impairment do not simply have difficulty in learning and/or remembering words (or sound patterns) but also have a different appreciation of concepts. Thus, language therapy may involve the teaching of concepts using practical, experiential methods at the same time as teaching sound patterns.

3. Linguistic Signs Do Not Exist in Isolation but Are Part of a System

Each sign has its place in an interrelated network of other signs and it is from this system that each sign gains its meaning. A commonly used illustration of this point is the system of colour terms. In English, *red* has meaning only in the context of the other terms in the colour spectrum. It is that colour which is not blue, yellow, orange, green and so on. In order to assimilate the full value of red the whole colour spectrum must be appreciated. In the absence of the rest of the colour terms, then, *red* has no meaning at all. This notion has profound implications for speech and language therapists and, indeed, anyone involved in language teaching. Jonathan Culler (1976) uses an amusing hypothetical example to illustrate this point in which a language teacher tries to teach a non-English speaking student 'brown' by presenting him with a hundred brown objects of varying types and spending several hours teaching the student that each object is 'brown'. On testing, the student does not appear to have grasped the concept 'brown' and so the teacher resolves to find five hundred brown objects and repeat the process the following day. He concludes:

> Fortunately, most of us would not adopt this desperate solution and would recognise what had gone wrong. However many brown objects we may show him, our pupil will not know the meaning of brown...until we have taught him to distinguish between brown and red, brown and tan, brown and grey, brown and yellow, brown and black. It is only when he has grasped the relation between brown and other colours that he will begin to understand what brown is. And the reason for this is that brown is not an independent concept defined by some essential properties but one term in a system of colour terms defined by its relations with the other terms which delimit it. (p. 25)

The essential point to grasp is that this principle applies not only to such easily exemplified phenomena as the colour spectrum but to every linguistic sign in the language. *No linguistic sign has value, or meaning, in its own right.* To appreciate fully the significance of this assertion, it is necessary to examine further the ways in which linguistic signs link to form a system.

4. Linguistic Signs Are Linked in Two Main Ways

Saussure distinguished two major types of relationship which exist between linguistic elements. First, there is the relationship which exists between opposing (or alternative) elements. *Opposing* used in this context does not refer only to opposite elements (such as hot and cold). Rather it refers to any element which may be substituted for another in any particular string of elements. For example, in the sentence 'This tea is hot', *hot* may be replaced by *cold* or *tepid* or *scorching*. Further, *tea* may be replaced by *coffee* or *water* or *drink*; *This* may be replaced by *My* or *Your* or *Aunt Lucy's*; and *is* may be replaced by *was* or *should be* or *isn't*, and so on. Making any of these changes would, of course, alter the meaning of the sentence but it would still make sense. The point is that there are connections between *hot, cold, tepid* and *scorching* as there are between *tea, coffee, water* and *drink* and so on. Saussure called the relations which exist between such elements *associative* but they are now more commonly referred to as *paradigmatic* (cf. *Sense Relations*, Chapter 2, this volume).

The notion of paradigmatic relations enables one to develop the concept that language exists as a network of interrelating signs, each one being dependent upon the others for its value. If, for example, the linguistic sign *hot* was removed from the system, the value of the other signs in the system linked to hot in a paradigmatic relationship would subtly alter. That is, the concept currently associated with the sound pattern 'hot' (or the *meaning* of hot) would be subsumed by the terms *warm, fiery, heated, scorching* and so on.

The other major relationship exists when linguistic elements are combined with one another. For example, in the string of linguistic signs 'The girl slid on the jelly-fish' each sign within the string is dependent upon the preceding and following signs for its meaning. 'The jelly-fish slid on the girl' has a distinctly different meaning. These latter relations Saussure called *syntagmatic* and they define the combinatorial possibilities of linguistic elements (cf. *Syntax*, Chapter 2, this volume). Saussure captured the distinction between syntagmatic and paradigmatic relations by stating that paradigmatic relations exist between items *in absentia*; whereas syntagmatic relationships exist between items *in presentia*. That is, paradigmatic relations hold between any linguistic sign in an utterance and a range of linguistic signs absent from the utterance: for instance, in the example above, 'This tea is hot', paradigmatic relations hold between *tea* and the absent items *coffee, water, lemonade, milk* and so on, whereas syntagmatic relations exist between all items present in an utterance 'this – tea – is – hot'.

Syntagmatic relations can also affect paradigmatic relations as although many paradigmatic relations exist in their own right (for example, *chair/table/bed'* etc., *apple/pear/banana etc.*) others do not and are dependent upon syntagmatic context. For instance, in the above example, 'This tea is hot', *hot* could be replaced by *Aunt Lucy's* which means that *hot* and *Aunt Lucy's* stand in a paradigmatic relationship with one another *in this particular syntagmatic context*.

If we now return to the problem for the child who confuses opposite terms, we can see that it is one of paradigmatic relations ('The tea is hot/cold'; 'This work is easy/hard'). As we have acknowledged that linguistic signs cannot be taught in isolation, one approach to remediating this problem might be to teach the two opposite terms together and introduce the child to, say, *hot* objects and *cold* objects so that she or he can see/feel the difference between them and learn *hot* and *cold*. It is possible, as was mentioned earlier, that this approach may result in the child being unable to remember which sound pattern matches which concept. An alternative approach, then, would be to take one term at a time and teach terms that are syntagmatically related to it, for example, *hot/fire/danger/burn/hurt; hot/sun/summer/holiday/beach/swim/tan*.

So far we have only discussed linguistic signs as if we were referring to *words* and it is important to recognise that, because a linguistic sign is composed of a concept and sound pattern, idioms such as *a red herring* and *a rolling stone* are also linguistic signs. Further, we have acknowledged that words combine to form larger units but they may also be broken down into their component parts – *anti/dis/establish/ ment/arian/ism* – which themselves break down into their component sounds. Each of these units exists in a system of paradigmatic and syntagmatic relations. For example, the word *helpless* may be divided into the root *help* and the suffix *less* (cf. *Morphology*, Chapter 2, this volume); *help* may be replaced by *use, need, hap*, etc. and less by *ful, ing, er*, etc. *Help, use, need, hap* and so on stand in a paradigmatic relation with one another, as do *less, ful, ing, er* and so on. The prefixes *un, dis, sub, re* and so on also stand in a paradigmatic relation with one another. The syntagmatic relations which exist between these units define the possible combinations, for example, *unhelpful, reusable, discontinuing* are possible combinations but **dishelpful, *reuseful, *subcontinuing* are not. (In linguistics, unacceptable forms are conventionally marked with an asterisk.) Turning to the sounds of language we can see that they, too, are linked by paradigmatic relations. In the word *hat*, for example, *h* may be replaced by *c, p, f, m* (and so on) to form *cat, pat, fat, mat; a* may be replaced by *i, u, o* (*hit, hut, hot*); and *t* by *d, m, g* (*had, ham, hag*). Further, each sound within a word is syntagmatically related to the preceding and following sounds to create meaning. If the order of sounds is changed, so is the meaning, for example, *pat, tap, apt*.

The notions of paradigmatic and syntagmatic relations, then, lead to what is now termed the *structuralist view* of language. That is, language is a structured network of interrelated signs but, in addition, consists of different *levels* and at each level the units contrast and combine with one another to form the larger units of the next level (sounds/parts of words/words/sentences/discourse). Thus, structural linguistics provides a framework which we may use to establish exactly where a language problem lies. We can take a sample of language and analyse it in an ordered and systematic way by looking at one level at a time and, having considered the overall picture, can decide upon priorities for therapy (see further Section III, this volume). The component levels of language are examined in more detail later and in Chapter 2 and so will not be covered further here.

The above discussion has outlined Saussure's theory of the linguistic sign. We have seen that the linguistic sign has two inseparable parts, concept and sound pattern, and that both parts are totally arbitrary. The idea that no linguistic sign has meaning in its own right has been illustrated by reference to the colour spectrum and further explained in the discussion of paradigmatic and syntagmatic relations. Language has been described as a highly complex system of interrelating linguistic signs, but the structure of language is only one aspect of it. The other aspects rest in Saussure's distinction between *langue* (language) and *parole* (speech). Until a clear distinction has been made between these two phenomena, it is not possible to appreciate fully Saussure's theory of language. Further, the distinction between speech and language is crucial to the work of speech/language professionals. It is this distinction that the following sections will examine.

Language versus Speech

As indicated in the outline of the speech circuit above, speech is a physiological act which results in the production of sound-waves. Sound-waves are physical phenomena which, although invisible to the naked eye, may be 'captured' by a tape recorder, or transmitted over a telephone line. In this sense then, speech may be said to have *substance*; a concrete, physical existence. Language does not have substance but exists as a *form*; it is an abstract, psychological phenomenon. Saussure's comparison of language and a game of chess helps to illustrate his distinction between substance and form.

The game of chess involves a chess-board, a set of pieces, a set of rules and two players, both of whom must know and abide by the rules of the game. Two people, then, go to play a game of chess and discover that one of the knights is missing. This does not deter them. They find a small square of cardboard, write *knight* on it and proceed with the game. The reason that the players so quickly find a solution to this problem is that they recognise that the *substance* of the knight (or any other piece) is unimportant. What is important is that the piece can be recognised as being different from the other pieces and both players know how it relates to the other pieces in the game (that is, the direction and type of movement that the piece can make).

The substance of speech is equally unimportant to the form of language. Take the word *knight*, for example. When a child says *knight*, the actual *sound* produced will be quite different from the sound produced when, for instance, an adult male says the word. Further, when an English person says *knight*, the sound will be different from the sound produced when a Scottish/Welsh/Irish/American/French person says it, and so on. Despite these differences in sound we (usually) recognise the word *knight*. In fact, our own pronunciations of *knight* may be slightly different each time we say it. None of these differences is important, however, *provided* that what is said cannot be mistaken for *not, nit, net, gnat, knife, nine, nigh, right, white, light* and so on. In other words, one individual can say *knight* (or any other word) in a perceptibly different way from another individual, *provided* that their pronunciation does not impinge upon the pronunciation of other words in that language. Thus it can be seen that, in the composition of the word, sounds carry the function of signalling meaning differences.

It is worth questioning at this point how we accept many variant productions of a word as 'the same'. If a child says 'mummy' and her father says 'yes, there's mummy'; the two *mummy* sound-waves will be perceptibly different, yet we understand both as the same linguistic sign. The reason for this is that the sound wave triggers in the brain a sound pattern. Although the sound wave has concrete, physical substance, the sound pattern is an abstract, psychological phenomenon with no physical reality. A sound pattern is a mental category. If we consider for a moment a more tangible type of mental category, for example *cat*, we accept that *persian, tabby, siamese* fall into the cat category. We know that *terrier, alsatian, dachshund* do not fall into the cat category but into the dog category. Returning to the sound pattern as a mental category, we know that the different sound waves produced when a man, a woman and a child say 'mummy' all fit our mummy sound pattern category. If one said 'muddy' it would not fit the same sound pattern category. Sound-waves have substance but sound patterns have only form.

The form of language may be compared to the rules of chess. Whilst the physical substance of the pieces is unimportant to the game, the rules are intrinsic to it and cannot, therefore, be changed or broken. One player cannot, for example, decide that his or her knights are invincible and unable to be 'taken' and expect their opponent to continue with the game. In the same way, an individual cannot decide that what everyone else refers to as a *house*, they are going to refer to as a *horse* and expect to be understood. These examples bring us to another aspect of the distinction between speech and language, which is that speech is an individual act whereas language is a social phenomenon.

The individuality of speech manifests itself in several ways. The act of speech requires only one person. An individual may choose to speak or not to speak. If the choice has been made to speak, the individual may choose *what* they wish to say – what linguistic signs they wish to use, simple or complex, polite or not, and so on – and *how* they wish to say it – whispering, shouting, adopting an accent, and so on. Any constraints upon what is said come from the social conventions of language. Further, the sound-waves that any person produces are highly individual, as evinced by the fact that we can quickly recognise the person on the other end of the telephone line without them having to identify themselves. The individuality of speech further distinguishes it from language.

The social aspect of language is not simply that language is used for social (or communicative) purposes but, more importantly, that language is a *socially created conventional system* which exists *outside* the individual. To return to the chess analogy, the rules of chess are predetermined; they exist before a game of chess is played and continue to exist when the game has finished. A chess-board may be set up in a living room, unused, but the game of chess is still 'there'. It is brought into existence when two people, who know the rules, sit down at the board and use the pieces.

In order for speech to communicate meaning, both speaker and listener must share the same set (or system) of linguistic signs. In this sense language may be compared to any other social institution, or system. Individuals must conform to the social conventions of the institution if they are to exist happily within it. Moreover, an individual cannot change a social system, such as language, without gaining the agreement of the majority of other users. This point has particular relevance for the issue of 'politically correct' language. For example, the terms Mr/Mrs/Miss are arbitrary and socially created. There is no *logical* reason to oppose the abolition of the title system or the introduction of the alternative two-term system Mr/Ms. However, because language is arbitrary, it is not logical and, thus, change in language requires consensus agreement based on systems of values rather than logic.

In summary then, language is an abstract, psychological phenomenon which has no substance but exists as a 'form'. *In its entirety* language does not exist within any one individual but in the shared knowledge of a linguistic community. To appreciate this point, one has only to consult a dictionary and see that there are many linguistic signs in our shared language which are not part of our personal language system. In this respect, language can be said to have a social aspect – the shared knowledge of the linguistic community, and an individual aspect – each person's own language system. Language embodies the social values of its linguistic community. Change in language arises through changes in conceptual understanding of the linguistic community. Advances in technology represent one type of change in conceptual understanding and the language develops to accommodate these advances. Social change, that is change in the attitudes or views of a community, is also reflected in language. A pertinent example for speech and language therapists is change, over recent years, in the terms used to refer to people with reduced intellectual capabilities: *the mentally handicapped; the educationally subnormal; the intellectually impaired*; and most recently *people with learning difficulties*.

Speech is a physiological phenomenon which results in the production of physical sound-waves. Sound-waves have substance – a concrete, 'real' existence. Speech is an individual act involving only one person and each speaker produces individual sound-waves. An individual can change the sound-waves they produce, for example by lowering or raising the pitch of the voice, or by changing accent. However, changes in speech are restricted by the form of language. We can understand the sound-waves produced by non-native speakers, for example, provided that their pronunciations do not prevent them from signalling meaning differences. Thus, as native English-speakers, we might understand a non-native pronunciation *theeng* as meaning *thing*, but be unsure as to whether *sheep* refers to *sheep* or *ship*.

Language, Speech and Hearing

The above discussion has distinguished between speech and language and at this point it will be useful to consider hearing. Hearing, like speech, is a complex physiological process involving integration of anatomical, physiological and neurological processes. In some respects, the hearing process can be compared to the transmission of morse code. The morse signal arrives as a series of dots and dashes which have no meaning until they are *decoded* by the operator. The hearing system receives the speech sound-wave and transforms it into a 'signal' which it then transmits to the brain. It does not interpret, or give meaning to, the signal. The brain decodes the signal and interprets its meaning (SP→C). In some respects we have no control over hearing – we hear whether we choose to or not. This lack of choice with regard to hearing is captured by Saussure's notion that the hearing process is *passive*. Speech is further differentiated from hearing, as a process, in that Saussure characterises speech as *active*.

Returning to the notions of *executive* and *receptive*, the speech circuit could be characterised thus: the speaker associates concept with sound pattern, that is *encodes* language (the *executive* part of the speech circuit). The encoded language is transmitted to the ear of the listener via the *active* process of speech. The speech signal is transmitted to the brain of the listener via the *passive* process of hearing. The listener's brain *decodes* the speech signal, that is, 'translates' sound patterns into concepts (the *receptive* part of the speech circuit). This clearly separates language encoding and decoding from speaking and hearing.

There is an aspect of language encoding and decoding that Saussure's theory does not appear to address. If language is a structured network of paradigmatically and syntagmatically related linguistic signs, how do we know which signs can be used together to form communicative sentences and which cannot? Saussure makes brief reference to some sort of 'language-organising faculty' but this does not enable us to answer this question. Without some idea of how we are able to formulate sentences, we are in a poor position to decide how best to help people who have difficulty in formulating sentences.

How Do We Combine Linguistic Signs into Communicative Sentences?

This is an appropriate point at which to consider Chomsky's contribution to language theory. Chomsky considers that the most important reason for studying language is the contribution that such study makes to our understanding of mental processes. His theories therefore extend beyond the bounds of linguistics *per se* and encompass much more general philosophical, psychological and sociological questions. There will be no attempt here to cover Chomsky's theories in any depth; for a good introduction the reader is referred to John Lyons's (1991) text *Chomsky*. There are two major aspects of his theories which have particular relevance for speech/language professionals. Chomsky opened up investigation into the nature of the rules which govern language and developed the theory of deep and surface structures. In addition, he introduced the distinction between competence and performance which is similar to, but subtly different from, Saussure's langue/parole distinction.

Chomsky's starting point is the *creativity* of language. Languages do not consist of a finite number of possible sentences which are duly learned and repeated by speakers of that language. Rather, the possible combinations of words are infinite and, indeed, language users are able to understand and produce an infinite variety of combinations. The question to be addressed is, how do we do this? Chomsky postulated that the nature of language is such that it enables us to create an infinite number of sentences from a finite set of rules – the grammar of language – and it is the grammar of language that we store.

Drawing on mathematical theory Chomsky wrote a grammar of language which he asserted best accounted for the way in which humans are able to produce an infinite variety of sentences. To exemplify, consider the simple mathematical formula $x + y = z$. The value of z will vary dependent on the values of x and y. As there is an infinite number of possible values for x and y, the formula $x + y = z$ generates infinite possible values for z. If we take the English sentence (S) 'Martha eats' this can be analysed as consisting of a noun phrase (NP) *Martha* and a verb phrase (VP) *eats*. In English declarative sentences, NPs must precede VPs; *'eats Martha' is an ungrammatical sentence. Thus, we can write the rule (or *formula*) S→ NP + VP. The NP consists of a noun (N) *Martha* and the VP consists of a verb (V) *eat* plus a tense marker *s*. So, we can also write the following rules: NP→N; VP →V + tense. Just from these three rules we can see that the 'formula':

1. S → NP + VP
2. NP → N (horses, flowers, John, people...)
3. VP → V + tense (run, bloom, cried, eat...)

allows for numerous combinations.

The sentence 'That silly Martha liked that awful Fred' can also be described as consisting of NP + VP. However, the NP here consists of a determiner (D) *that*, an adjective (Adj) *silly* and a noun *Martha*; and the verb phrase consists of the verb *like* plus the tense marker *ed*, and another NP *that* (D) *awful* (Adj) *Fred* (N). The rules underlying this sentence construction could, therefore, be described as follows (bracketed items are optional):

1.   S → NP+VP
2.   NP → (D) + (Adj) + N
3.   VP → V + tense/person (+ NP)
4.   NP → (D) + (Adj) + N

and they may be represented by the following tree-diagram:

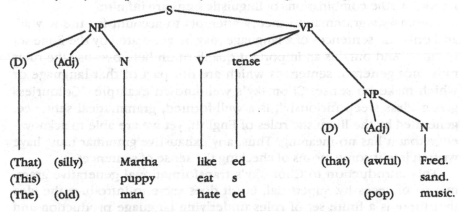

(D)	(Adj)	N	V	tense	(D)	(Adj)	N
(That)	(silly)	Martha	like	ed	(that)	(awful)	Fred.
(This)	(puppy)		eat	s			sand.
(The)	(old)	man	hate	ed		(pop)	music.

These rules, which describe the structure of sentences, Chomsky calls *phrase structure* (PS) rules. Phrase structure grammar is only part of Chomsky's theory of transformational generative grammar. The core of the theory is the notion of *transformations*, which leads to the concepts of deep and surface structure. Chomsky suggests that there are two different kinds of structure in language: deep structure and surface structure. Phrase structure rules generate the deep structure of sentences, which embodies their meaning. Deep structure (or *kernel*) sentences are active, affirmative and declarative in nature. Not all surface structure sentences are active, affirmative and declarative; for example, there are negative sentences, 'Martha did not like Fred'; questions, 'Did Martha like Fred?'; commands, 'You must like Fred, Martha'; and so on. Chomsky suggests that transformations may be applied to the deep structure sentences to provide various surface structures. Transformations involve movement or deletion of existing *constituents* in the deep structure and/or the addition of new constituents to this structure. For example, passive transformation changes the deep structure 'Martha kissed Fred' into the surface structure 'Fred was kissed by Martha'. Where a passive transformation occurs the meaning (or deep structure) remains the same, that is, 'Martha kissed Fred'. Thus, the idea of a deep and a surface structure captures the interrelatedness of meaning between active and passive sentences. The distinction between a deep and a surface structure also accounts for our ability to acknowledge two interpretations of ambiguous sentences: 'Martha likes Fred more than me': 'Martha likes Fred more than I do'; or 'Martha likes Fred more than she likes me'? That is, one surface structure can be seen to have two possible deep structures (or meanings).

By having rules that can be applied again and again (*recursive rules*) the grammar is able to generate sentences such as 'This is the woman, who wrote the letter, that got left in the tray, that belonged to Jim...'. It is sentences such as these that linguists tend to use to exemplify the fact that we have a finite number of linguistic signs and rules for their combination but the combinations of linguistic signs are infinite.

Chomsky's grammatical theory attempts to account for the way all, and only, the sentences of a language may be generated by the finite set of rules. 'And only' is an important qualification here because the rules must not generate sentences which are not part of that language or which make no sense. Chomsky's well-known example, 'Colourless green ideas sleep furiously', is a well-formed, grammatical sentence, generated by the linguistic rules of English, yet we are able to acknowledge that it has no meaning. Thus, any exhaustive grammar must have written into it some means of checking the sense of sentences.

This introduction to Chomsky's transformational generative grammar is, of necessity, superficial, but it does serve to introduce the idea that there is a finite set of rules underlying language production and reception which allows us to create and understand an infinite variety of sentences. It cannot be claimed that these rules have any 'psychological reality' – that is, we cannot assume that the rules proposed by Chomsky match the processes which our brains use to organise language. Nevertheless, it is safe to assume that language production and reception is in some sense rule-governed and that our 'knowledge' of language includes knowledge of these rules – the grammar of our language.

Competence and Performance

Chomsky calls the individual's knowledge of grammar their *linguistic competence*. Use of the word *knowledge* in this context is not intended to imply that linguistic knowledge is the same as other sorts of knowledge. Knowing that Britain is part of Europe is an example of one type of knowledge: factual, overt knowledge that has been taught, or learned. The grammatical knowledge that we have of our native language is different from this and could be described as *covert* knowledge. We are able to use language whether or not we are aware of the fact that it can be analysed into noun phrases and verb phrases. We are able to make judgements about the grammaticality of sentences without necessarily knowing why some are ungrammatical or *how* we know that they are.

The sentence 'She saw himself in the mirror', for example, would be judged as ungrammatical by the majority of English speakers, and, if asked, they may be able to say precisely why. Yet, we only consult our grammatical knowledge when placed in the situation of being required to do so, otherwise it is just 'there' and we use it without even being aware that we do. Chomsky refers to this type of knowledge as *intuitive* and considers that grammatical theory can justifiably be based on native speaker intuitions.

Linguistic competence, then, describes language knowledge, but not language use. Chomsky calls use of language *performance*. Performance is subject to many psychological variables such as memory, attention, fatigue, emotional state and so on. Any of these variables may affect an individual's performance and result in their making 'errors' such as hesitations, false starts, repetitions and unfinished sentences. Chomsky insists that these errors are performance errors and do not constitute linguistic incompetence. An individual's linguistic competence Chomsky sees as 'perfect'; performance errors arise through the imperfections of human functioning. For example, an individual's linguistic competence might generate the sentence 'Would it be all right if we met half an hour later?'. In performance this might be produced as 'Would it be, er, would it be all right if, er, if we met, mmm, later – er, half an hour?' Thus, performance does not necessarily reflect linguistic competence.

At the beginning of this chapter it was stated that the theories of Saussure and Chomsky are not entirely incompatible. By way of a summary to this section on Chomsky, it seems appropriate to bring the two theories together within the context of current linguistics.

Langue/Parole and Competence/Performance

Saussure characterises language as a network of interrelated linguistic signs and identifies different levels in language. Within linguistics there are subdisciplines which study these different levels:

phonology – the study of the ways sounds contrast and combine in languages to create meaning differences;

morphology – the study of internal word structure;

syntax – the study of the ways in which words combine to form larger units;

semantics – the study of meaning in language.

Different linguists view the *grammar* of language in different ways. Most consider morphology and syntax as constituting the grammar of a language whilst others see grammar as including semantics and still others as also including phonology.

Chomsky criticised Saussure's theory of language for its weakness in accounting for sentences. In Saussure's view sentences arose through the individual choosing which linguistic signs to combine and his theories did not extend to explaining how the individual did so. The view that combination of linguistic signs into sentences arose through individual choice led Saussure to account for sentences as part of parole, that is, outside language. Chomsky found this view unsatisfactory and went on to account for sentence production in language. His early work focused specifically on morphology and syntax but later included semantics and phonology within the grammar of language. Thus a major difference between Saussure's langue and parole and Chomsky's competence and performance is where sentence formulation is placed. Saussure accounted for sentence formulation within parole (speech) whereas Chomsky firmly placed sentence formulation within an individual's linguistic competence.

There is also a subtle distinction between parole and performance. In defining parole, Saussure accounts for what speech is: a physiological process which produces sound-waves. Chomsky goes further with performance by considering the content of parole and drawing attention to the psychological variables which can affect spoken output. Thus in the term 'performance', we have a sense of the physiological phenomenon of parole being mediated by psychological variables such as attention, memory, emotional state and so on. Performance, then, is not simply the physiological act of speech but reflects the ongoing formulation of language as speech is being produced.

Within langue, Saussure identified the two aspects of language execution (expression) and language reception (understanding). Chomsky's theory of transformational generative grammar focuses heavily on language execution and has been criticised for its neglect of language reception. This emphasis on language execution has had a direct, and some would say deleterious, effect on clinical work, which will be discussed later. At this point we will accept that there are two aspects to language – expression and reception – and that both are of equal importance.

Viewed from a chronological perspective, Chomsky can be seen to have absorbed and developed the concepts of langue and parole. At first glance linguistic competence may appear to include only the individual aspect of langue. That is, Chomsky describes *individual* linguistic competence. But the shared nature of langue becomes evident in the identification of rules governing the combination of linguistic signs. Using Saussure's chess analogy: the rules of chess are shared by the chess-players in a community; in order to play chess one must learn the rules. The rules governing language are shared by the linguistic community. A child, or a foreign-language learner, must 'tap into' the shared rules of the linguistic community in order to 'play the language game'. Individual linguistic competence, then, may be described as the knowledge of the shared rules of the linguistic community.

In summary, the notions of langue and parole lead to a clear distinction between language and speech. Linguistic competence might be described as the individual's knowledge of langue and the rules governing combinations of linguistic signs. The notion of performance encapsulates an individual's execution of language through the medium of speech. We will now turn to the applications of linguistic theory in clinical work.

The Contributions of Linguistics to Clinical Work

There are four main areas in clinical work in which linguistics has had a major impact:

- linguistics provided the crucial distinction between speech and language which enables us to differentiate between speech/hearing impairments and language impairments;
- linguistics has provided a framework for the assessment and diagnosis of speech and language disorders;
- linguistic theories and methods of investigation have contributed to the study of language acquisition;
- linguistic principles are used in clinical work to inform treatment planning.

The following paragraphs will consider each of these areas in turn.

Speech, Hearing and Language Impairments

The identification of language as a psychological phenomenon distinct from the physiological processes of speech and hearing facilitates the broad differential diagnosis between speech and hearing impairments and language impairment. The complex physiological process of speech involves integration of neurological, physiological and anatomical systems. Impairment in any of these systems may result in an inability to produce adequate speech sound-waves. For example, the child who is born with a cleft palate has an anatomical anomaly which, if uncorrected, may result in the production of unclear speech. Individuals who are unable to produce clear (or intelligible) speech are described as having a *speech production disorder*. It is quite possible that an individual may have a speech production disorder with no accompanying language impairment.

Speech sound waves do not only have to be produced clearly, they must also be received (or heard) clearly. Hearing, like speech, is a complex physiological process. Any impairment in the neurology and/or physiology and/or anatomy of the hearing system may result in inadequate transmission of speech sounds. An individual who has a major impairment in their hearing system is described as having a *profound hearing loss*, or *deafness*, and, of course, will be unable to hear most sounds, not just speech. Individuals with less serious damage to their hearing system are described as having a *hearing impairment*. A break-down in the hearing system may result in a faulty signal, or no signal, reaching the brain. If no signal gets through then there is nothing for the brain to decode and language, as identified above, will not develop. It is important to consider, however, that it is the sound pattern that may not be accessible to the deaf individual but that conceptual understanding will still develop. Thus there is a link between deafness/hearing impairment and language but it is not simply that a deaf person will have a language impairment, rather that deaf language may be different from hearing language.

Some individuals have no disruption to their hearing system but have difficulty in understanding language. For these people, the signal reaches their brains but, to a greater or lesser degree, they are unable to decode it. Individuals who have difficulty in decoding language are referred to as having a *receptive language impairment* or *difficulty with language comprehension*. Some individuals acquire brain damage (through a stroke, for example) and lose their part of their 'language-decoding faculty'. This observation has led linguists, psychologists and speech/language professionals to infer that a *developmental receptive language impairment* (developmental indicating present from birth), which may not be explained by hearing loss, may be the result of some impairment in the brain. Cognitive psychologists and psycholinguists attempt to specify more precisely the exact nature of impairment by identifying the psychological processes involved in language reception and expression. Some of these issues are discussed in Chapters 6, 7, 8, 11 and 15.

It is perhaps logical to assume that if an individual is unable to receive (or decode) language then they will also be unable to produce (or encode) language. In other words, one might assume that language reception will precede language expression. In practice, it is sometimes the case that an individual with an expressive language impairment also has some degree of receptive language disability. However, the relation between reception and expression is unclear and is not necessarily a parallel. Individuals who have difficulty in encoding language are referred to as having an *expressive language impairment*.

Chomsky's distinction between competence and performance alerts us to the dangers of inferring the extent of an individual's linguistic competence from the evidence provided by their performance. To evaluate fully an individual's linguistic ability we must attempt to assess their competence through means other than simply observing their performance (see Chapter 7, this volume). Further, as all humans produce language which contains errors, when is the decision to be made that one individual produces too many and has a language impairment'? The clinician is thus faced with the task of deciding which errors are within 'normal' limits and which constitute a language impairment. In addition, once a language impairment has been diagnosed, a further decision must be made regarding which errors are performance errors and which reflect underlying competence defects. Errors which arise through performance deficits may require that remediation concentrates on improving psychological variables such as memory and attention, whilst competence deficits may require teaching of specific rules of language. In practice, it is difficult to separate performance and linguistic competence and clinicians often have to plan programmes which cover both the more general psychological processes involved in attending, sequencing, memorising etc., and provide opportunities for grammatical rules to be acquired.

In summary, language may be described as having two aspects, expressive and receptive, and people with a language impairment may have difficulties in the expression and/or reception of language. Speech production disorders and hearing impairment may exist with or without language impairment. Deaf language should be viewed as different from hearing language rather than viewed as deficient, but deaf individuals may have a language impairment which exists in addition to their deafness rather than being caused by it. With these broad distinctions in mind we will now consider the linguistic framework of language levels which allows us to describe more specifically the language impairment.

Framework for Assessment and Diagnosis

Until the 1970s, clinicians had no clearly defined way of describing language. From the early 1970s, linguistics has had a major impact on clinical work because it has provided terminology and a methodology for the description of language. Clinicians now routinely take a sample of language and analyse it systematically by looking at one level of language at a time. So, for example, one might look at the sample of language and analyse the way in which the individual makes use of the sounds in the language (phonological analysis), ignoring syntax; or one might ignore the sound system and analyse the individual's use of word order (syntactical analysis) and so on. This method of analysis of language impairment is generally referred to as the *linguistic-descriptive* approach. The chapters in Section II reflect this approach. Each chapter discusses issues relating to assessment of a particular level of language and evaluates currently-available assessment procedures. Thus, these chapters clearly indicate the value of the linguistic-descriptive approach in the identification and assessment of speech and language impairments. All chapters in this book indicate that it is important also that linguistic-descriptive analysis contributes to clinical decision-making in a wider framework of clinical knowledge. Some of the broad issues relating to this point are outlined below.

Linguistic Levels Interact

In the 1980s it became apparent that there were potential dangers in looking at one level of language at a time to the exclusion of others. Each level of language interacts with other levels and deficits in one level of language may create deficits at other levels. For example, phonological analysis may reveal that a child produces no consonants at the ends of words (referred to as *Word Final Consonant Deletion*). Lack of word final consonants will affect the child's language at the morphological level. That is, the child with no word final consonants will not indicate plurals (*shoe* and *shoes* will both be *shoe*); past tense (*play* and *played* will both be *play*); possessives (*Lee* and *Lee's* will both be *Lee*); and so on. In turn this may affect the child's syntax. For example, a child may use phrases such as 'we did go, we did play'; or 'yesterday, we play ball' to indicate past tense. And, undoubtedly, lack of word final consonants will affect the child's language at the level of semantics (meaning) as, for example, *back, bad, bag, badge, ban, bap, bat* may all be produced as 'ba'. Thus, it is most important for clinicians to ensure that, having analysed a language sample in terms of its component levels, the sample is 'put back together again' to evaluate the effects of deficits in one level of language on other levels of language.

Explaining interaction between levels in this way assumes a certain 'hierarchy' in the structure of levels. That is, phonology → morphology → syntax → semantics; phonology is the lowest level and semantics the highest. It is important to be aware that this is a *description* of language which provides a framework that we may utilise to analyse language and provides a language that we can use to talk about language (a *metalanguage*). We cannot assume that this is the way in which language is organised in our brains. The way in which our brains organise and/or process language is an issue of longstanding and ongoing research and debate. The two main opposing views in this debate are captured in the terms *bottom-up* and *top-down*. Bottom-up exponents suggest that our brains analyse language by starting with the smallest units in language (sounds), building these up into larger units (parts of words/words/phrases/clauses/sentences). Top-down exponents suggest that our brains take in large units (sentences) and break these down into smaller units (clauses/phrases/words/parts of words/sounds). Thus it is equally possible that deficits in higher levels may contribute to deficits in lower levels. For example, a lack of knowledge of morphological markers (such as plurals, past tense, possessives etc.) may contribute to the absence of word final consonants. The important point is that linguistic levels *interact* and interactions may be uni-directional, bi-directional or multi-directional.

An overview of the whole language sample is perhaps particularly important when analysing children's language. Crystal (1987a) reviews research which indicates that while normally developing children are acquiring language, gains in one aspect may result in losses in another aspect. Evidence for 'trade-offs' between phonology and syntax is most common. Similar effects have been shown with language-impaired children (see also Chapter 12, this volume). Crystal (*op. cit.*) analogised language processing capacity to a bucket 'into which a certain amount of linguistic water has been poured. The bucket gets larger, as the child develops; but in the case of the language handicapped child, there is a series of holes at a certain level. As the child's language level rises, and reaches the holes, there is a stage when any extra water poured into the bucket will cause some of the water already present to overflow via the holes..... An extra 'drop' of phonology (syntax, semantics etc) may cause the overflow of a 'drop' of syntax (semantics, phonology etc)' (p. 20). This knowledge is clearly pertinent to the assessment of language impairment but also has implications for evaluation of therapy. Clinicians need to be aware that progress in one level of language may temporarily co-occur with apparent retrogression in another level.

Clinical Diagnoses Need To Take Account of Non-Linguistic Factors

Prior to linguistic influence, speech and language therapy was heavily influenced by the medical model. Diagnosis itself is a medical term and classification of language impairment was placed in the medical model of aetiological explanation (cause) (see also Chapter 13). Thus, diagnoses would be framed in terms of identifiable aetiologies such as *language disorder associated with autism; language disorder associated with learning difficulties*. This classification system apparently identified a cause for the language disorder which was helpful to carers. In addition, categorisation of individuals as *autistic* or *physically handicapped* or *hearing impaired*, for example, facilitated the provision of resources for those individuals. A problem with the medical model, however, is that it implies that there are characteristics of language impairment specific to each group. That is, it implies that all people with physical handicap will have similar language impairments and that their language impairments will be different from those of the group of people with, say, hearing impairment.

The linguistic approach to the classification of language disorders does almost exactly the opposite of the medical model. The linguistic approach ignores medical factors and classifies language impairment solely on the basis of the language characteristics of each individual. Thus whilst the linguistic approach provides a more detailed and informed characterisation of linguistic breakdown, it has been criticised for ignoring important associated information. Speech and language therapists therefore need to acknowledge this weakness and utilise the linguistic approach within the broader framework of their knowledge which takes account of medical, environmental, cognitive, social, psychological and physical factors.

Linguistic-Descriptive Analysis Should Be Placed in the Broader Context of Communication

Another criticism of the linguistic approach is that it has tended to focus on language and language deficits to the exclusion of other aspects of communication. For example, Chomsky's theory considers linguistic competence on the one hand, and linguistic performance, as affected by psychological variables (memory, fatigue, attention, etc.), on the other, but there are other variables which affect performance such as relative status of speaker and listener, situation, topic and levels of socially acceptable behaviour. These latter variables cannot simply be dependent upon the performance of the individual because they conform to certain rules, yet the status of these rules is unclear. In some respects they might be considered to be part of linguistic competence because word and structure choice can be closely related to many of them. For example, 'dunno, what d'you think?' and 'I'm not entirely sure, what's your opinion?' are both grammatical, appropriate utterances in certain situations, but equally, both are inappropriate in other situations. Knowing which types of language are appropriate in which situations is part of our language knowledge, and Hymes (1970) suggested that this total language knowledge may be referred to as *communicative competence*. Whilst it is difficult to write rules to generate contextually appropriate and feasible sentences, there are theories of grammar which attempt to account for language as a social and communicative phenomenon (for example, Dik's *Functional Grammar*, 1978; and *Halliday's Systemic Grammar*, see Berry, 1975).

More recently the field of *pragmatics* has come to prominence in clinical work. Pragmatics is concerned with identifying and analysing all factors which affect communicative competence. The subject-matter of pragmatics is thus vast and includes *non-verbal communication*: eye contact, facial expression, gesture, body posture and proximity, etc.; *communicative functions*: questioning, explaining, joking, commanding, etc.; *communicative context*: relationships between communicative partners, formality of situation, etc.; *conversational context*: rules of initiation, turn-taking, topic maintenance, topic change etc.

There is some debate as to how pragmatic aspects of communication relate to language structure (see also Chapter 9, this volume). There are three main views which are summarised in Figures 1.2, 1.3 and 1.4 below. (For detailed discussion of these views see McTear and Conti-Ramsden, 1992.)

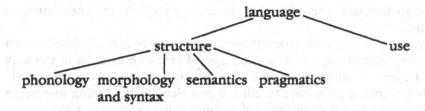

Figure 1.2 Pragmatics is viewed as another level of language

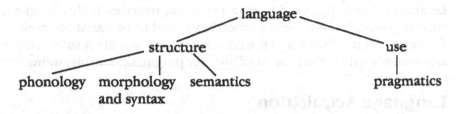

Figure 1.3 Pragmatics is viewed as the study of language use

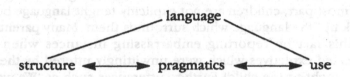

Figure 1.4 Pragmatics is viewed as relating language structure and language use

As this text takes as its framework a structural view of language, for the purposes of convenience, pragmatics is treated as if it were another level of language (Figure 1.2). Thus Chapter 8 is entitled 'Assessment of Pragmatics'. Notwithstanding this, many of the chapters in Sections II and III highlight the importance of pragmatics in all aspects of clinical work and thus Figure 1.4, which characterises pragmatics as relating language structure and language use, more accurately captures the predominant view throughout this text.

With regard to the assessment of language impairment, pragmatics draws our attention to the context and focus of assessment. That is, from a pragmatic perspective the typical clinical assessment situation provides a context which will affect the performance of the individual being assessed. A true picture of the individual's linguistic capabilities may not emerge because of the constraints of the assessment situation. Further, a structural linguistic approach to assessment tends to lead us to focus on deficit and inability and perhaps to ignore ability. That is, whilst focusing on the syntactic content of an individual's language we may unwittingly overlook her/his ability to communicate meanings, whether this be through unusual use of syntax or through other channels such as gesture.

Pragmatics is rapidly establishing its importance in the field of speech and language therapy with an upsurge of research interest in the area and a corresponding increase in the literature. Texts which specifically apply pragmatic principles to clinical practice are beginning to emerge (McTear and Conti-Ramsden, 1992; Smith and Leinonen, 1992). Many clinicians have always taken the more 'holistic' approach to communication impairment promoted by pragmatics and welcome the justification that theoretical pragmatics provides for their approach (see Smith and Leinonen, 1992, pp. 44–51, for a historical overview). Nevertheless, currently-available assessment procedures tend to be based on levels of language and it is thus left to the clinician to evaluate the results of these assessments within the context of broader pragmatic considerations.

Language Acquisition

Before evaluating the contribution of linguistics to the study of language acquisition, it is worth considering the term 'language acquisition'. We refer to language acquisition rather than language *learning* because, for the most part, children are not explicitly taught language but somehow 'pick up' the language which surrounds them. Many parents will testify to this fact by reporting embarrassing instances when their child repeated expletives which were unwittingly uttered by the parent and not taught to the child! Further, utterances such as 'We wented shops today' are typical of the speech of very young children, yet such utterances are unlikely to have been overheard or taught. Thus, children are said to acquire language rather than learn it. It is also worth noting that children acquire the language of the community in which they live rather than the language to which they 'were born'. So, if a Chinese child is adopted by Indian parents and brought up in an Indian community, that child will acquire an Indian language and not Chinese. Children, then, acquire the language that they are exposed to, and we may infer from this that the first prerequisite for language acquisition is that the child be exposed to a language. This is an important point for speech and language professionals. Where language acquisition does not appear to be proceeding at the usual rate, the clinician will need to evaluate the opportunities that the child has had to acquire language. That is, to what extent has the child been exposed to language?

Observing that children are not taught language but 'acquire' it does not tell us how they do it. The only honest answer to the question 'How do children acquire language' is 'No one knows'. Language processing (encoding and decoding), as we have seen, occurs in the brain and as we have no direct access to the workings of the brain, we have no means of specifying, with certainty, how language acquisition occurs. It is therefore necessary to theorise. Explanatory theories of language acquisition are not solely the domain of linguists. Linguistics describes language and, thereby, what is acquired, but language use is a human function and so is of interest to psychologists, sociologists, biologists and philosophers. Thus several disciplines have contributed to, and enriched, our current understanding of language acquisition. As might be anticipated, the field of language acquisition is vast and there will be no attempt here even to overview explanatory theories. Recently, several books have been published in the area and the reader is referred to these (Foster, 1990; Harris, 1990; Ingram, 1989; Naremore and Hopper, 1990; Stilwell Peccei, 1994). In addition to these books which cover the 'normal' course of language acquisition, the reader is referred to Bishop and Mogford's book *Language Development in Exceptional Circumstances* (1988).

Linguistics and Language Acquisition

Linguistics provides a framework of analysis and methodologies for describing the 'normal' course of language acquisition. Examining how children go about acquiring language involves observing children in the process of language acquisition and recording or describing the language that they produce and (appear to) understand at any particular stage in their development. Several such studies exist (see Ingram, 1989 for a historical overview). Those which examine the whole development of one child are referred to as 'diary' studies because they involve the investigator making regular (weekly) notes of the child's linguistic behaviour. Cross-sectional studies take language samples from large numbers of children at certain ages (such as 9 months, 18 months, 2 years, 3 years and so on) which are then analysed in order that characteristic linguistic behaviours for each age may be established. These studies provide data on the 'normal' course of language development. At a broad level all children may be said to go through similar initial stages of development (see Foster, 1990; Ingram 1989). Some time between the ages of 4 and 10 months children begin to 'babble', at which time they seem to be experimenting with their vocal apparatus to see what sounds they can make. Between the ages of 10 months and 19 months, they go through the 'one-word' or holophrastic stage, when they utter single words which can be interpreted as representing several meanings. The next stage involves putting two words together and continues to the age of approximately 3 years. From this stage onwards the complexity of linguistic structures used by children increases steadily and they acquire vocabulary at a surprisingly fast rate.

Naturally, it would be a daunting task to attempt to describe the entire process of language acquisition. However, the framework of structural linguistics enables researchers to focus on one level of language at a time. For example, Crystal, Fletcher and Garman (1979) developed a profile of the development of sentence structure (Language Assessment, Remediation and Screening Procedure [LARSP]) and Grunwell (1985) a profile of the development of language sounds (Phonological Assessment of Child Speech [PACS]; Developmental Assessment). However, not all levels of language are equally amenable to observational analysis and description. Chapter 7, this volume, discusses the problems involved in establishing developmental norms for language comprehension and Crystal (1987b) draws attention to the fact that methodological inadequacies have resulted in a gross underestimation of the expressive vocabularies of small children (see Chapter 8). Nevertheless, the developmental profiles which do exist are very useful to the clinician, as they provide norms of development against which the performance of children who have a language impairment may be measured and the reader is referred to Ball (1992) and Crystal (1992) who discuss language profiling in some detail. Developmental profiles enable clinicians to establish whether the language produced by such children is characteristic of a delay in development, or shows signs of deviant development. For example, a language sample may be elicited from a 4-year-old, measured against a norm-referenced profile, and the comparison may reveal that the child's language is characteristic of a normally developing 3-year-old, indicating language delay. Alternatively, certain aspects of the sample may be judged age-appropriate whilst others are characteristic of earlier stages of development, indicating uneven language development which is in some cases more characteristic of disorder than delay. If some characteristics of the child's language do not match any developmental norms then the diagnosis may be developmentally-deviant language.

Linguistics Principles Inform Treatment Planning

The chapters in Section III of this book illustrate the ways in which linguistic principles inform treatment planning in the fields of developmental dysfluency: developmental speech and language disorders and acquired speech and language disorders. The following paragraphs will, therefore, simply indicate some of the influences that trends in linguistics have had on intervention.

In the 1970s therapy was heavily influenced by structural linguistics. Drawing on assessment procedures which allowed us to identify areas of deficit in syntactic production, therapy programmes were devised which aimed to teach specific syntactic structures in carefully graded steps which mirrored the 'normal' development of language. In some cases, the focus on production of correct linguistic structures resulted in programmes which were devoid of communicative purpose and required the client to produce language which was situationally inappropriate. For example, the following sample interaction was given at the beginning of one language programme as an exemplification of how to use the programme:

Clinician: What colour is the dog?
Child: Black and white.
Clinician: No, say 'The dog is black and white'.
Child: The dog is black and white.
Clinician: Good.

The task itself requires the child to respond to questions to which the clinician already knows the answer and thus has little communicative interest for either party. Further, it will be clear to the reader that 'black and white' is a more natural response to the question 'what colour is the dog?' than 'the dog is black and white' (see also Chapter 13, this volume). Dissatisfaction with such programmes has grown and, since the mid-1980s, under the influence of pragmatics, communicative purpose has become a central tenet of intervention. There has been a reacknowledgement that the basic aim of therapy is to facilitate an individual's ability to communicate effectively and that effective communication is unlikely to be facilitated through precise repetition of correct linguistic structures.

Just as something was lost in clinical practice through strict adherence to linguistic principles at the cost of consideration of a broader perspective, it is important that the value of linguistic knowledge is not lost in the current swing towards a more pragmatic approach. Pragmatic principles do not exclude the use of knowledge of language structure. For example, having identified that a child does not use a specific syntactic structure in their expressive language, it is possible to manipulate the therapeutic environment so that the child has opportunities to acquire the structure in a natural setting. It is likely that, in the future, published intervention procedures will guide our efforts to achieve appropriately communicative intervention. In the meantime, we will need to use our ingenuity in the application of linguistic knowledge within a firmly established pragmatic framework.

Summary

This chapter provides an introduction to the subject-matter of linguistics and the role of linguistics in clinical work. By examining the theories of Saussure in some depth, we have established that speech and language are separate phenomena and that language could be described as a structured system of interrelated, arbitrary linguistic signs. Although less space has been allocated to Chomsky, this should not be taken to imply that his theory is less worthy of consideration. His description of linguistic competence provides us with a greater understanding of what children have to acquire and what adults have to maintain. The distinction between competence and performance shows us that we cannot infer the extent of an individual's language knowledge from the speech they produce. Speech and language therapists need to draw on all areas of their broad-ranging knowledge to diagnose and appropriately manage clients with impaired communication. Linguistic knowledge facilitates our efforts to do so.

Acknowledgements

Thanks to Ali Tempest for taking the time to read through and comment on this chapter as it stood in the the the first edition. Thanks to Pam Grunwell for her helpful comments on the final draft of this chapter. Remaining shortcomings are my own responsibility.

References

Ball, M. (1992). *A Clinician's Guide to Linguistic Profiling*. London: Whurr Publishers.
Berry, M (1975). Introduction to Systemic Linguistics, Vols 1 & 2. London: Batsford.
Bishop, D. and Mogford, K. (1988). *Language Development in Exceptional Circumstances*. Edinburgh: Churchill Livingstone.
Chomsky, N. (1957). *Syntactic Structures*. The Hague: Mouton.
Crystal, D. (1981). *Clinical Linguistics*. Vienna: Springer-Verlag.
Crystal, D. (1987a). Towards a 'bucket' theory of language disability: taking account of interaction between linguistic levels. *Clinical Linguistics and Phonetics* 1, 1, 7–22.
Crystal, D. (1987b). Teaching vocabulary: the case for a semantic curriculum. *Child Language Teaching and Therapy* 3, 40–56.
Crystal, D. (1992). *Profiling Linguistic Disability*, 2nd edn. London: Whurr Publishers.
Crystal, D., Fletcher, P. and Garman, M. (1979). *Language Assessment, Remediation and Screening Procedure*. Reading, UK: University of Reading.
Culler, J. (1976). *Saussure*. Glasgow: William Collins.
Denes, P.B. and Pinson, E.N. (1993). *The Speech Chain*, 2nd edn. New York: W.H. Freeman.
Grunwell, P. (1985). *Phonological Assessment of Child Speech*. Windsor: NFER-Nelson.
Foster, S.H. (1990). *The Communicative Competence of Young Children*. London and New York: Longman.
Harris, J. (1990). *Early Language Development*. London: Routledge.
Hymes, D. (1970). On communicative competence. In: J.J. Gumperz and D. Hymes (Eds) *Directions in Sociolinguistics*. New York: Holt, Rinehart & Winston.
Ingram, D. (1989). *First Language Acquisition: Method, Description and Explanation*. Cambridge: Cambridge University Press.
Lyons, J. (1991). *Chomsky*, 3rd edn. London: Fontana.
McTear, M. and Conti-Ramsden, G. (1992). *Pragmatic Disability in Children*. London: Whurr Publishers.
Naremore, R.C. and Hopper, R. (1990). *Children Learning Language*. New York: Harper & Row.

Saussure, F. de (1916). *Course in General Linguistics*, trans. R. Harris (1983). London: Duckworth .

Smith, B.R. and Leinonen, E. (1992). *Clinical Pragmatics*. London: Chapman & Hall.

Stilwell Peccei, J. (1994). *Child Language*. New York: Routledge.

Chapter 2
Terminology

KIM GRUNDY

Introduction

In the previous chapter a distinction was drawn between *speech* and *language*. This distinction is reflected in the two disciplines of Phonetics, the scientific study of speech; and Linguistics, the scientific study of language. One prerequisite for scientific study is that all features of the subject under investigation are precisely identified and labelled, a necessity which frequently gives rise to a daunting body of 'technical' terms. Once study of the subject is undertaken, such terms are quickly learned and use of them facilitates communication between people working in the field. Terminology is, in fact, no different from any other vocabulary – it is simply vocabulary specific to a particular area of knowledge.

The field of phonetics is sub-divided into three main areas: articulatory, acoustic and auditory. Linguistics also has a number of sub-fields. As was discussed in Chapter 1, different *levels* of language can be identified and each level provides a focus for linguistic description and analysis. The sounds used by a language are the subject-matter of phonology; morphology examines the internal structure of words, and syntax the way in which words combine to form sentences. Semantics studies meaning in language and pragmatics is concerned with the relationship between language structure and non-linguistic factors in human communication.

The main aim of this chapter is to introduce many of the phonetic and linguistic terms used in later chapters of this text and/or likely to be encountered in clinical work. Each section will thus take one of the above areas, outline the subject-matter, define some of the main terms and refer the reader on to later chapters in this volume as appropriate. Clearly, a single chapter could not provide an exhaustive introduction to clinical phonetic and linguistic terminology. A list of suggested additional reading is therefore included at the end.

Phonetics

ARTICULATORY PHONETICS studies the way in which human beings use

34

their vocal (articulatory) apparatus to produce (articulate) speech sounds. Most speech sounds are made by interfering with the free passage of an airstream initiated by the lungs. In normal breathing the airstream passes freely from the lungs, through the trachea (windpipe), larynx (voice box), oral cavity (mouth) and/or nasal cavity (nose) and back again. As there is no major obstruction to this continual breath cycle, it creates little or no sound. Articulatory phonetics is concerned with observing and describing the movements of the vocal organs which interrupt the airstream to create speech sounds.

Vocal apparatus refers to the organs which may be used to produce speech sounds. Because breath streams are a requisite part of speech sounds some phoneticians include lungs and diaphragm as part of the vocal apparatus. More commonly, speech organs are considered to be the larynx and those organs and structures situated above the larynx (supralaryngeal). The air passages above the larynx are known as the **vocal tract**. A specific organ involved in the production of a particular speech sound is called an **articulator**. Articulators may be **active** or **passive**. Active articulators are those which move in the production of a speech sound, for example, the tongue. A passive articulator remains still whilst the active articulator moves towards it, for example, the hard palate. Figure 2.1 shows the conventional diagram used to display the speech organs.

Classification of Speech Sounds

Consonant sounds are usually described using three main parameters:

1. The movement of the vocal folds during production of the sound. Vocal fold vibration is called **phonation** or **voicing**. Consonant sounds are thus classified as either **voiced** or **voiceless**. To feel the difference between a voiceless sound and a voiced sound, place your fingers on your larynx (Adam's apple) and say *s* (a voiceless sound) then *z* (a voiced sound).
2. The use of the articulators in the production of a sound. (The adjectives derived from each articulator are listed on Figure 2.1). The point at which the articulators are closest together during the production of the sound is called **place of articulation**.
3. The way in which the articulators are used to produce sound. There are several basic ways in which sound may be created at most places of articulation. For example, a pair of articulators may meet, totally preventing the air from passing between them, for a fleeting time or for a longer time; or they may be brought close together to form a very narrow gap through which the air can pass; or less close leaving a wider gap. These different ways of using articulators to create sound are called **manners of articulation**.

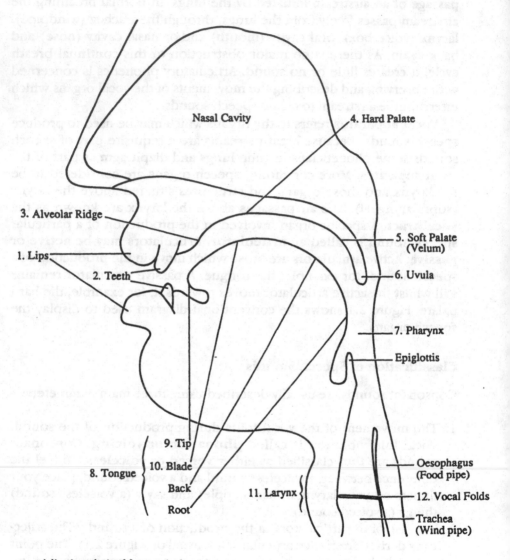

Nasal Cavity

4. Hard Palate

3. Alveolar Ridge

5. Soft Palate (Velum)

1. Lips

2. Teeth

6. Uvula

7. Pharynx

Epiglottis

9. Tip

10. Blade

8. Tongue {

Back

Root

11. Larynx {

Oesophagus (Food pipe)

12. Vocal Folds

Trachea (Wind pipe)

Adjectives derived from articulators

1. Lips: labial
2. Teeth: dental
1 & 2. Lips and teeth:
         labio-dental
3. Alveolar ridge: alveolar
4. Hard palate: palatal
5. Soft palate: velar

6. Uvula: uvular
7. Pharynx: pharyngeal
8. Tongue: lingual
9. Tongue tip: apical
10. Tongue blade: laminal
11. Larynx: laryngeal
12. Vocal folds: glottal

Figure 2.1: Diagrammatic representation of the speech organs

Different vowel sounds are made by using the tongue and lips to make the vocal tract different shapes. The parameters for classifying vowels are therefore:

1. The position of the highest point of the bulk of the tongue. Two-dimensional axes are used for this: **front** to **back** of the mouth and near to or far from the roof of the mouth. The poles of this latter axis are **close** or **high** for when the tongue is very near the roof of the mouth; and **open** or **low** for when the tongue is far away from the roof of the mouth. For example, the vowel in *car* /ɑ/ is classified as an open back vowel (or a low back vowel) whereas the vowel in *be* /i/ is classified as a close front vowel (or a high front vowel).
2. The shape of the lips, which is described on an axis from **rounded** to **unrounded** or **spread**. For example, the vowel in *to* /u/ is rounded whereas the vowel in *be* /i/ is spread.

The International Phonetics Association (IPA) produced a system of symbols and diacritics which may be used to represent most of the speech sounds so far discovered. Figure 2.2 shows the International Phonetic Alphabet (first published in 1889). The top section charts place of articulation in the vertical columns against manner of articulation in the horizontal columns for sounds made on a **pulmonic** airstream (an airstream initiated by the lungs). The symbol to the left of any pair of symbols represents the voiceless sound and the symbol to the right represents the voiced counterpart. Some languages use other airstream mechanisms in addition to a pulmonic airstream. It can be seen that the symbols for sounds produced on non-pulmonic airstreams (clicks, implosives and ejectives) are charted in a separate box below the pulmonic consonants.

Vowel symbols are charted below non-pulmonic consonants on a schematic representation of the highest point of the tongue during articulation of each vowel. As indicated below the vowel diagram, where symbols appear in pairs, the one to the right represents a vowel produced with rounded lips and the symbol to the left represents a vowel produced with the same tongue position but with spread lips.

The 'other symbols' section below the vowel diagram shows pulmonic consonants which need further explanation than could be provided within the pulmonic consonant chart. The **diacritics** charted in the bottom right-hand corner are used to supplement the information conveyed by the main symbols. Suprasegmentals are discussed below.

Phonetics training enables the clinician to recognise and produce each of the sounds on the IPA chart. At the same time the symbols and diacritics conventionally used to represent each sound are learned. Clinicians are thus able to write down (**transcribe**) any stretch of speech in a systematic and consistent way (see Chapter 3). **Phonetic transcriptions**

38

THE INTERNATIONAL PHONETIC ALPHABET (revised to 1993)

CONSONANTS (PULMONIC)

	Bilabial	Labiodental	Dental	Alveolar	Postalveolar	Retroflex	Palatal	Velar	Uvular	Pharyngeal	Glottal
Plosive	p b			t d		ʈ ɖ	c ɟ	k g	q ɢ		ʔ
Nasal	m	ɱ		n		ɳ	ɲ	ŋ	N		
Trill	ʙ			r					R		
Tap or Flap				ɾ		ɽ					
Fricative	ɸ β	f v	θ ð	s z	ʃ ʒ	ʂ ʐ	ç ʝ	x ɣ	χ ʁ	ħ ʕ	h ɦ
Lateral fricative				ɬ ɮ							
Approximant		ʋ		ɹ		ɻ	j	ɰ			
Lateral approximant				l		ɭ	ʎ	L			

Where symbols appear in pairs, the one to the right represents a voiced consonant. Shaded areas denote articulations judged impossible.

CONSONANTS (NON-PULMONIC)

Clicks	Voiced implosives	Ejectives
ʘ Bilabial	ɓ Bilabial	' as in:
ǀ Dental	ɗ Dental/alveolar	p' Bilabial
ǃ (Post)alveolar	ʄ Palatal	t' Dental/alveolar
ǂ Palatoalveolar	ɠ Velar	k' Velar
ǁ Alveolar lateral	ʛ Uvular	s' Alveolar fricative

VOWELS

```
          Front          Central           Back
Close    i y ─────── ɨ ʉ ─────── ɯ u
            ɪ  ʏ               ʊ
Close-mid e ø ─── ɘ ɵ ─────── ɤ o
                        ə
Open-mid   ɛ œ ── ɜ ɞ ── ʌ ɔ
              æ         ɐ
Open          a ɶ ───── ɑ ɒ
```

Where symbols appear in pairs, the one to the right represents a rounded vowel.

OTHER SYMBOLS

ʍ Voiceless labial-velar fricative   ɕ ʑ Alveolo-palatal fricatives
w Voiced labial-velar approximant   ɺ Alveolar lateral flap
ɥ Voiced labial-palatal approximant   ɧ Simultaneous ʃ and x
ʜ Voiceless epiglottal fricative
ʢ Voiced epiglottal fricative   Affricates and double articulations can be represented by two symbols joined by a tie bar if necessary.
ʡ Epiglottal plosive

k͡p t͡s

SUPRASEGMENTALS

ˈ	Primary stress	ˌfoʊnəˈtɪʃən
ˌ	Secondary stress	
ː	Long	eː
ˑ	Half-long	eˑ
̆	Extra-short	ĕ
.	Syllable break	ɹi.ækt
ǀ	Minor (foot) group	
ǁ	Major (intonation) group	
‿	Linking (absence of a break)	

TONES & WORD ACCENTS

	LEVEL			CONTOUR	
e̋ or ꜛ	Extra high	ě or ˅	Rising
é ˥	High	ê ˄	Falling
ē ˧	Mid	e᷄ ˈ	High rising
è ˩	Low	e᷅	Low rising
ȅ	Extra low	e᷈	Rising-falling
↓ Downstep		↗ Global rise	
↑ Upstep		↘ Global fall	

DIACRITICS

Diacritics may be placed above a symbol with a descender, e.g. ŋ̊

Voiceless	n̥ d̥	Breathy voiced	b̤ a̤	Dental	t̪ d̪
Voiced	s̬ t̬	Creaky voiced	b̰ a̰	Apical	t̺ d̺
Aspirated	tʰ dʰ	Linguolabial	t̼ d̼	Laminal	t̻ d̻
More rounded	ɔ̹	Labialized	tʷ dʷ	Nasalized	ẽ
Less rounded	ɔ̜	Palatalized	tʲ dʲ	Nasal release	dⁿ
Advanced	u̟	Velarized	tˠ dˠ	Lateral release	dˡ
Retracted	i̠	Pharyngealized	tˤ dˤ	No audible release	d̚
Centralized	ë	Velarized or pharyngealized	ɫ		
Mid-centralized	ě	Raised	e̝ (ɹ̝ = voiced alveolar fricative)		
Syllabic	ḷ	Lowered	e̞ (β̞ = voiced bilabial approximant)		
Non-syllabic	e̯	Advanced Tongue Root	e̘		
Rhoticity	ɚ	Retracted Tongue Root	e̙		

Figure 2.2: The International Phonetic Alphabet (Revised to 1993). Reproduced by kind permission of the International Phonetics Association

are placed in square brackets [ ] (cf. **phonemic transcription** below). Transcriptions which are relatively detailed, that is, which make use of the full range of symbols and diacritics, are termed **narrow transcriptions**, those which are less detailed are termed **broad transcriptions**. Accurate recording of disordered speech often requires narrow transcription and in some cases even the full range of IPA symbols and diacritics is inadequate for the clinician's purposes. In 1983 the Phonetic Representation of Deviant Speech Committee (PRDSC) published a list of additional phonetic symbols which supplemented the IPA chart and enabled clinicians to transcribe disordered speech more accurately. Recently, members of the International Clinical Phonetics and Linguistics Association (ICPLA) revised and extended the PRDS symbols and brought their presentation into line with the revised IPA chart. Figure 2.3 presents the extIPA (extended IPA) symbols. In addition to these, Ball, Esling and Dickson (1994) produced a list of symbols to facilitate the transcription of aspects of voice quality. Figure 2.4 presents these voice quality symbols.

Student speech and language therapists learn to identify the articulatory movements involved in the production of native speech sounds. They also learn how to produce non-native speech sounds. The skill of being able to produce this range of speech sounds enables clinicians to imitate accurately the speech of people with speech disorders, thereby gaining a true feel for their articulatory movements and a deeper insight into possibilities for change. The process of learning these skills provides a valuable appreciation of the difficulties faced by individuals who are struggling to achieve their native sounds.

Articulatory phonetics training also provides clinicians with the necessary skills to analyse and transcribe the speech of any individual referred for therapy. Transcriptions provide records which are used to analyse and assess the progress of an individual and may further be used as data for research (see further Chapter 3). The combination of these phonetic skills with knowledge gained from training in anatomy and physiology, neurology and speech pathology enables the clinician to differentially diagnose speech disorders, predict the outcome of the disorder (prognose) and formulate a management plan based on systematic investigation (see also Chapter 15).

ACOUSTIC PHONETICS studies the speech sound-waves, produced by human articulatory movements, as they travel between the mouth of the speaker and the ear of the listener. Sound-waves are difficult phenomena to come to grips with as they have no substance and cannot be seen. A sound wave is a set of movements or disturbance. If a pebble is dropped into a calm pool of water, ripples can be seen on top of the water radiating out from the point at which the pebble fell. If you click your fingers, the clicking movements set the air molecules surrounding your fingers into vibration and create ripples of movement (waves) through

extIPA SYMBOLS FOR DISORDERED SPEECH
(Revised to 1994)

CONSONANTS (other than those on the IPA Chart)

	bilabial	labiodental	dentolabial	labioalv.	linguolabial	interdental	bidental	alveolar	velar	velophar.
Plosive		p̪ b̪	p̟ b̟	p̪ b̪	t̼ d̼	t̪ d̪				
Nasal			m̪	m̟	n̼	n̪				
Trill					r̼	r̪				
Fricative median		f̪ v̪	f̟ v̟		θ̼ ð̼	θ̪ ð̪	ħ̪ ɦ̪			ʩ
Fricative lateral+median								ⱡ ⱡ		
Fricative nareal	m̃							ñ̥	ŋ̥̃	
Percussive	ʬ ʬ						ʭ			
Approximant lateral					l̼	l̪				

DIACRITICS

labial spreading	s̪	strong articulation	f̬	denasal	m̃
dentolabial	v̪	weak articulation	v̥	nasal escape	ṽ
interdental/bidental	n̪	reiterated articulation	p\p\p	velopharyngeal friction	s̃
alveolar	s̪	whistled articulation	s̟	ingressive airflow	p↓
linguolabial	d̼	sliding articulation	θs	egressive airflow	!↑

CONNECTED SPEECH

(.)	short pause
(..)	medium pause
(...)	long pause
f	loud speech [{f loud f}]
ff	louder speech [{ff laudɚ ff}]
p	quiet speech [{p kwaɪət p}]
pp	quieter speech [{pp kwaɪətə pp}]
allegro	fast speech [{allegro faːst allegro}]
lento	slow speech [{ lento sloʊ lento}]
crescendo, ralentando, etc may also be used	

VOICING

pre-voicing	˳z
post-voicing	z˳
partial devoicing	z̥
initial partial devoicing	z̥
final partial devoicing	z̥
partial voicing	s̬
initial partial voicing	s̬
final partial voicing	s̬
unaspirated	p⁼
pre-aspiration	ʰp

OTHERS

(◌̈) indeterminate sound	() silent articulation (ʃ)	
(V̈) indeterminate vowel	(()) extraneous noise ((2 sylls))	
(Pl) indeterminate plosive	* sound with no symbol available	
(Pl.vls) indeterminate voiceless plosive, etc	(to be described elsewhere)	

© 1994 ICPLA

Figure 2.3: extIPA Symbols for Disordered Speech (Revised to 1994). Reproduced by kind permission of the International Clinical Phonetics and Linguistics Association

VoQS: Voice Quality Symbols

AIRSTREAM TYPES

Œ	oesophageal speech	Ƕ	electrolarynx speech
Ю	tracheo-oesophageal speech	↓	pulmonic ingressive speech

PHONATION TYPES

V	modal voice	F	falsetto
W	whisper	C	creak
V̬	whispery voice (murmur)	V̰	creaky voice
V̤	breathy voice	C̤	whispery creak
V!	harsh voice	V!!	ventricular phonation
V̰!!	diplophonia	V̤!!	whispery ventricular phon.
V̪	anterior or pressed phonation	W̱	posterior whisper

SUPRALARYNGEAL SETTINGS

L̝	raised larynx	L̞	lowered larynx
Vᶜᶜ	labialized voice (open round)	Vʷ	labialized voice (close round)
V̈	spread-lip voice ·	Vᵛ	labio-dentalized voice
V̺	linguo-apicalized voice	V̻	linguo-laminalized voice
Vˤ	retroflex voice	V̪	dentalized voice
V̳	alveolarized voice	V̳ʲ	palatoalveolarized voice
Vʲ	palatalized voice	Vˠ	velarized voice
Vᵝ	uvularized voice	Vˤ	pharyngealized voice
V̰ˤ	laryngo-pharyngealized voice	Vᴴ	faucalized voice
Ṽ	nasalized voice	V̷	denasalized voice
J̞	open jaw voice	J̝	close jaw voice
J̦	right offset jaw voice	J̧	left offset jaw voice
J̪	protruded jaw voice	Θ	protruded tongue voice

USE OF LABELED BRACES & NUMERALS TO MARK STRETCHES OF SPEECH AND DEGREES AND COMBINATIONS OF VOICE QUALITY

[ˈðɪs ɪz ˈnɔˑməl ˈvɔɪs {3V! ˈðɪs ɪz ˈveri ˈhɑˑʃ ˈvɔɪs 3V!} ˈðɪs ɪz ˈnɔˑməl ˈvɔɪs wʌns ˈmɔˑ {L̝1V! ˈðɪs ɪz ˈles ˈhɑˑʃ ˈvɔɪs wɪð ˈloʊəd ˈlærɪŋks 1V!L̝}]

© 1994 Martin J. Ball, John Esling, Craig Dickson

Figure 2.4: VoQS: Voice Quality Symbols (1994). Reproduced by kind permission of the copyright holders

the air which radiate out from that point in a similar way to the ripples surrounding the pebble in water. However, sound waves and water waves are different in that, first, the water waves radiate out in one plane only – across the surface of the water – whereas sound waves radiate out in all directions creating a sphere of movement surrounding the sound source. Second, only **pure tone** sound-waves (such as are created by striking a tuning fork) have a simple wave pattern comparable to the water wave. Sound-waves in general, and speech sound-waves in particular, create very complex patterns of air molecule movement.

The movements of air molecules set in motion by a sound-wave cannot, of course, be seen by the human eye. The study of speech sound-waves, therefore, involves the use of various instruments which utilise the energy created by the sound-wave to produce a visual representation of it. Acoustic phonetics is a complex field and advanced study of the subject requires some knowledge of physics and mathematics. However, clinicians who have a basic understanding of the principles and terms used within the field will find that they are able to apply the information provided through research experiments in their approach to treatment planning (see further Chapter 3).

AUDITORY PHONETICS is concerned with the way in which speech sounds are perceived by the listener. Speech sound-waves enter the ear and are transformed into neural impulses which are transmitted to the brain via the auditory nerve. The anatomical structure and innervation of the outer, middle and inner ear and the physiological processes involved in transmitting the sound-wave to the brain are somewhat outside the mainstream of this text (the reader is directed to the reading list at the end of this chapter for texts which address this area). However, there is an important distinction to be made between the processes involved in registering sounds in the brain and the processes which (are assumed to) occur once the sounds have reached the brain. Auditory phonetics is mostly concerned with the latter phenomena.

Audition refers to the physiological process of hearing. Study of this process is well advanced and a number of instruments have been developed for measuring an individual's **auditory acuity** (ability to hear). **Audiology** is the clinical study of the hearing process and is now a well-established discipline; **audiometry** is the clinical measurement of audition.

In auditory phonetics *audition* is contrasted with **speech perception**. Speech perception is concerned with what happens to the speech signal once it reaches the brain. How do humans *decode* the acoustic signals and extract from them linguistic meaning? As the processes involved in decoding speech take place in the brain they are, of course, not observable, extremely complex and, as a result, are poorly understood. Hypothesising about what the processes might be involves taking into account several levels of human functioning and requires reference to several other disciplines such as psychology, neurology, neuro-psychology and audiology. There are certain aspects of the speech perception process which are particularly relevant to people working with individuals who have speech and/or language disorders (see further Chapter 4).

Perceiving speech requires first that the individual can *hear* speech. The distinction between speech perception and audition may be better appreciated when the effects of deafness are compared with the effects of brain damage. Children who are born deaf do not develop speech because they cannot hear speech; if they could hear speech they would learn to interpret it and would learn to speak. The child who is born with damage to the brain resulting in misinterpretation of speech signals does not have a *hearing* problem. Speech signals *do* register in that child's brain but he or she is unable to learn how to gain meaning from them. Similarly, adults who suffer brain damage, through stroke or accident, do not lose their sense of hearing but may lose the ability to interpret speech signals.

Auditory discrimination refers to the ability to perceive differences between speech sounds.

The distinction between audition and perception is clearly pertinent to the clinician. Individuals who have a hearing loss may need to be referred for surgery or to have a hearing aid fitted. In contrast, individuals who have speech perception difficulties may benefit from perceptual training or from having language transmitted to them through non-auditory channels, such as the visual channel utilised by manual and graphic signing systems (see further Section III).

Phonetics versus Phonology

Phonetics is concerned with the human capacity to produce and perceive all and any of the speech sounds of the world. Phonology studies the nature of the sound systems of human languages and the limited system of sounds used by a particular language to convey meaning.

Since the 'raw material' of both phonetics and phonology is essentially the same thing – vocal sound – it is difficult, initially, to appreciate the distinction between the two disciplines. It may be helpful to compare language with a picture. To paint a picture you do not need to use the full range of colours available in paint form. All that is necessary is that the colours used are different enough to contrast with one another to allow the overall image to be perceived. In language, it is not necessary to use all of the speech sounds that the human articulatory apparatus is capable of producing. More than one sound is necessary as a single sound used to apply to everything would carry no meaning at all, just as a single colour conveys no image other than that invoked by the colour itself. A painter uses a range of colours, a language uses a range of sounds. The way in which the painter organises and combines the colours produces a distinctive painting. The organisation and combination of the chosen speech sounds produce a distinctive language. Any group of linguistic elements which forms a potentially endless group is called an **open class**; this term contrasts with **closed class** which refers to a finite group of items. So, whereas phonetics is concerned with the 'world supply' of speech sounds (an open class); phonology is concerned with the range of sounds used by a particular *language* (a closed class) and, therefore, is an area of *linguistic* study.

Speech sounds have physical reality. The movements of the vocal organs used to produce a speech sound may be observed and described. Speech sounds may be heard and tape-recorded. **Phonemes** are abstract linguistic units. They do not have physical existence in the same way that speech sounds do. Take, for example, the utterance 'That darn' cat!' The final *t* in *cat* may be said in a number of different ways:

it may be aspirated [tʰ] or unreleased [t'] or affricated [tˢ] or ejected [t'] or replaced with a glottal stop [ʔ] for example.

Regardless of which of these pronunciations of *t* is used, the sound uttered is recognised as representing *t* and the meaning of the word remains: *carnivorous quadruped that has long been domesticated* (OED). If, however, we were to replace the *t* with *p – cap*; or *n – can*; or *b – cab*; we recognise different words with different meanings. Speech sounds that signal meaning differences in this way are called phonemes. None of the above *t* sounds is a phoneme in the English language because none of them signals a meaning difference. Because *t* can be said in so many different ways and still be recognised as *t*, it is clear that *t* itself does not have actual physical existence but is made to exist through one or other of the *t* sounds. Different pronunciations of a phoneme are called **allophones**; [tʰ t' tˢ t' ʔ] are all allophones of the /t/ phoneme. (To keep speech sounds and phonemes clearly distinguished from one another, it is conventional to place speech sounds in square brackets [ ] and phonemes in slant brackets / /.)

Breaking speech down into its constituent speech sounds, or language into its component phonemes, is referred to as **segmental analysis**. There are, however, certain vocal effects (such as whispering, hoarseness, nasalisation, high pitch and so on) and articulatory postures (such as curling the tongue tip back, protruding the lips etc.) which may be extended over more than one segment. These features come under the general heading of **suprasegmentals** and may be divided into **paralinguistic** and **linguistic**. Paralinguistic suprasegmental features are not generally used to convey linguistic meaning although they may be used to add to the effect of an utterance. Whispering, for example, indicates that the speaker does not wish to be overheard but does not change the linguistic meaning of what is said. Linguistic suprasegmental features are usually referred to as **prosodic features** and they serve to indicate meaning differences. For instance, placing stress on a particular word within an utterance can change the meaning of that utterance. For example, 'She didn't break the *window*,' implies that she broke something else, whereas '*She* didn't break the window,' implies that someone else broke it. (See further Chapter 10.)

Distinctive feature refers to any phonetic characteristic of a group of sounds which serves to distinguish that group from another group of sounds. For example, [t] and [s] involve the same *place of articulation* – the alveolar ridge – and neither sound involves *voicing*. The difference between them is that in [t] the tongue tip makes firm contact with the alveolar ridge which is then sharply broken allowing the breath to rush out, whereas in [s] the tongue tip moves very close to the alveolar ridge and a continuous breath stream passes between the two. In other words, the two sounds differ in *manner of articulation*. Sounds made in the same manner as [t] are called **plosives** and sounds made in the same manner as [s] are called **fricatives**. Plosion and frication are examples of distinctive features. [t] and [k] are both voiceless plosives; the difference between them is that [t] is produced by bringing the tongue tip into firm contact with the alveolar ridge (an **alveolar** sound) whereas [k] is produced by bringing the back of the tongue in firm contact with the velum (a **velar** sound). [t] and [k] therefore differ in *place of articulation*. Alveolar and velar are further examples of distinctive features. [t] is a *voiceless alveolar plosive* whereas [d] is a *voiced alveolar plosive*. The difference between them is therefore that [t] is a voiceless sound whereas [d] is a voiced sound. Voiced and voiceless is another example of a distinctive feature.

Assimilation, Co-articulation and Elision

The allophones of /t/ used in the above example, may occur when the word *cat* (or any other word ending in /t/) is spoken in isolation or within an utterance. When spoken within certain utterances, however, there are other pronunciations which may occur. These pronunciations may involve other English phonemes but do not, in fact, affect meaning. For example, in the utterance 'Empty the can please', unless each word is articulated unnaturally clearly, the last two words may be produced as /kam pliz/; and in the utterance 'They can go tomorrow', 'can go' may be produced as /kaŋ gəʊ/. This phenomenon is the result of a process termed **assimilation**. The word final /n/ has, in both cases, assimilated to the word initial phoneme of the following word. Assimilation is an effort-saving device: it is easier to say /kam pliz/ than /kan pliz/.

Co-articulation is closely related to assimilation. Speech is a dynamic, fluid process and the production of any one sound will be influenced by sounds adjacent to it. For example, in the utterance 'too cool' the first consonant of *cool* [k] will be produced with rounded lips due to the influence of the rounded vowels which precede and follow it. In the utterance 'three keys' the [k] of *keys* will be produced with spread lips, again due to the influence of the preceding and following vowels. **Anticipatory co-articulation** is the term used when an articulatory posture is affected by the sound following it. (The articulators *anticipate* the posture of the upcoming sound.) **Perseverative co-articulation** is the term used when an articulatory posture is affected by the sound preceding it. (The posture *perseverates* into the next sound.) Co-articulatory processes are studied in experimental phonetics and co-articulation is used to explain assimilation. (See also Chapters 4 and 15.)

Another effort-saving device is **elision**. In certain contexts, certain phonemes may be missed out altogether: elided. For example, in the utterance 'He started singing and they all left', the final /d/ of *and* is likely to be elided (/an ðeɪ ɔl lɛft/) . In some contexts elision and assimilation operate together, for example, *handbag* is often produced as /hambag/; the /d/ of *hand* is elided, and the /n/ of *hand* assimilates to the articulatory posture of the /b/ of *bag* and is produced as /m/. Assimilation and elision only occur in specific contexts such as the above. There is, therefore, a finite set of rules governing assimilation and elision in any language. Speech and language therapists need to be aware of these rules when analysing the speech of individuals presenting with unclear speech because, if a 'connected speech' sample (as opposed to a single word sample elicited through picture naming for example) is taken, analysis of individual words must take into account assimilatory and elision processes.

Sound System

As discussed above, phonemes are abstract units and are realised through speech sounds. The range of speech sounds used by a particular language may be organised into groups according to the phonemes they represent. For example the *t* sounds [tʰ tˈ tˈ tˈ ʔ] (and so on) form a group represented by the phoneme /t/. This organisation of speech sounds into phoneme groups is called the sound system, or **phonological system** of the language. Clinicians can make use of their knowledge of the phonological system of their language in situations where they do not need to record all the phonetic details of an individual's speech. On these occasions, clinicians may make a **phonemic transcription** and record the speech heard using only the phonemic symbols of their language.

Accent is the term used to refer to the varieties of pronunciation which occur in any language (cf. **Dialect**, below). Variety arises through speakers living in different geographical locations (**regional accent**) and/or within different social groups (**social accent**). Some accents may be judged to be 'nicer' than others, but such judgements must be recognised as having their basis in personal taste and accepted values, because all accents are equally capable of communicating meaning. The 'standard' accent in English is **received pronunciation** or RP (*received*, in this case, meaning *acceptable*) and is that accent used by the upper classes in English society and by many educated people. Clinicians need to be sensitive to the accent of each individual they work with in order that they do not try to 'correct' pronunciations which arise through the accent.

Minimal pair is a term used to refer to two words which differ from one another by one phoneme only. For example, *box* and *fox*; *bat* and *hot*; *bat* and *bag*; *sin* and *in*. A group of words in which each word differs from each other word by only one phoneme is called a minimal set. For example, *locks, rocks, docks, mocks, box, fox, shocks, woks* (etc.) is a minimal set as is *ban, badge, bap, bang, bat, back* (etc.) and *park, peek, poke, pike, pack, pick, peck* (etc.). Minimal pairs and sets may be used in treatment programmes for speech disorders (see Section III).

Phonotactics is a term used in phonology to refer to the way in which a language combines phonemes to make words. All languages use their phonemes in a finite set of combinations and **phonotactic rules** describe the permissible combinations in a particular language. There are two aspects to the study of phonotactics. First, it examines **syllable structure**. In phonology, a **syllable** must have a *nucleus* which is called a *vowel*, and may or may not have other elements which are called **consonants**. (Conventionally, vowels are represented by a capital v thus: V, and consonants are represented by a capital c thus: C.) Syllables which have no consonant at the end (CV, CCV, etc.) are called **open syllables** and those which have a *closing* consonant (CVC, CCVC, CVCC, etc.) are called **closed syllables**. **Cluster** refers to the combination of two or more consonants which may occur at the beginning or end of syllables.

The other aspect of phonotactic analysis involves establishing which particular phonemes may occur at each position in the syllable structure. In English, for example, /ŋ/does not occur at the beginning of syllables (**syllable-initially**) */ŋ-/, but does occur at the end of syllables (**syllable-finally**), for example, *thing*: (/θɪŋ/). Also in English, nasals do not occur as the first phoneme of a cluster in syllable-initial position, */mp-/ */nt-/; but do occur in that combination syllable-finally, for example; *stamp*: /stamp/; *went*: /wɛnt/.

Speech and language therapists draw on phonetic and phonological knowledge in the management of individuals presenting with impaired speech. An appreciation of the distinction between phonetics and phonology contributes towards the clinician's ability to differentially diagnose between articulation disorder and phonological impairment and enables the clinician to formulate principled treatment programmes appropriate to the individual concerned (see further Chapters 3, 4 and 5 and Section III).

Syntax and Morphology

(a) The cheese sandwiches are in the fridge.
(b) *Sandwiches cheese the in fridge the are.
(c) She washed herself.
(d) *She washed himself.

As native speakers of English, we know that sentences (a) and (c) are acceptable English sentences whereas sentences (b) and (d) are not. The fact that we are able to make these decisions suggests that we have acquired rules regarding permissible word combinations in our language. **Syntax** is the study of the rules which govern word combination in language. Rules describing acceptable word combinations are called **syntactic rules**.

As well as having knowledge about acceptable ways of putting words together to make sentences, we also have knowledge about acceptable ways of forming words. For example, we know that *unhelpful* is an acceptable English word and that **fulhelpun* is not; *washed* is an acceptable past tense form, **goed* is not. The study of internal word structure is called **morphology** (see further **Morpheme**, below). Rules describing word formation in a language are called **morphological rules**.

Syntax and morphology interrelate to some extent. In some instances, the syntactic relationships between words govern the morphological rules. In example (d) above, **She washed himself* is unacceptable because use of the feminine pronoun *she* means that the feminine reflexive pronoun *herself* must be used. This interdependence between syntax and morphology suggests that they 'belong' together more than other levels of language. Some linguists subsume the two areas under the heading of **grammar**.

In this sense of the word, the grammar of a language may be studied and analysed without taking into account *phonology* (the sounds of the language); or *semantics* (the meaning of the language). For example, in English:

(i) [çi çɛ d çi wox kʌmɪn]; *she said she was coming*; and,
(ii) *colourless green ideas sleep furiously*,

are both grammatical sentences as they conform to the syntactic and morphological rules of the language, despite the fact that (i) is not pronounced in an acceptable way and (ii) does not make sense.

Units of analysis in grammar are called **grammatical units** and may be arranged in order from biggest to smallest thus: *sentence–clause–phrase–word–morpheme*. This organisation is called **rank structure** or **scale**. Each unit will comprise one or more units of the other ranks.

In the above definitions of syntax, morphology and grammar, the word used to describe sentences or words that are possible in a language is *acceptable*. Acceptable is the term used in linguistics to describe utterances which native speakers would judge to be 'normal'. Use of the term 'acceptable' dispenses with notions of 'correctness'. Modern linguistic grammar aims to describe comprehensively the language in current usage and not to prescribe 'correct' usage. These grammars are thus called **descriptive grammars** and may be contrasted with the **prescriptive grammars** of 'traditional' linguistics which attempt to *impose* rules on language users. A descriptive grammar which attempts to include all the syntactic and morphological rules of a language is called a **reference grammar** (for an example see Quirk *et al.*, 1972).

Morpheme

Some words may be divided into smaller component parts. For example, *unhelpfully* may be divided into *un- help- -ful -ly*. Each of these parts may be shown to take part in regular and recurrent patterns in the English language:

un-	*like*	*help-*	*ing*	*-ful*	*useful*	*-ly*	*quietly*
	deniable		*s*		*mindful*		*uselessly*
	seen		*less*		*wonderful*		*evenly*

These component parts may or may not have *lexical meaning* (see below **Semantics**) and they may or may not occur in isolation, but because they can be shown to take part in these patterns they have what is called **grammatical significance**. They are, in fact, the smallest units of grammatical significance and are called **morphemes**.

Morphemes are abstract units and should not be confused with affixes, suffixes and prefixes (see Chapter 1) or syllables (see **Phonotactics**, above). In the above examples, each component morpheme may be given physical form: that is, it may be spoken or written (or signed). Now consider the past tense of the verb to *think*. '*Thought*' has two morphemes, one which enters into a pattern with the other forms of the verb *to think* – *thinks, think, thinking*; and another which enters into a pattern with other past tense forms – *walked; rained; smiled*. So, although *thought* may not be divided into two distinct parts it is still said to have morphemes. Morphemes are conventionally encapsulated in curly brackets, for example, *went* is composed of the two morphemes {go} and {ed}.

When a word *can* be divided into morphemes which may be written or spoken, each morpheme is called a **morph**. Some morphs which have the same grammatical significance as one another are, however, pronounced differently from one another. For example, in *cats*, *dogs* and *borses*, the plural morpheme {s} is pronounced /s/, /z/ and /ɪz/ respectively. These differences in pronunciation occur systematically according to the phonological context in which the morph occurs. In the case of English plurals, /s/ occurs after voiceless sounds; /z/ occurs after voiced sounds; and / ɪz/ occurs after the fricatives /s z ʃ ʒ / and the affricates /tʃ dʒ/. The study of rules governing the pronunciation of morphs is called **morphophonology**. The label given to variant pronunciations of the same morph is **allomorph**. Thus the English plural morph {s} has three allomorphs: /s/, /z/ and /ɪz/.

Overgeneralisation is a term used in language acquisition studies to describe children's over-use of grammatical rules. Normally developing children often pass through a stage when they apply certain grammatical rules in more contexts than would an adult. For example, the words: **goed, *wented, *jumpeded;.*bestest, *badder* are characteristic of this stage of development. This stage may occur later, or persist longer, in children with language impairments.

In any language there are variations in syntactic structure, word formation and lexical items which are used by people living in different parts of the country and/or belonging to different social groups. These different varieties of language are called **dialects**. A variety which arises within a specific geographical location is a **regional dialect**, a variety which occurs within a particular social group is called a **social dialect** and a variety which exists within a particular culture is called a **cultural dialect**. Regional, cultural and social dialects interact and speakers of any particular regional or cultural dialect will recognise varieties within that dialect which reflect the social status of the speaker.

As there are often gross differences between dialects which may prevent speakers of one dialect from understanding speakers of another, countries often adopt one variety which all members of the country understand. In England, there is one variety of English – **Standard English** – which is used in educational literature, by the media, by prominent public figures and so on. It should be recognised, however, that Standard English originated as just one of many different varieties of English and that it has gained importance for social and political reasons only. In linguistic terms, Standard English is not 'better' than any other dialect of English because all dialects are equally capable of communicating meaning amongst speakers of that dialect.

Grammatical analysis has become a routine part of the clinician's work (see further Chapter 6). Such analysis enables clinicians to identify which aspects of syntax and morphology an individual needs to (re)acquire to convey their meaning adequately. Grammatical theory also provides a framework which may be used to investigate an individual's ability to understand specific syntactic and/or morphological structures (see further Chapter 7).

Semantics

Semantics is the study of meaning in language. Linguistics considers meaning from several different aspects.

Lexeme/Lexicon

The vocabulary of a language is termed the **lexicon**. The minimal distinctive unit within the lexicon is called a **lexeme**. In linguistics lexemes are conventionally written in small capitals. In an abstract sense, *imitates, imitated, imitator, imitation* may be said to be different forms of the same word. The differences between the four words are *grammatical*, in that they are composed of different morphemes and have different possibilities of syntactic occurrence; and *phonological*, in that they are composed of different phonemes. What they share is an underlying abstract unit of meaningfulness which is the lexeme IMITATE. The term 'lexeme' may thus be differentiated from the grammatical word and the phonological word and provides us with a more useful label than *word* when we are discussing vocabulary. By this definition, idiomatic phrases are also lexemes. The phrase *take off*, for example, is composed of two grammatical words but is one lexical unit which can have the same meaning as the alternative lexeme IMITATE.

Some individuals have difficulty in producing lexical items as and when required and this phenomenon is referred to as **word-finding difficulty** (see further Chapter 8).

Sense Relations

The alphabetical listing of lexemes in dictionaries can leave one with the impression that words exist as separate units which have nothing to do with one another. We may also be left with this impression if we see lexemes as labels for objects, entities, states etc. Labelling does account for one aspect of the meaning of a lexeme. The lexeme CHAIR, for example, refers to the object *chair*. In linguistics, this type of relationship is termed **reference**. The object *chair* is the **referent** for the lexeme CHAIR. However, if we consider the lexemes CHAIR, BANANA, WATCH and BED, we can see that there is a link between CHAIR and BED, which does not exist between CHAIR and BANANA, or CHAIR and WATCH. CHAIR and BED fall into the group of lexical items called FURNITURE. The relationship between CHAIR and BED is one of **hyponymy**; they are both **hyponyms** (or are **co-hyponyms**) of the **super-ordinate** lexeme FURNITURE. Hyponymy is one example of the **sense relations** which interconnect lexical items. Two other sense relations are **antonymy** (oppositeness) and **synonymy** (sameness). HOT and COLD are **antonyms**; WARM and TEPID are **synonyms** (but see below, **Sentence Meaning**). Hyponymy, antonymy and synonymy are examples of the **paradigmatic** relations which exist between linguistic units (see further Chapter 1).

A group of lexical items within which words define one another and interrelate in ways such as the above is called a **semantic field**. The semantic field most commonly used for exemplification is that of *colour*. Each colour term depends upon the other colour terms for its definition: the lexeme RED, for example, refers to the colour which is not orange or purple, yellow, blue or green and so on.

Collocation is another type of sense relation which accounts for the fact that some lexical items habitually co-occur in sentences. For example, *safety* frequently co-occurs (*or* collocates) with *first/match/pin; bank* with *manager/statement/account*. Collocation can also affect meaning; for example, consider the meaning of *match* when collocated with (a) *safety*, (b) *football*, and (c) *perfect* (see also **Sentence Meaning**, below). Collocational relations are an example of the **syntagmatic** relations which exist between linguistic units (see further Chapter 1). Collocational relations are often used in therapy programmes, particularly with adults who have lost their ability to produce lexical items as and when they want to. Clinicians are often able to 'cue' the individual to produce the required word by themselves uttering a word/words which collocate(s) with it. For example, a person who is struggling to come up with the word *tea* may well utter it when cued with 'a nice cuppa_'. (See further Section III.)

Lexemes which have the same orthographic (written) and phonological (sound) form, but different meanings, are called **homonyms**. For example, ROSE can be a flower, or the past tense of rise. In some cases homonymy is only partial. For example, BOUGH and BOW are spelled differently but have one phonological form /baʊ/. Lexemes such as BOUGH and BOW, with the same phonological form but different orthographic forms, are called **homophones**. The reverse also occurs; LEAD, for example, may be pronounced /lid/ meaning the verb or /lɛd/ meaning the metal. Lexical items sharing one orthographic form but which have different phonological forms are called **homographs**.

Whilst acquiring language, children often go through a stage when they use one lexical item to refer to a wider range of referents than would an adult. For example, *daddy* is often used by small children when referring to any adult male. This phenomenon is termed **over-extension**. The contrasting term **under-extension** applies when the child uses one lexical item to refer to a narrower range of referents than an adult. For example, cup may be used by a child to refer to her or his own personal cup but not to refer to any other cup. The over- and under-extension of lexical items may occur later, or persist longer, in children with language impairment (see further Chapter 8).

Sentence Meaning

There is a limit to which lexical items have meaning in their own right.

The meaning of those lexemes which have concrete referents may be demonstrated by pointing to, or describing, or showing a picture of, the referential object. However, consider the two terms WARM and TEPID. In the example above these lexemes were said to be synonyms. If we put them into a sentence such as 'The water was warm/tepid', they are synonymous. If, on the other hand, we put them into the structure 'She received a warm welcome', or 'She received a tepid welcome', the two sentences could not be said to have the same meaning and therefore the two lexemes WARM and TEPID are not synonymous in this particular syntactic context. Meaningfulness of individual lexical items is, there-fore, dependent upon the context in which they occur. Further, mean-ingfulness is also dependent upon the syntactic arrangements of words: for example, 'The girl surprised her mother'; 'Her mother surprised the girl'. Ultimately, then, meaningfulness is a property of whole sentences rather than being a property of individual linguistic units within the sentence.

An awareness of how lexical items come to have 'meaning' guides clinicians in their approach to vocabulary teaching and treatment plan-ning for individuals who have word-finding difficulties. In addition, knowledge of the ways in which words interrelate can be used in the selection of lexical items to be integrated into therapy programmes (see also Chapters 1, 11 and 13).

Pragmatics

Pragmatics is the study of factors which govern the way communicators make use of language, world knowledge and social convention to convey and interpret meaning. In pragmatics, language is seen as a tool which we use to communicate information to one another. In any **communicative interaction** (conversation, sermon, play, commentary and so on) there are other factors which contribute to the communi-cative message, over and above the **linguistic content** of that message. The above sections have defined linguistic content as phonological, grammatical and semantic. Pragmatics examines the ways in which the meaningfulness of linguistic content may be modified by non-linguistic factors.

An **utterance** is a unit of speech which is preceded and followed by silence or a change of speaker and about which no linguistic judgements have been made. Utterance may be contrasted with the term *sentence* which is a grammatical unit composed of one or more clauses. In the above discussion on semantics, we have seen that the meaningfulness of individual lexical items often depends upon syntactic context. The meaning of an utterance *always* depends upon the **situational context** in which it occurs.

Situational context refers to the whole, non-linguistic background which contributes to the meaningfulness of an utterance. This includes the immediate situation in which a communicative interaction takes place, and the roles of the participants. For example, the utterance; 'We are gathered here today to celebrate the joining of two people in the union of marriage' is an appropriate utterance when used by a registrar in a wedding ceremony. However, the same utterance would be considered either inappropriate, or intending humour, if uttered in response to the question' 'Why are all you people standing outside that building?'.

Situational context also includes knowledge of what has been said prior to that utterance. For example, 'She went there yesterday' is meaningless unless both speaker and hearer know who *she* is and where *there* was. Lastly, situational context incorporates any world knowledge, beliefs and assumptions held by the participants which may be relevant to the interpretation of the utterance. To use the above example, if we take *she* to be the speaker's mother; the utterance will have different significance if *there* was a Buckingham Palace Garden Party, than if *there* was the doctor's surgery.

Speech act theory is an approach to the study of utterances and provides terminology for describing some aspects of situational context. **Speech act** is a term used to refer to a communicative event involving a speaker and listener(s). Specifically, a speech act has four basic components, namely:

1. the **utterance act**: saying something;
2. the **propositional act**: referring to something and saying something about it;
3. the **illocutionary force** of the utterance: the intention behind what is said, for example, making a statement or joke, asking a question, directing someone to do something, and so on; and
4. the **perlocutionary effect** of the utterance: the effect of the sum total of the above on the actions, thoughts or beliefs of the listener(s); for example, verbal response, physical action, change of view and so on.

So, for example, (1) a speaker may say 'It's hot in here'; (2) referring to a place and stating something about the condition of that place; (3) the speaker may intend this utterance as a simple (if superfluous) statement of fact; alternatively, (3) he or she may use the utterance to induce the listener to open a window, turn down a fire, offer a drink and so on. If the listener does, in fact, (4) open a window, then the perlocutionary effect is an act of compliance. (Note: *speech act* is often used loosely to refer to illocutionary force in much of the literature).

Pragmatic terminology is discussed in more detail in Chapter 9 and the influence of pragmatics on clinical work is evident in all chapters in this book.

Metalanguage

Linguistic **metalanguage** is a language which is used to talk about language. All the terminology used in this book contributes to the metalanguage of linguistics. In the previous chapter it was stated that everyone has knowledge of their language but that the knowledge we have is covert or intuitive knowledge which we do not consult unless we are called upon to do so. As children we acquired our language without being aware that it could be said to made up of words, that words are made up of sounds and are combined to form sentences. We had to learn what was meant by *word, sentence, sound, noun, verb* and so on. As student speech and language therapists are introduced to linguistics they rapidly acquire its metalanguage and utilise it in their work.

Over the past ten to fifteen years there has been increasing interest in the question of when children begin to develop **metalinguistic awareness**. That is, at what age do children begin to show an awareness of the language that they are acquiring? Research suggests that true metalinguistic awareness does not develop until around 7 years of age. For example, prior to that age, children asked to think of a 'long' word might say *train* and when asked to think of a 'short' word might say *caterpillar* indicting that they have little awareness that words can be separated from the referents with which they are associated. This is an important point for speech and language therapists: if a child has no concept for *word*, for example, intervention which requires her or him to reflect on words may prove to be unsuccessful.

Just as different levels of language have been identified above, so different levels of metalinguistic awareness are identified. For example, **metaphonological awareness** refers to overt knowledge that words are made up of different sounds, that some words 'rhyme', that changing a sound in a word can make a different word and so on. Children need to develop metaphonological awareness in order to learn to read and write. **Metacommunicative awareness** refers to conscious knowledge of rules of communication such as: people take turns when they speak, some language is only appropriate in certain situations, what is polite and what is impolite and so on.

Clinicians need to be cognisant of their own metalinguistic awareness in order to make appropriate use of linguistic metalanguage in the clinic situation. The development of metalinguistic skills may be an appropriate aim for intervention with some clients (see further Chapters 12, 13, 14).

Psycholinguistics

As the term suggests, **psycholinguistics** is a field of study where psychology and linguistics meet. The previous chapter identified language as a psychological phenomenon. That is, language processing (encoding and decoding) occurs in the brain. Linguistics identifies, analyses and describes language but it does not seek to *explain* the processes involved in language production and reception. Explanation is the domain of psychology. Cognitive psychologists attempt to explain how we process information. Neuropsychologists seek to identify specific areas in the brain which are responsible for different human behaviours. Recently a branch of neuropsychology has developed: **cognitive neuropsychology**. Cognitive neuropsychologists test the validity of cognitive models of information processing through observing the behaviours of brain-damaged individuals. Models of language processing draw on linguistic descriptions of language and cognitive neuropsychologists attempt to identify the psychological processes which allow us to understand and express language. Research in this area is rapidly expanding and speech and language therapists are increasingly referring to cognitive neuropsychological models of language processing in clinical work. It would be neither feasible nor appropriate to attempt to discuss these models here but cognitive neuropsychological assessment is addressed in Chapters 6, 7 and 8 and Chapter 11 addresses the application of such models in intervention.

Summary

The analysis of language in terms of its component levels provides clinicians with a framework which may be utilised in the management of individuals with speech and/or language impairments. Any individual with a speech/language impairment experiences difficulty in communicating with others either because they cannot make themselves understood, or because they cannot fully understand spoken language. In Chapter 1 of this volume, speech impairment was differentiated from language impairment and the broad distinction was drawn between expressive and receptive language impairments. Another broad distinction exists in speech pathology between **acquired** and **developmental** impairments; acquired impairments occur as a result of disease or injury, developmental impairments are present from birth.

Using the framework provided by structural linguistics, the features of the presenting language impairment can be further specified. The clinician is able to record a sample of language and then, by focusing on one level at a time, analyse it to ascertain precisely where the breakdown occurs. Several assessment procedures exist to aid the clinician in this task. Each chapter in Section II of this volume looks at one level of language and discusses the purpose, value and methods of assessing that aspect of an individual's communicative ability. Clinicians also draw on their knowledge of the structure and functions of language in the planning and execution of therapy programmes. In Section III, each chapter looks at one area of speech/language impairment and examines the role of linguistics in the management of individuals presenting with that particular type of impairment.

Acknowledgements

I would like to thank Geoffrey Campion and Eva Leinonen for their helpful comments and suggestions for the first edition version of this chapter; and Pam Grunwell for eagle-eyed copy-editing and helpful discussion on the final draft for the current edition. Remaining shortcomings are my own responsibility.

Suggested Additional Reading

Phonetics

Ball, M. (1993). *Phonetics for Speech Pathology*, 2nd edn. London: Whurr Publishers.
Cruttenden, A. (1994). *Gimson's Pronunciation of English*, 5th edn. London: Edward Arnold.
Ladefoged, P. (1993). *A Course in Phonetics*, 3rd edn. Fort Worth: Harcourt Brace Jovanovich.

Phonology

Clark, K.J. and Yallop, C. (1990). *An Introduction to Phonetics and Phonology*. Oxford: Blackwell.
Grunwell, P. (1987). *Clinical Phonology*, 2nd edn. Beckenham: Croom Helm.
Stoel-Gammon, C. and Dunn, C. (1985). *Normal and Disordered Phonology in Children*. Baltimore: University Park Press.

Syntax and Morphology (Grammar)

Crystal, D., Fletcher, P. and Garman, M. (1989). *The Grammatical Analysis of Language Disability*, 2nd edn. London: Edward Arnold.
Graddol, D., Cheshire, J. and Swann, J. (1987). *Describing Language*. Oxford: Oxford University Press.
Quirk, R., Greenbaum, S., Leech G. and Svartvik, J. (1972). *A Grammar of Contemporary English*. London: Longman.
Yule, G. (1985). *The Study of Language*. Cambridge: Cambridge University Press

Semantics

Aitchison, J. (1987). *Words in the Mind: an Introduction to the Mental*

Lexicon. Oxford: Blackwell.

Dromi, E. (1987). *Early Lexical Development*. Cambridge: Cambridge University Press.

Hurford, J.R. and Heasley, B. (1983). *Semantics: a Coursebook*. Cambridge: Cambridge University Press.

Pragmatics

Gallagher, T.M. (Ed.) (1991). *Pragmatics of Language: Clinical Practice Issues*. London: Chapman & Hall .

McTear, M. and Conti-Ramsden, G. (1992). *Pragmatic Disability in Children*. London: Whurr Publishers.

Smith, B.R. and Leinonen, E. (1992). *Clinical Pragmatics* London: Chapman & Hall.

Processes of Speech and Hearing

Borden, G.J., Harris, K.S. and Raphael, L.J. (1994). *Speech Science Primer: Physiology, Acoustics and Perception of Speech*, 3rd edn. Baltimore: MA: Wilkins & Wilkins.

Denes, P.B. and Pinson, E.N. (1993). *The Speech Chain*, 2nd edn. New York: W.H. Freeman.

Instrumental Phonetics

Borden, G.J., Harris, K.S. and Raphael, L.J. (1994). *Speech Science Primer: Physiology, Acoustics and Perception of Speech*, 3rd edn. Baltimore: MA: Wilkins & Wilkins.

Code, C. and Ball, M. (1984). *Experimental Clinical Phonetics: Techniques in Speech Pathology and Therapeutics*. London: Croom Helm.

Denes, P.B. and Pinson, E.N. (1993). *The Speech Chain*, 2nd edn. New York: W.H. Freeman.

Psycholinguistics

Ellis, A.W. and Young, A.W. (1988). *Human Cognitive Neuropsychology*. Hove: Lawrence Erlbaum.

Metalinguistics

Gombert, J.E. (1992). *Metalinguistic Development*. London: Harvester Wheatsheaf.

Communication Impairment

Crystal, D. and Varley, R. (1993). *Introduction to Language Pathology*, 3rd edn. London: Whurr Publishers.

Syder, D. (1992). *An Introduction to Communication Disorders*. London: Chapman & Hall.

Section II

Linguistics and assesment of speech and language impairment

Chapter 3
Assessment of Speech Production

SUSANNA EVERSHED MARTIN AND ALLEN HIRSON

Introduction

Productive versus Phonological Assessment

The observer of both qualified and student speech and language therapists is aware of the possible confusion between assessment from the phonological versus the speech production standpoint. In this volume Grunwell discusses phonological assessment. It is important to emphasize that neither is exclusive of the other. Understanding lies in grasping the fact that the *terms* applied to describe the type of assessment being used are not necessarily closely defining. Thus, when Grunwell (1985a) entitles her procedures *phonological*, she is not thereby implying that they will ignore characteristics of speech production; on the contrary, she argues that assessment is inadequate if it fails to account for the interaction between pronunciations *per se*, and their phonological values. The point at which 'production' and 'phonological' assessments meet (and possibly clash!) is in the speech data. The standpoints from which those data are viewed depends on the information being sought at the time, and may be either phonetic in orientation, that is, concerned with *what* is being produced, or phonological in orientation, which is concerned with the systematic and structural *values* to which pronunciations are being put. It is, as it were, a difference between a 'bottom-up' or 'top-down' approach, the former being that taken in speech production assessment. Assessment of speech production is seldom complete without reference to other levels of speech and language output processing (for discussion of the relationship between phonological, phonetic and articulatory levels of speech output see Hewlett, 1990). Here, the focus lies at the productive level. It should not be concluded that phonological use is ignored, merely that a phonological focus lies outside the brief of this chapter.

The Contribution of Phonetics

In assessment, investigators draw on their understanding of phonetics, without which they would be ill-equipped to describe, identify and

61

classify speech, or to judge anything but gross 'errors'. Some aspects of
the contribution of phonetics to clinical science are given in Chapter 2.
Articulatory, acoustic and *auditory* phonetics may all contribute to
assessment; the first and last must certainly be used, and acoustic
phonetics is increasingly required. It is sometimes wrongly supposed
that phonetics is merely to do with 'fixing' the data for later analysis,
whereas in reality phonetic thinking and skills are exploited in all levels
of clinical intervention. Assessment of speech production draws directly
from all three branches of phonetics and from phonology. A single example of two phonetically different sounds which are relevant in English
phonology will serve to illustrate phonetic thinking.

The listener hears, at the beginning of two stressed syllables, [pʰ] and
[b̥], and transcribes these narrowly. Both are recognised visually by
complete lip closure and auditorily by the presence of plosion. Knowledge of the IPA (see Chapter 2) provides the symbols and the conventions
for marking aspiration and devoicing. The transcriber is further aware
that, for plosive production, velic closure is present and a three-stage
mechanism of complete oral closure, raised intra-oral pressure and
release has been used in production on an outgoing pulmonic airstream.
Instrumental measurement may verify these judgements. Spectrographic
evidence will confirm the presence of plosion and the differences of
timing, delayed voice onset time for [pʰ] showing as a relatively late start
of the voicing bar within the following segment. Observation of formant
patterns will confirm articulatory placement, the vowel context and the
absence of nasal resonance. Measurement of absent nasal airflow may
also be used to confirm spectrographic evidence of oral airflow.

Finally, within the framework of the entire corpus of data, and in the
knowledge of the speaker's linguistic intention, the analyst may judge
the articulations to be appropriate allophonic realisations of the English
plosive phonemes /p/ and /b/.

Definitions of Speech Production Disorders

Disorders arising from vocal tract anomaly are self-defining, being
caused by abnormalities of vocal tract anatomy. Common amongst these
are congenital clefts of lip and palate, which cause disturbances of resonance, oral air pressure capacity and the coarticulation of oral and nasal
productions. Characteristics of other disorders belonging within this
category depend on which structures are affected and to what extent.

Dysarthria refers to a collection of motor speech disorders in which
impairment originates in the central or peripheral nervous system. In
the words of Darley, Aronson and Brown (1975), 'the term encompasses
coexisting motor disorders of respiration, phonation, resonance and
prosody. It will also encompass single-process impairments, such as
cranial nerve XII involvement....' Thus, depending on the extent and site

of the neural lesion, involvement may be confined to one area, or widespread throughout the vocal tract. Speech manifestations of dysarthria depend on the nature of neural damage; for classification of flaccid, spastic, ataxic dysarthria and so forth, the reader is referred to standard texts such as *Motor Speech Disorders* by Darley, Aronson and Brown (1975).

Dyspraxia is known by a variety of labels, including 'articulatory dyspraxia', 'verbal dyspraxia' and 'developmental apraxia of speech'. For the sake of simplicity the term is reduced here, but the preferred understanding of this reduction is 'developmental articulatory dyspraxia'. It is defined as a motor programming disorder of neurogenic origin, involving loss of volitional control and impaired ability to plan, combine and sequence sound production. The presenting characteristics are confusing and diverse. Jaffe (1984) states that dyspraxia is defined by 'a symptom cluster....Not *all* symptoms *must* be present; no *one* characteristic or symptom *must* be present; and the typically reported symptoms are not *exclusive* to (dyspraxia).' As it is in dyspraxia that agreed description is most wanting, the definition remains for the present broadly based.

Learned misarticulations: In the absence of the foregoing three disorders there remains the possibility that children acquire immature or faulty articulations which persist. They may be learned from a parent or sibling, in which case persistence is reinforced. Where a single misarticulation is present, for example [ɬ,ʒ] for /s, z/, with no identified organic or environmental cause, this too, may be regarded as a learned misarticulation, especially where other articulations are accurate.

Assessment of Production

Aims of Assessment

Assessment aims to verify the presence or absence of external factors (to use the term in Harris and Cottam, 1985) contributing to the presenting speech disorder. It should explain its nature, determine a hierarchy of contributing factors, enable planning of remediation and predict the outcome of intervention. The assessment procedures discussed below are suitable for investigating the three main disorder clusters defined above.

Components in Assessment

Assessment must look to several sources of information including:

1. the speech data, a corpus of recorded speech;
2. non-speech data gained from clinical observations, data about the speaker which cannot be found from speech data alone, e.g. from language assessment, behavioural observation, etc.;

3. reports from other professionals, e.g. of ENT procedures, psychological assessment, etc.;
4. the case history.

Whilst the purpose of assessment is to explore in some depth the first two of these four components, which rely on one another to provide any explanation of disorder, assessment is incomplete if it fails to include all four elements. It is taken for granted in this context that the reader will understand the need to include the other two. Neither analysis of the corpus of speech data nor other clinical observations are mutually exclusive. One is seldom complete without the other; analysis alone, however thorough, cannot *explain the data*, cannot account for the processes of production of which the speech data are the end product. Analysis of the speech data provides the answer to 'What is produced?', but assessment is incomplete without an answer to 'Why is speech produced in this way?'

Only clinical examination, including observation of the speaker's behaviour during speech production, can answer this. For further discussions of the description and explanation of disordered speech the reader is referred to Harris and Cottam (*op. cit.*), Hawkins (1985), Hewlett (1985) and Grunwell (1985b), and Chapters 5, 13 and 15, this volume. The resources available to the clinician for collecting speech data and speaker information may be:

1. predetermined/published procedures, for example articulation tests, which involve 'fixed' and often quantitative assessment and are frequently termed 'formal assessments';
2. procedures not dependent on any published, recommended or standardised protocol, sometimes termed 'informal assessments'.

Selectivity in Assessment

In some cases it is necessary, at least in the initial stages of management, to assess for all levels of breakdown. In others, the investigator starts with a clear 'signpost' into assessment, which then serves less to inform diagnosis than to establish the details of involvement, and to form the basis for remediation. It is in cases where the point of origin of the disorder is less clearly 'signposted', and several aspects of speech assessment require attention, that skill is needed in selecting appropriate assessment.

Listed below are many items of potential interest in investigating production disorders, but this does not imply that the assessor is bound to include all of them. Attention is given only to aspects judged to be of greatest informative value, but this is not to say that other aspects are ignored. Assessment of the same individual at a later stage may reveal other facets which require closer scrutiny. Clinicians should be aware of all aspects of potential breakdown, including the neurological, neuroanatomical, neurophysiological, neuromotor, psychological and linguistic bases. Through education and experience, skill is acquired in selecting those procedures most capable of granting insight.

The order presented here places speech data before the clinical observations; in reality both co-occur. Speech data are collected early, setting the requirement for further clinical observation. Sometimes non-speech observations are made first, in which case it is important not to prejudice judgement of the nature of speech production in the individual concerned. The two parts of assessment overlap considerably because, whilst data collection is made, the clinician is simultaneously observing the speaker's behaviour.

The Speech Data

Phonetic analysis of a corpus of data supplies the following:

(i)   the sounds used by the individual;
(ii)   the distribution and stability of production;
(iii)   the phonetic relationship between productions and targets (including comparison of airstream mechanisms, voice, place, manner, resonance features, etc.);
(iv)   prosodic features;
(v)   features of phonation;
(vi)   timing of speech, including fluency;
(vii) the age appropriateness of productions.

An adequate sample of speech data should include connected speech if it is to provide the means of insight into all of these. In addition, further information can be gained from assessing the child's ability to produce modelled utterances. In theory, at least, and depending on neuromuscular development, the child who has no failure at the articulatory levels should be capable of accurate modelling; if such is the case, a phonological explanation of the disordered speech is indicated (see further Chapter 13). Assessment of modelling single consonant articulations may be regarded as belonging to clinical observations, being outside 'true speech' as the manifestation of language, but the connection between the child's ability to reproduce articulations, singly and in nonsense syllables, has relevance to both the articulatory capability and phonological values. If the data contain no instance of production of [s], for example, the fact that the child can be stimulated to produce [s] outside linguistic usage weakens the case for an articulatory explanation. Conversely, if the data contain [ç] and the child's response to stimulation to produce [s] is [ç], disruption not of intent but of articulatory execution should be suspected. This is putting the case at its simplest; the interactions between the levels of processing can present far greater complexities than such a simple interpretation implies.

Phonetic Transcription and Recording Speech Data

The analysis of data is dependent on consistent and accurate recording. The need for good practice in phonetic transcription is paramount; records should be truly representative of pronunciations, and should not be corrupted by 'normalisation' through the transcriber's phonology. The transcriber of clinical data is frequently confronted by productions which are not catered for by the *International Phonetic Alphabet*, and must be prepared to invent symbols, to annotate transcriptions, and draw on a wide range of diacritics. Extensions to the IPA (Ball *et al.*, 1994) suggest extra symbols for use in transcribing disordered speech (see Chapter 2). The need for attention to detail in transcription may be illustrated by a single example here (see Grunwell, 1982; 1985a for further discussion).

> /s/ and /θ/ are produced by a child as [ʂ] and [θ], that is, both voiceless dental fricatives, but grooved and slit respectively. If the transcriber is able to record this difference, then the phonological contrast, which exists in a pair such as *sin* versus *thin*, and which is being signalled by the child as [ʂɪn] versus [θɪn], has been appreciated. If, however, both are transcribed as [θ] realizations, then the data will imply a loss of phonological contrast. The two solutions will have different implications: the first will imply that phonetic adjustment of an existing contrast is required, the second that remediation will be aimed at acquisition of a new contrast.

High-standard phonetic transcription requires skill and is time-consuming, but an impressionistic attitude towards the child's pronunciation should be maintained. Transcription may be greatly enhanced by the practice of making high-quality recordings. The use of both audio- and video-recordings is recommended in all data collection; a good quality tape recorder should be regarded as essential clinical equipment.

The accepted wisdom is that transcription of data should be simultaneous with utterance but this is of limited practicality for accurate transcription, particularly if the clinician is to communicate 'naturally' with the child. The suggestion made by Grunwell (1985a), that recruitment of the child's carer or another professional to interact with the child while the therapist concentrates on transcription, is in fact seldom feasible. Providing that transcription is carried out soon after the recording is made, the use of recordings must be regarded as an acceptable compromise. Amorosa *et al.* (1985) report higher levels of inter-transcriber agreement when recordings were used, suggesting that the value of visual contact with the speaker is outweighed by that of repeated opportunities for listening. However, general annotation of the recordings, including time codes associated with specific events, may also be of value for delayed transcription and subsequent analysis.

Articulation Tests

Data collection frequently includes the use of 'articulation tests'. These are useful so long as no inferences are made beyond those which are directly served by them. 'An articulation test can only test what it tests' is a truism, the implications of which are not always appreciated. In discussing data collection for phonological analysis, several authors stress the need for representation of a *full range* of consonant pronunciations, both singly and in clusters, in different word positions (Ingram, 1981; Grunwell, 1982; 1985a; Crystal, 1987). The same may be said from the standpoint of phonetic/productive assessment which, though it assumes an 'opposite' approach, requires the same information. Articulation tests provide one method of collecting data which are standard and gives a quantitative evaluation. In the two tests most widely used in the UK, *The Edinburgh Articulation Test* (EAT) (Anthony *et al.*, 1971) and *The Goldman-Fristoe Test of Articulation* (GFTA) (Goldman and Fristoe, 1969), the material chosen for elicitation represents a balance of phonetically different targets, but neither is fully representative of all possible productions of single and clustered English consonants. Furthermore, neither can account for contextual variability, as only one response for each item is recorded at each administration. It is possible, therefore, in the case of a child whose productions are markedly variable, to achieve different results at each administration. Perhaps, then, it is necessary to add to the above, 'on the occasion on which it is administered'.

The ideal for all speech assessment is 'naturalness', by which is meant that the sample for analysis should be spontaneous, connected speech, collected under conditions which do not place inhibitions on use of language. The naturalness of speech obtained by naming pictures (as in both EAT and GFTA) is questionable; further constraints may arise, in both tests, from the cultural bias of certain vocabulary items. The practicality of the naturalness ideal, which prescribes spontaneous conversational speech, is discussed by Grunwell in *Phonological Assessment of Child Speech (PACS)* (Grunwell, 1985a) and *PACS Pictures* (Grunwell, 1987). Problems of providing a gloss and transcription arise which render single-word data sampling a viable compromise, so long as the more natural connected speech level is not ignored. Of the two tests, GFTA contains both connected speech and 'stimulability' (ability to model) subtests, which go further in providing a fuller data sample. The Qualitative Assessment of EAT goes some way to comparing the child's productions with the norms found in articulatory development. Neither

test, however, can be regarded as fully adequate to serve clinical requirements, and the clinician may therefore need to collect supplementary
data.

Standard procedures are none the less valuable. First, the data
remain 'fixed' for subsequent assessment which measures change;
second, an 'articulation age' may be useful in demonstrating to other
professionals the need for therapy. The ease and speed of administration
speaks further in favour of such tests, and their use as a guide, whether
or not closer scrutiny is required, is surely valid.

Non-standard/unpublished procedures are often termed 'informal',
which would seem to suggest a lack of reliability. The 'formality' or
'informality' of procedures lies more in the principled nature of the
collection, transcription and analysis of data than in *which* approach is
taken. Providing sound principles are strictly followed, 'informal' assessments can be reliable, and if the same principles are reapplied in
reassessment, then results gained will faithfully reflect progress.

Other Features in Productive Assessment

In Chapter 10, Wells, Peppé and Vance explore the linguistic assessment of
prosody. Attention here has largely been at the segmental level. However,
if one requirement of analysis is that it should account for the influence of
phonetic context, then units of analysis larger than single segments must
be considered. Disruption of production causes disturbances not only of
coarticulation of discrete units, but also of syllable and word combinations. Many individuals are intelligible provided utterances are short but
are less so in longer utterances. A possible interpretation of this observation is that a hierarchy of constraints exists for such speakers; selection
of sounds and planning and executing their articulation is relatively easy if
only a limited set is involved. Once the complexities of programming
continuous speech flow are added, functioning breaks down. Many levels
exist between single words and fluent, modulated sentence production;
more, possibly, than current models suggest (Borden, Harris and Raphael,
1994). Prosodic features such as pace, timing, volume, stress and intonation may all be disrupted in individuals with disorders attributable to
different levels of breakdown. The degree of disturbance in dyspraxic
speakers interacts with utterance length and complexity, connected
speech being more unintelligible than expected on the basis of articulation testing alone (see, for example, Rosenbek and Wertz, 1972).

Research has also been carried out into the relationship between stuttering and dyspraxia, notably by Rosenbek (1980). Van Riper (1982)
proposes that stuttering may be defined as 'disruption of the simultaneous and successive programming of muscular movements required
to produce a speech sound or its links to the next sound in a word'. This
is remarkably similar to descriptions of dyspraxia. Though the end product

may be different, in that those diagnosed as having either a stutter or dyspraxia may *behave* differently, there can be a remarkable similarity in the *type* of speech produced. That both must be regarded as the result of a disruption of speech production is undisputed; what remains uncertain is whether the explanation of stuttering requires modification of proposed production models, or whether, at least in some cases, it can be fitted into current models which aim to explain dyspraxic disruption. Even if in future the two can be merged unequivocally within the same level of breakdown, it is likely, given their different manifestation, that different approaches to the assessment of both will remain appropriate (see Miller, this volume).

Also in this volume, Myers explores the relationship between developmental psycholinguistics and dysfluency, including psycholinguistic, psychosocial and psychophysiological considerations. Though integration of processing should be stressed, no direct reference to these additional factors has been made here. This is not to suggest their relevance is ignored; indeed their influence is potent, markedly so in the generation of dysfluency. Without appreciation of these factors we cannot begin to formulate an explanation for why one child, with an observable organic predisposition to speech breakdown, acquires speech and language without difficulty, whereas acquisition for another, with no identifiable organic basis, is severely disrupted. Chiat and Hirson (1987), taking a psycholinguistic approach to *developmental dysphasia* (language impairment which is present from birth), allude to the different perspectives resulting from different approaches:

> Developmental dysphasia has been described and analysed from numerous points of view....Because of the boundaries between the disciplines involved, the descriptions and explanations they offer have been treated as separate and mutually exclusive. There has been little attempt to investigate interrelations between observations made by different disciplines such as psychology and linguistics, or to pursue their implications for language processing....

If there is any sense in the notion that speech and language processing is continuous then the same must be true for the approaches taken to all disorders. Myers's broadly-based approach to dysfluent speech integrates linguistic and psychological stances. In the assessment of production disorders, speech data analysis is essential but must be viewed, especially where dysfluency exists, within the broader canvas of linguistic usage and psychological functioning.

The Severely Impaired Child

For children with severe communication handicaps such items as articulation tests may not apply. Instead of assessing what is being produced, because this is so limited, assessment will aim to explain why speech production is so difficult, and to ascertain the potential for

speech remediation. Clinical observations will be essential to complete
the investigation of all productive disorders, but for the children
concerned these data may be the primary source of information. Pre-
speech assessments are available which can be useful with such children
(e.g. Kiernan and Reid, 1987; Coope *et al*, 1982; Evans-Morris, 1982).

Clinical Observations

An explanation for such disorders of pronunciation as emerge from
analysis of the data, whether they be errors of substitution, omission or
distortion, must be sought. The analysis may have allowed for tentative
explanation of why the speech is as it is, particularly if articulatory
modelling has been included, but further assessment is required to
verify dyspraxic, dysarthric or vocal tract anomalies. The potential for
developing normal production is dependent on both structural normality and normality of articulatory movement, the latter depending on
both 'higher level' motor planning constraints and on intact 'lower level'
motor-neural transmission. Assessment outside the speech data is
concerned, then, with examining:

(i)   the vocal tract structures, for any presenting anomaly;
(ii)   movement of the vocal organs, for (a) dysarthric and (b)
        dyspraxic involvement.

Examination of Oral Structures

In some cases, such as when cleft palate is present or suspected, outside
referral may be required. Whether or not other professionals are
involved, no assessment of speech production can be complete without
knowledge of the state of the vocal tract. Such factors as overall proportions of the face and jaw, shortening of the frenum, size and appearance
of the tongue, presence and alignment of dentition and so forth are
observable directly by the speech therapist. Observation of the 'hidden'
structures such as the nasal tract and larynx may require the cooperation
of ENT. The space available here precludes any detailed formulaic procedure but these are well documented elsewhere (e.g. St Louis and
Ruscello, 1981). Again, 'informal' procedures are viable, and many therapists will have developed their own techniques and 'check-lists' for
examining oral structures.

    If structure is thoroughly examined and found to be normal, then the
lowest level of involvement (i.e. vocal tract anomaly) can be eliminated. (It
should also be noted that many normal speakers have vocal tracts which
present structurally as 'abnormal'.) To imply the converse, that abnormal
structure eliminates higher involvement, is clearly false. Dysarthric speakers frequently present with structures which are abnormal in appearance.

For example, the tongue to or from which the nerve supply is damaged may be of normal size proportionate to the mouth, but may *appear* larger, as it has to adopt a certain stance. Likewise, absence of dentition may arise from inability to perform habitual mouth cleaning leading to decay, rather than structural anomaly *per se*. Interpretation of oral examination observations is essential and can only be made by reference to other components of the entire assessment procedure. In the examination of oral structures two possible contributions to the explanation of disorder may be revealed: (i) the vocal tract is structurally anomalous *per se*; (ii) structures are 'different' due to higher level involvement. Which is the true explanation may be immediately apparent, as in known cleft palate, or where there is obvious spastic/flaccid oro-facial musculature. In less obvious cases, closer scrutiny may be required of the way in which speech muscles function, and not merely of their structural configuration.

Assessment of Vocal Tract Movement

Absence of structural anomaly cannot guarantee normal articulatory movement. The dyspraxic child will seldom present with any physical signs of articulatory disorder, and in cases of mild dysarthria oral examination may reveal no significant findings. Conversely, in children where a structural 'fault' has been found, the assessment must be capable of determining two things. First, if the child is bypassing the fault and articulating adequately, then assessment needs to determine how this is being achieved. Second, if no compensatory movements have been acquired, then it should estimate the potential for achieving viable production. Remediation may require surgical or prosthetic intervention, or, in severe cases, alternative means of communication. Again, no exhaustive discussion of the means and procedures which may be adopted in assessing vocal tract movement is possible here. (Protocol assessments include those proposed by Dabul, 1979; Blakeley, 1980; Robertson, 1982; Enderby, 1983; Wertz, Lapointe and Rosenbek, 1984; Huskins, 1987.) Instead each disorder is treated separately and such items as should be included are outlined.

In cases involving **structural anomaly** articulatory movements at and around the site of the fault should be noted. To illustrate this by examples, in the case of a child with high palatal arch and small tongue the ability of the tongue to reach the arch is observed. Where such movements are clearly possible as evidenced by the presence in the speech data of lingual plosives, then the manner in which closure is achieved by compensatory movements should be identified. Where palatal shortening or cleft is found, again any compensatory movements should be noted and velic valving ability is assessed by noting any failure to achieve nasal closure.

Assessment for velo-pharyngeal competence may be carried out in a number of ways. The speech data will have revealed, in the case of insufficient valving, hypernasality and/or absence or distortion of pressure consonants, both in 'real speech' and modelled productions. Here the assessment must discover whether valving is achievable outside language use, which has positive implications for therapy by, for example, observing the child's capacity to blow, or by instrumental flowrate/nasality measurement. If no adequate velic closure is achievable either in speech or in non-speech movement, then observation of the deficiency of movement via lateral X-ray filming may be indicated to assess the need for surgical intervention.

In a case of suspected **dysarthria**, or where there is known neural transmission involvement, investigation is aimed at discovering which musculature is affected and to what extent. Assessment of articulatory movement needs to embrace the whole vocal tract. All of the following may be evaluated: breath capacity and control; initiation of phonation; onset and cessation of voicing; velic valving; ability to achieve oral closure/approximation by the tongue and lips; the ability to imitate lateral and vertical tongue movements; speed and accuracy of articulatory placement and strength of articulatory movement. Furthermore, functions such as coughing, swallowing and sucking may need to be considered, particularly where assessment is aimed at estimating potential for speech production in severely affected children.

If **dyspraxia** has to do with the inability to perform voluntarily that which is possible involuntarily, then the key to its discovery must lie in assessment aimed at eliciting volitional movement. The assessment of movement outside language and of the comparison between automatic vocal tract movement and structured, modelled movement is paramount. Dyspraxic children may be capable, for instance, of licking their lips to remove crumbs, but quite unable to perform this movement if asked to do so. In assessing movement of the articulators in the search for dyspraxia, a number of tasks such as licking the lips, elevating the tongue tip and performing lateral movements of the tongue may be presented. Whilst some children with dyspraxia may evince a marked struggle in carrying out such movements, others will be able to do so quite readily, though speed and accuracy may be affected. In the latter case the differential diagnosis between mild dysarthria and dyspraxia may be contentious and no clear picture may emerge without reference to other aspects of assessment. Where no difficulty exists in making these movements, then the ability to vary movement may be absent; the rapid movement towards and away from the same and/or different articulatory targets may be disturbed. In the dyspraxic child, for whom executing isolated volitional movements is possible, it may be that only by including testing of diadochokinetic rates is his or her motor planning capacity sufficiently taxed to reveal the dyspraxia. Assessing diadochokinetic rate may also be valuable in assessing for dysarthria, but the quality of movement in these two disorders differs. For the dysarthric child changing from one target to another may be possible *of itself* but speed, accuracy and strength of movement may be disturbed. In the dyspraxic child speed is disturbed, and altering direction of movement may evidence struggle behaviour, or may be impossible.

Findings should be supported by observation of movements other than those of the articulators and breathing mechanisms. Whilst structural anomaly is frequently isolated, both articulatory dyspraxia and dysarthria may be part of more widespread impairment. The vocal tract should, therefore, never be regarded as isolated from the rest of the body; indeed, in cases where the results of assessing the movements of the vocal tract are equivocal, and speech symptomatology presents a confusing picture, these other movements may be crucial in reaching a working diagnosis.

Instrumental Assessment

Assessment as presented above relies on the direct observations by the assessor of the child, mediated only by the phonetic and related skills of the assessor. For this purpose, the only electronic equipment routinely incorporated into the assessment is audio- and video-recorders, used primarily for *post hoc* inspection of the data in order to produce a detailed and accurate record of the complex speech behaviour. Although good quality recordings are significantly better than none at all, this method of data analysis has two limitations. First, the observations are subjective, and even the most skilled assessor is subject to phonological bias. Second, there are details of the speech, captured by recordings, which cannot be easily extracted or isolated by the unassisted human ear.

With the aid of a number of analytic tools, clinical observations may be corroborated and refined in order to produce a more complete – and objective – profile of the speech data, and hence enable a more searching probe into the disorder. In the example cited at the beginning of this chapter, the aspiration of the voiceless bilabial plosive in English [pʰ] may be confirmed spectrographically, and the voice onset time (VOT) between the burst and the onset of vocal fold vibration may be measured and compared with that in the voiced counterpart, [b] (see also Chapter 4).

Many of the professionals whose reports may be crucial in the overall assessment of the child may similarly depend upon instrumental equipment, and all of these devices have developed in leaps and bounds over the past ten years. An audiologist may use computer-based pure tone or impedance audiometry; an otolaryngologist or voice therapist may use stroboscopy and video technology (Harris and Collins, 1989); and an ENT surgeon may employ nasendoscopy to examine the larynx or parts of the vocal tract.

The therapist (and his or her phoniatrician colleagues elsewhere in Europe) is also increasingly using technology to augment assessment. Recording technology has come a long way since the bulky reel-to-reel tape recorders and crude microphones of the 1960s; digital audio tape (DAT) recorders and high-quality video recorders have been minia-turised and data generated by devices such as the laryngograph (the *PCLx*™) may be captured in digital format, giving the assessor access to very high-quality speech data. Over the next few years it is likely that these and other records may be combined on CD-ROM (multimedia format) so that different aspects of the speech sample may be easily cross-referenced.

Baken (1987) and Code and Ball (1984) describe a large number of techniques that may be used to: (a) capture data, and (b) subject these data to a variety of detailed analyses. Techniques for the direct tracking of articulatory movements such as electropalatography (Hardcastle and Morgan, 1982; Gibbon and Hardcastle 1989; Nicolaidis, Hardcastle and Gibbon, 1992) or videofluoroscopy (McCurtain, 1990), directly record aspects of articulation; and laryngography (Abberton, Howard and Fourcin, 1989) provides details of vocal fold vibration. Such direct assessment of vocal fold activity, or computer-based acoustic pitch-esti-mation devices such as *Visi-Pitch*™ (Horii, 1983) may also be invaluable tools for examining and/or providing feedback of the contours of funda-mental frequency underlying intonation (Curtis and Schultz, 1986; Sataloff *et al.*, 1990; see also Chapter 10, this volume). In parallel with such records of articulatory and phonatory behaviour, nasometry enables monitoring of velopharyngeal control (Dalston, Warren and Dalston, 1991; Van Denmark *et al.*, 1985; Besar, Kelly and Greenhalgh, 1989; Besar, Kelly and Manley, 1990; Mirlohi, Kelly and Mauley, 1994) and devices such as the *Aerophone*™ also permit detailed analysis of airflow (see, for example, Draper, Ladefoged and Whitteridge, 1960; Frøkjær-Jensen, 1992).

Until recently, such equipment was to be found exclusively in univer-sity or research establishments, but clinicians now frequently use such instrumentation to provide a more complete assessment in the hospital or clinic setting. Video, audio and laryngographic records may now be cut and pasted using waveform editors to isolate crucial utterances for analysis, and/or to re-present these to the client in order to explore his or her phonological system. Narrow transcriptions may be matched frame by frame with electropalatographic or laryngographic records, and details of the acoustic signal may then be subjected to detailed spec-trographic and other analyses using devices such as the PC-based CSL (*Computer Speech Laboratory*)™ or *Speech Workstation*™, the MacIn-tosh-based *Soundscope* ™ or *Waves+* on the powerful UNIX platform.

The complexity of sound spectrography, and allied techniques such as linear predictive coding (LPC) used to track changes in vocal tract resonances, highlights the complex segmenting performed by the human listener making even the broadest transcription. Detailed acoustic analysis of speech features may involve description in terms of frequency, amplitude and time, and this may be achieved using sound spectrography. A selection of the extensive spectrographic research into normal and pathological speech may be found in Baken and Daniloff (1987). In short, it is no mean feat for the therapist cum speech scientist to identify the boundaries of phones in the continuum of speech. Using instrumentation to provide a 'still photograph' mitigates against the ephemeral nature of speech (see also Miller, this volume).

Methods of automatic speech recognition tackle this problem of segmenting speech in ingenious ways, and speech and language therapy is now benefiting from such technology, for example, via IBM's *SpeechViewer*™ (Maulet, 1990; IBM SpeechViewer Guide, undated; Ryalls, Michallet and LeDorze, 1994). Originally devised for use with deaf children, this system now incorporates visual feedback applications for people with a wide range of speech pathologies. Using games formats with attractive and accessible graphic images, the production of vowels may be compared with models, and two or more vowels contrasted directly. Practical and theoretical difficulties with visual feedback are discussed further by de Bot (1983), Weltens and de Bot (1984), and Hirson and Fawcus (1991). One of the problems of this method is the use of arbitrary norms (or simply the therapist's productions), and it is only the more sophisticated systems such as *SpeechViewer* that enable the creation of appropriate models for the patient/client to replicate. This, in turn, provides the therapist with the necessary basis for working with people with markedly different pitch ranges, dialects or other speech and language variables (see Chapter 10, this volume).

Finally, it should be stressed that the bewildering range of analytic tools are useful only to the extent that they are used appropriately. High-fidelity recordings still require proper placement of the microphone, laryngograph electrodes or airflow masks, appropriate setting of recording levels and so forth. In addition, which data are collected and the most appropriate type of analysis for addressing particular clinical or research questions is theory-driven. Cleft palate may call for airflow measurements or nasometry; inappropriate prosodic structures or voicing control may call for laryngography; and the articulation of vowel contrasts may require LPC or spectrographic formant analysis to highlight a particular aspect of the speech production. Ultimately, the most powerful type of analysis will be that which is motivated by the clinical judgement and theoretical insight of the assessor.

The sources of speech analysis equipment referred to in this chapter are provided in the Appendix.

Diagnosis of Disorders of Production

Interpreting Assessment

If assessment is to be of value to diagnosis and management, then simply carrying it out is insufficient! Interpretation must be made by drawing together the strands of information gained from the entire investigation. Only then are provisional explanations possible and remediation planned. It is impossible to extend in the abstract to all the possible interpretations of findings which could be made, given the manifold nature of the assessment procedure. Each child, even within each assumed category, will present with different combinations of features in each area of the investigation. The investigator must refer back to the definitions and descriptions of disorders and weigh the findings against them. Few difficulties arise in diagnosing vocal tract anomaly involvement. Greater subtlety may be required in delineating dysarthria from dyspraxia, and articulation from phonological disorder. Where doubt is present, it may be appropriate to form a working hypothesis and keep an open mind towards selecting new dimensions for investigation at a later date. In all cases, clinicians should be willing to amend original diagnoses; there is no shame in starting from a tentative position which is later altered, particularly given the frequent difficulty of reaching a certain conclusion. Indeed, great danger lies in a rigid adherence to opinion. Furthermore, 'mixed' disorders are commonplace so, for example, a child presenting with identifiable dyspraxia may be simultaneously dysarthric. Initial assessment frequently reveals factors attributable to one type of disorder but, as assessment and remediation progress, other layers of involvement unfold. This is particularly so where the presenting picture is complex and shows weak or subtle signs of contributing factors. For example, the investigator should not be misguided into assuming that in a case of identified cleft palate, the presence of dyspraxia and/or dysarthria may be eliminated. The synergistic nature of all levels within the speech/language process, both in input and output, must be remembered, and is particularly relevant when considering developmental disorders.

The Developmental Dimension

The discussion so far has focused mainly on children. The question arises as to whether the same principles can be applied in the field of acquired disorders, and whether the same definitions of disorder are viable. The answer must be that in a broad sense the processes involved in the speech production are no different in the adult and child, because the same structures for both reception and production, and the same neural integration, are common to both. The procedures in assessment of acquired and developmental disorders are essentially the same, with certain obvious provisos which account for abilities such as reading. Furthermore, the definitions proposed are equally applicable to adults with acquired disorders and to children (see Chapter 15, this volume). However, it should be recognised that, in development, there is a dimension which is not present in the adult, namely that the child *is in the process of acquiring language* in its entirety. The normal adult is, by virtue of maturity, fully developed at all levels: anatomical, physiological, neurological, perceptual, phonological, syntactic and so forth. The normal child has yet to achieve integrated functioning through experience, experimentation and learning. The adult with an acquired speech disorder confined to a single area retains capacities within other areas. Though this is not to suggest that effects other than those directly attributable to the specific area of damage may not be found, the very fact that these preserved areas of functioning have been fully developed previously presents a situation which is different from that found in the child. If integration of functioning of the whole is important in the adult speaker, how much more so is it in the child during the process of acquisition, which is itself so delicately balanced? The presence of disorder, in upsetting this balance, creates disturbances that may spread far beyond the primary site of dysfunction. Miller, in this volume, refers to 'knock-on' effects, and an example of the effect on the whole of an isolated disorder is readily found in the child with severely impaired hearing. The disorder, at the lowest level of input, has profound implications for the acquisition of all language functioning; disordered reception bars the way to perception and so fails to allow integrated phonological acquisition, which in turn distorts production and so forth throughout the chain. If such 'feed-forward' in the system is clearly apparent in deaf speakers, could not a reversal to 'feed-back' (as opposed to 'feedback') be present in the types of disorder being considered here? At the lowest levels of output, disturbed *experience* of movement and of proprioceptive and kinaesthetic feedback may be potent in disturbing phonological acquisition. It should not, then, be surprising to find mixed characteristics in the same child, nor should these necessarily be regarded as conflicting. Until greater clarity in the definition and delineation of disorders is achieved, particularly those within areas which are not 'directly observable', such thoughts as these must remain speculative. It is, however, in failing to address the need for explanation and accepting that explanations may necessarily be uncertain in children who present with no gross, observable organic and/or neurological symptoms, that the dangers of labelling, and attributing explanation to labels given, arise.

Perception and Speech Production

Where 'feed-back' and 'feed-forward' are referred to earlier, the single crude example of a child with impaired hearing is given to illustrate the need to think in terms of overall integration. To address output levels as the point at which assessments begin is not to suggest that input is ignored. It is standard clinical practice to include a hearing test in investigating the causes of speech production failure. This is frequently only pure-tone, air conduction audiometric testing, often in screening form, which may only extend to bone conduction and speech audiometry if specifically requested. Furthermore, interpretations put on such results are frequently open to question. A case was recently encountered in which a child with a conductive loss of 35dB in both ears was described as having 'normal hearing'; another child, with a 20dB bilateral loss was regarded by an ENT registrar as having 'good hearing'. It is hoped that such judgements are peculiar to non-speech experts. The need to avoid getting 'stuck' at the lowest levels of input must lead the investigator into regions beyond conduction to auditory perception. The perception of speech and its assessment is the subject of the next chapter.

Conclusion

This chapter has endeavoured to present a résumé of the factors which are of concern to the investigator of speech production disorders. Whilst difficulties are encountered in establishing the relationship between phonetic capacity and phonological ability, and between input and output modalities, it has been stressed that the investigator of speech and language disorder should always be aware of that relationship. Furthermore, we must remain alert to complementary aspects of the investigation from the articulatory, auditory and acoustic standpoint. Crystal (1987) proposes a 'bucket' theory of language disability in discussing the interrelationship of levels of processing. In so doing, he warns that to 'remember at the same time' is not the same as to 'take into account'. As the search for clearer understanding continues it is valuable to heed this warning, remaining ever aware of the complex task which is undertaken in assessment, and to counteract the tendency to compartmentalise areas of speech and language functioning.

References

Abberton, E.R.M., Howard, D.M. and Fourcin, A.J. (1989). Laryngographic assessment of normal voice: a tutorial. *Clinical Linguistics and Phonetics* 3(3), 281–296.

Amorosa, H., von Benda, U., Wagner, E. and Keck, A. (1985). Transcribing phonetic detail in the speech of unintelligible children: a comparison of procedures. *British Journal of Disorders of Communication* 20, 281–287.

Anthony, A., Bogle, D., Ingram, T.T.S. and McIsaac, M.W. (1971). *The Edinburgh Articulation Test*. Edinburgh: Churchill Livingstone.

Baken, R.J. (1987). *Clinical Measurement of Speech and Voice*. London: Taylor & Francis.

Baken, R.J and Daniloff, R.G. (1987). *Readings in Clinical Spectrography of Speech*. San Diego: Singular Publishing.

Ball, J.B, Code, C., Rahilly, J. and Hazlett, D. (1994). Non-segmental aspects of disordered speech: developments in transcription. *Clinical Linguistics and Phonetics* 8(1), 67–83.

Besar, S.S., Kelly, S.W. and Greenhalgh, P.A. (1989). Nasal airflow measurement using a compensated thermister anemometer, Part I: System description and qualitative analysis. *Medical & Biological Engineering & Computing* 27, 628–631.

Besar, S.S., Kelly, S.W. and Manley, M.C.G. (1990). Nasal airflow measurement using a compensated thermister anemometer, Part II: Computer signal processing and quantitative analysis. *Medical & Biological Engineering & Computing* 28, 127–132.

Blakeley, R.W. (1980). *Screening Test of Developmental Dyspraxia*. Oregon: C.C. Publishing.

Borden, G.L., Harris, K.S. and Raphael, L.J. (1994). *Speech Science Primer: Physiology, Acoustics and Perception of Speech*. Baltimore: Williams & Wilkins.

Chiat, S. and Hirson, A. (1987). From conceptual intention to utterance: a study of impaired language output in a child with developmental dysphasia. *British Journal of Disorders of Communication* 22, 37–64.

Code, C. and Ball, M. (1984). *Experimental Clinical Phonetics: Techniques in Speech Pathology and Therapeutics*. London: Croom Helm.

Coope, J., Anerne, P., Crawford, N., Herring, J., Jolliffe, J., Levy, D., Malone, J. and Crystal, D. (1982). *Profiling Linguistic Disability*. London: Edward Arnold.

Crystal, D. (1987). Towards a 'bucket' theory of language disability taking account of interaction between linguistic levels. *Clinical Linguistics and Phonetics* 1, 7–23.

Curtis, J. and Schultz, M. (1986). *Basic Laboratory Instrumentation for Speech and Hearing*. Boston/Toronto: Little, Brown.

Dabul, B.L. (1979). *Apraxia Battery for Adults*. Leicester: Task Master Teaching Aids.

Dalston, R.M., Warren, D.W. and Dalston, E.T. (1991). Use of nasometry as a diagnostic tool for identifying patients with velopharyngeal impairment'. *The Cleft Palate–Craniofacial Journal* 28(2), 329–346.

Darley, F.L., Aronson, A.E. and Brown, J.R. (1975). *Motor Speech Disorders*. Philadelphia: Saunders.

de Bot, K. (1983). Visual feedback of intonation, I: Effectiveness and induced practice behavior. *Language and Speech* 26(4), 331–350.

Draper, M.H., Ladefoged, P. and Whitteridge, D. (1960). Expiratory pressures and air flow during speech. *British Medical Journal* 18, 1837–1843.

Enderby, P.M. (1983). *Frenchay Dysarthria Assessment*. San Diego: College Hill Press.

Evans-Morris, S. (1982). *Pre-speech Assessment Scale*. New York: J.A. Preston Corp.

Frøkjær-Jensen, B. (1992). Data on air pressure, mean flow rate, glottal input and output energy, aerodynamic resistance, and glottal efficiency for normal and healthy voices. *Proceedings of the XXII World Congress of the International Association of Logopedes and Phoniatricians*, Hanover.

Gibbon, F. and Hardcastle, W. (1989). Deviant articulation in a cleft palate child following late repair of the hard palate: a description and remediation procedure using electropalatography (EPG). *Clinical Linguistics and Phonetics* 3(1), 93–110.

Goldman, R. and Fristoe, M. (1969). *Goldman–Fristoe Test of Articulation*. Circle Pines: American Guidance Service.

Goldman, R., Fristoe, M. and Woodcock, R. (1970). *The Goldman–Fristoe–Woodcock Test of Auditory Discrimination*. Circle Pines: American Guidance Service.

Grunwell, P. (1982). *Clinical Phonology*. London: Croom Helm.

Grunwell, P. (1985a). *Phonological Assessment of Child Speech (PACS)*. Windsor: NFER-Nelson.

Grunwell, P. (1985b). Comments on the term 'phonetics' and 'phonological' as applied in the investigation of speech disorders. *British Journal of Disorders of Communication* 20, 165–170.

Grunwell, P. (1987). *PACS Pictures*. Windsor: NFER-Nelson.

Hardcastle, W.J. and Morgan, R.A. (1982). An instrumental investigation of articulation disorders in children. *British Journal of Disorders of Communication* 17, 47–65.

Harris, T. and Collins, S. (1989). The Voice Clinic: tools of the trade. *College of Speech Therapists Bulletin* No. 448, 6–8.

Harris, J. and Cottam, P. (1985). Phonetic features and phonological features in speech assessment. *British Journal of Disorders of Communication* 20, 61–74.

Hawkins, P. (1985). A tutorial comment on Harris and Cottam. *British Journal of Disorders of Communication* 20, 75–80.

Hewlett, P. (1985). Phonological and phonetic disorders; some suggested modifications to the current use of the distinction. *British Journal of Disorders of Communication* 20, 155–164.

Hewlett, P. (1990). Processing of development and production. In: Grunwell, P. (Ed.), *Developmental Speech Disorders*. Edinburgh: Churchill Livingstone.

Hirson, A. and Fawcus, R. (1991). Visual feedback in the management of dysphonia. In: Fawcus, M. (Ed.), *Voice Disorders and their Management*, 2nd edn. London: Chapman & Hall.

Horii, Y. (1983). Automatic analysis of voice fundamental frequency and intensity using a Visipitch. *Journal of Speech and Hearing Research* 26, 467–471.

Huskins, S. (1987). Diagnostic check lists. In: *Working with Dyspraxics*. Bicester: Winslow Press.

IBM SpeechViewer Guide (undated). *Personal System/2 SpeechViewer™: A Guide to Clinical and Educational Applications*. IBM (USA) Corporation Publication.

Ingram, D. (1981). *Procedures for the Phonological Analysis of Children's Language*. Baltimore: University Park Press.

Jaffe, M.B. (1984). Neurological impairment of speech production: assessment and treatment. In: Costello, J. (Ed.), *Speech Disorders in Children*. San Diego: College Hill Press.

Kiernan, C.C. and Reid, B.D. (1987). *Preverbal Communication Scale (PVC)*. Windsor: NFER-Nelson.

Maulet, M. (1990). Une experience d'utilisation de SpeechViewer aupres de patients atteints de deficience auditive profonde: analyse, applications et limites. In: McCurtain, F. (Ed.), *Proceedings of the European Voice Technology Seminar*, pp. 48–52. London: National Hospitals College of Speech Sciences.

McCurtain, F. (1990). Application of magnetic resonance to the diagnosis of vocal tract disorders. In: Welch, G. (Ed.), *Proceedings of the Fourth International Symposium of Care of the Professional Voice (UK)*. London: Ferens Institute of Laryngology.

Mirlohi, H.R., Kelly, S.W. and Mauley, M.C.G. (1994). A new technique for assessment of velopharyngeal function. *Medical & Biological Engineering & Computing* 32(5), 562–565.

Nicolaidis, K., Hardcastle, W. and Gibbon, F. (1992). Bibliography of electropalatographic studies, Parts 1 and 2. *Speech Research Laboratory University of Reading Work in Progress* 7, 28–106.

Robertson, S. (1982). *Dysarthria Profile*. Private publication.

Rosenbek, J.C. (1980). Apraxia of speech relationship to stuttering. *Journal of Fluency Disorders* 5, 223–253.

Rosenbek, J.C. and Wertz, R.T. (1972). A review of fifty cases of developmental apraxia of speech. *Language, Speech and Hearing Services in Schools* 3, 23–33.

Ryalls, J., Michallet, B. and LeDorze, G. (1994). A preliminary evaluation of the clinical effectiveness of vowel training for hearing-impaired children on IBM's SpeechViewer. *The Volta Review* 96, 19–30.

Sataloff, R.T., Spiegel, J.R., Carroll, L.M., Darby, K.S., Hawkshaw, M.J. and Rulnick, R.K. (1990). The clinical voice laboratory practical design and clinical application. *Journal of Voice* 4(3), 264–279.

St Louis, K.O. and Ruscello, D.M. (1981). *The Oral Speech Mechanism Screening Examination*. Baltimore: University Parks Press.

Van Denmark, D., Bzoch, K., Daly, D., Fletcher, S., McWilliams, B.J., Pannbacker, M. and Weinberg, B. (1985). Methods of assessing speech in relation to velopharyngeal function. *Cleft Palate Journal* 22, 281–285.

Van Riper, C. (1982). *The Nature of Stuttering*. New Jersey: Prentice Hall.

Weltens, B. and de Bot, K. (1984). Visual feedback of intonation II: Feedback delay and quality of feedback. *Language and Speech* 27(1), 79–88.

Wertz, R.T., Lapointe, L.L. and Rosenbek, J.C. (1984). Motor speech evaluation. In: Wertz, R.T., Lapointe, L.L. and Rosenbek, J.C. (Eds.), *Apraxia of Speech in Adults: the Disorder and its Management*. New York: Grune & Stratton.

Appendix: Commercial Sources of Selected Equipment for Speech Assessment and Analysis

AEROPHONE™ II: F J Electronics, Ellebuen 21, Vedbaek, Denmark.

CSL™ (COMPUTER SPEECH LAB): Wessex Electronics, 114–116 North Street, Downend, Bristol BS16 5SE, UK. (Also: Kay Elemetrics Corporation, 12 Maple Avenue, PO Box 2025, Pine Brook, NJ 07058-2025, USA).

ELECTROPALATOGRAPH (EPG): Reading University, Department of Linguistic Science, Whiteknights, PO Box 218, Reading RG6 2AA, UK.

LARYNGOGRAPH (PCLx™): Laryngograph Ltd, 1 Foundry Mews, Tolmer Square, London NW1 2PE; Rothenberg's *ELECTROGLOTTOGRAPH*: available from F.J. Electronics, Ellebuen 21, Vedbaek, Denmark.

NASAL ANEMOMETER: University of Kent, Canterbury CT1 7NZ, UK distributed worldwide by Millgrant Wells Ltd, PO Box 3, 7 Stanley Road, Rugby, CV21 3UF, UK.

NASOMETER 6200™: Wessex Electronics, 114–116 North Street, Downend, Bristol BS16 5SE, UK.

KAY PALATOMETER™: Wessex Electronics, 114–116 North Street, Downend, Bristol BS16 5SE, UK.

SOUNDSCOPE™ II: Millgrant Wells, Ltd, PO Box 3, 7 Stanley Road, Rugby, CV21 3UF, UK.

SPEECHVIEWER™ II: Papworth Ability Services UK, Unit D3A, Telford Road, Bicester, Oxfordshire, OX6 OTZ, UK.

SPEECH WORKSTATION™: Loughborough Sound Images plc, Loughborough Park, Ashby Road, Loughborough, Leicestershire LE9 3NE. Also available from: Millgrant Wells Ltd, PO Box 3, 7 Stanley Road, Rugby, CV21 3UF, UK.

VISIPITCH™: (6087AT//6095/6097): Wessex Electronics, 114–116 North Street, Downend, Bristol BS16 5SE, UK.

WAVES+™: Entropic Research Laboratory, Sheraton House, Castle Park, Cambridge CB3 OAX, UK.

Chapter 4
Assessment of Speech Perception

KEVIN BAKER AND KIM GRUNDY

Introduction

It is no coincidence that this chapter is placed between those on the assessment of speech production and the assessment of phonology. Speech perception may be viewed as the bridge between the physical reality of speech sounds discussed in the preceding chapter and the psychological concept of the phoneme discussed in the next. Before addressing assessment in this chapter it is necessary to identify precisely what we mean by speech perception. Thus we will consider the relation between hearing and perception; research into sound perception and how it relates to the perception of speech; and research on the development of speech perception in the child. Having offered some theoretical background we will then evaluate procedures for the assessment of speech perception.

Hearing and Auditory Perception

When we hear, sound-waves enter the outer ear and are transmitted through the middle ear to the inner ear where they are transformed into neuro-electric impulses which are in turn transmitted to the brain. Thus, hearing simply means that air-pressure vibrations (sound-waves) are being transformed into another form of energy. In this sense we could say that a tape recorder 'hears'. A tape recorder transforms sound waves into electro-magnetic vibrations. The tape recorder can 'hear', but it cannot perceive. It would be perfectly feasible to carry out a pure-tone audiometric assessment on a tape recorder to find out how faithfully a sound is recorded and this would tell us how well the recording mechanism is working. It would convince us that the tape recorder's 'hearing' is okay.

Human perception of speech is something more than hearing sounds which have been made by another human's vocal apparatus. The inner ears of mynah birds and budgerigars are physiologically very different to ours, yet they are able to hear and mimic speech sounds (Dooling and Brown, 1990). These birds hear the distinctions needed to reproduce the speech sounds but we would not say that they process the sounds phonetically or that they can *understand* speech.

Hearing is a necessary prerequisite for auditory perception, but perception also implies that we can make sense of what we hear, whether it is speech or the creak of a door in a horror film. In a sense then, it is like looking at a two-dimensional picture and 'understanding' that it is a representation of a three-dimensional scene. What we hear is a complex mix of all the sound-making events in the environment. Our auditory system has evolved to unravel this mix and work out effectively what kind of events are happening.

The outer, middle and inner ear, auditory nerve and brain do this by doing much more than simply transforming sound energy into neuro-electric impulses. When listening to Miles Davis playing trumpet in a jazz ensemble, for example, there are at least two perceptual feats we can perform. First, we can listen to the different levels of complexity in the sounds at any one point in time and focus on the harmony of the instruments, the intonation or timbre of individual notes, and the quality of the recording. Second, we can follow these sounds across time and listen to the melodies each instrument is playing (while ignoring other sounds) and we can also make connections between different sections of the musical score. Furthermore, we are able to switch our attention between these activities with incredible ease. The fact that we can shift our attention between aspects of the acoustic signal means that our auditory system is able to create different perceptual 'objects' in our minds which reflect aspects of what is happening in the real world.

Whether we like or dislike a piece of music is often related to our musical knowledge and experience of other pieces. A music critic would perhaps be most interested in the phrasing and accent of the melodies and harmonies which make each piece of music unique. Past knowledge and experience contribute to our perception and understanding of all sound. Some car mechanics can listen to the sound of an engine running and accurately locate and diagnose a fault. Similarly, we can describe speech as being perceived and understood at different levels in relation to past knowledge and experience. Warren (1970) recorded a political speech, removed the first /s/ in the word 'legislatures' and then replaced it with either a cough or a 1000 Hz tone. When presented as part of continuous speech, nine out of ten listeners did not report anything missing or strange in the speech. In effect they had perceptually restored the missing phoneme. Samuel (1981) continued this line of work and found that phonemic restoration was more likely when the word was long, when it was a real word as opposed to a non-word, and when it was a commonly used word. It is hard to say how much our linguistic expectations of speech are involved in perception but the research by Warren and Samuel clearly shows an effect of higher level knowledge on lower level perception.

Speech perception is a psychological phenomenon and cannot be directly observed, and our knowledge of the processes involved in speech perception is limited. We can only guess at the answers to many of the questions we would like to ask about speech perception. For example, how do we cope with the variability in the speech signal? Does our auditory system process speech in the same way as non-speech sounds? Is every part of the speech signal processed? Whilst neurological exploration is one way to investigate the auditory system, another paradigm for reseach is to describe accurately the functional characteristics of the auditory system. In other words, what is it, exactly, that the auditory system actually does?

Research in Hearing and Auditory Perception

Historically, our thinking about the auditory system has been powerfully influenced by an approach which attempts to reduce complex problems down to a collection of simpler ones. This 'reductionist' approach has produced two influential legacies. The first has led us to think of sound as being made up from smaller and more simple units. This, in turn, has produced a second legacy encouraging us to view the auditory system as breaking a sound down into these hypothetical units ready to be passed up to the brain to be recombined into meaningful perceptions. Problems arise when we try to apply this reductionism to the perception of complex and variable sounds such as speech. This can be seen in the two different research paradigms described below, *psychophysics* and *speech science*.

Psychophysics: When we concern ourselves with the psychophysics of sound, we consciously restrict ourselves to measuring things like the smallest detectable differences in the frequencies and/or amplitudes of pure tones. The idea behind this is to effect a tightly controlled environment in which accurate experiments and measurements can be carried out. Such detailed observations lead us to describe how the mechanics of the inner ear and the neuro-electric functioning of the auditory nerve deal with such information. It would appear, however, that in having evolved to deal with naturally occurring complex sounds, the auditory system does not treat artificially simple sounds any differently. It is not simply a matter of describing the characteristics of the auditory system in dealing with acoustically *simple* sounds, and then progressing on to more complex sounds. For the auditory system there is no distinction between simple and complex sounds because they are ultimately dealt with perceptually, and not acoustically. A common criticism of the psychophysical approach is that it has proved to be far too restrictive, resulting in a description of auditory behaviour specific only to situations in the laboratory (Handel, 1989; Jenkins 1985).

As an example of what a psychophysicist is faced with, consider Figure 4.1 as a visual analogue of some sounds used in an experiment. When listening to the acoustic version of Figure 4.1 (a) it is easy to understand that you would hear two beeps separated by a gap of silence. When listening to Figure 4.1 (b) you would expect to hear a 'beep, buzz, beep'. However, the perception is more likely to be 'a single beep *passing through* a buzz'. That is, you perceive something which you expect to happen in the real world. It is rare that some sounds stop at exactly the same time as other sounds start, but sounds happening over the top of others is a common event. In this situation our knowledge of acoustic events pushes us to a kind of perceptual restoration of the beep in the midst of the buzz, resulting in the perception of the beep passing through the buzz.

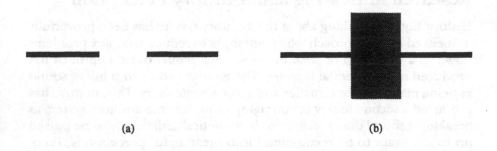

(a)   (b)

Figure 4.1: Visual analogues of simple sounds: (a) is perceived as two beeps separated by a silence. Following a psychophysics approach, you expect to hear (b) as two beeps separated by a buzz, but you perceive a single beep passing through a buzz.

Traditionally, psychophysics has had a hard time trying to explain how we perceive this kind of ambiguous auditory *scene* because it has followed a path of inquiry which has distanced itself from the real world. A more appealing explanation is arrived at by looking at this situation in a more *ecologically valid* way. That is, it makes much more sense to explain that our auditory system has evolved and developed in an environment where sounds like those in Figure 4.1 (b) usually mean that one sound has occurred *over* another rather than there being three separate sounds (Bregman, 1990; Gibson, 1966; Handel, 1989).

Speech science research begins with the phonetic and linguistic aspects of speech sounds. Questions which concern researchers in this tradition include: *What is the speech unit? How do we segment speech into phonemes? How do we discriminate speech sounds?* In our day-to-day lives we tend to think of speech as being made up of words, words of syllables, and syllables of phonemes. Trained speech and language therapists and phoneticians can pick out these speech segments and describe even slight variations in their production, which suggests to us that these segments may be observable and measurable in some way. Unfortunately, establishing this has proved very difficult.

The first spectrographs of speech gave us a useful and simplified way of looking at sound energy. But it was soon apparent that the speech signal cannot simply be divided into a linear sequence of segments occurring one after the other and corresponding to phonemes or even syllables. Not only was the speech signal found to be non-linear, but the acoustic information for each phoneme seemed to depend on its context. For example, the formant transitions for the /ɑ/ in [bɑ], [dɑ] and [gɑ] are acoustically different for each syllable (as you can see in Figure 4.2), but we perceive the second 'sound' of these utterances as a perceptually equivalent /ɑ/.

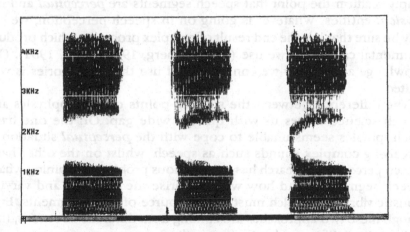

Figure 4.2: Spectrographic representation of the syllables [bɑ], [dɑ] and [gɑ] Spoken by a 30-year-old male native English speaker.

To explain this acoustic variation in similar phonemic segments it has been necessary to refer to *coarticulation* (see Chapter 2). Coarticulation is the effect that the articulation of the preceding and following sounds have on a phoneme, e.g. the sounds /b/, /d/ and /g/ are all articulated in different ways and thus affect the articulation of a following /ɑ/. If we recorded someone saying /bɑ/ and /dɑ/, then spliced the recordings to isolate the vowels, swapped them around and joined them back to the consonants, they would no longer be recognisable as /bɑ/ and /dɑ/. The reason for this is that the /ɑ/ in each phoneme is acoustically different.

Having referred to coarticulation to account for the non-linear nature of speech sounds, it would follow that we could simply quantify the acoustic variations due to coarticulation. But again this has proved a very elusive target. Consequently, we enter a frustrating circularity, not being able to define segments or coarticulation without reference to the other, and end up with no objective description of either (cf. Chapter 15).

In addition to discrete perceptual segments not being immediately apparent in the sound signal and the acoustic structure of each phoneme being dependent on the context, it also became apparent that there is variation within each phoneme in the same context even when produced by the same speaker. Every time a speech segment is uttered it comes out slightly differently and there appears to be little straightforward correspondence between the patterns in the sound signal and the sounds we perceive.

Handel (1989) suggested that one explanation for this uncomfortable state of affairs may be that we are looking at speech with the wrong kind of representation. For Handel and many other researchers, the three problems of *linearity, context* and *variabilility* in the speech signal simply reaffirm the point that speech segments are *perceptual* and not *physical* entities. Whatever is going on in speech perception, we can only be sure that it is the end result of complex processes which produce the mental categories we use (Hammarberg, 1976; Repp, 1981). Our knowledge about how we construct and use these categories is very limited.

The difference between the starting points of psychophysics and speech science leaves us with quite a wide gap. On the one hand psychophysics seems unable to cope with the *perceptual* situation of perceiving complex sounds such as speech, whilst on the other hand speech perception research has a continuous problem explaining what a speech segment is and how we categorise the complex and varying acoustic vibrations which must be the source of these segments. Even though these two approaches are coming from different directions, they both tend to follow a reductionist paradigm.

One way around the problems of reductionism is to think about auditory perception in a more ecologically valid way. By this, we mean thinking about how we perceive speech in the real world. Our acoustic environment is invariably noisy and ever changing but we still manage effortlessly to segregate the sound information of one event from another. For example, we have all heard the sound of trees rustling in the wind at the same time as a car 'vrooming' past. An acoustic-perceptual explanation of these events could be described thus: the array of frequencies in the acoustic signal from the trees rustling change at the same time and rate, determined by the vibrations of the branches and leaves, forming a coherent *stream* of sound-information; this is distinct from the sound-stream of the vibrations of the car's engine and moving parts which would be changing at different times and rates. Or, put another way: because the sources of the sound-events are different they produce different acoustic structures and consequently we are able to perceive the events differentially and as separate from each other. Bregman (1990) has described such an approach as 'Auditory Scene Analysis', in a historical reference to research in vision perception.

Auditory Scene Analysis

Bregman (*op. cit.*) argues that there are two forms of perceptual segregation: 'primitive stream segregation' and 'schema-based stream segregation'. Primitive stream segregation is an innate ability which allows us to segregate gross differences in sound, such as the sounds of engines from trees. These basic skills enable us to function in the acoustic world and lay the building blocks for learning to perceive more complex sounds. Schema-based stream segregation is the result of the learning process and involves the learnt control of attention. Without schema-based stream segregation we would not be able to identify whether a sound came from a large or small tree swaying in the wind, or to distinguish a broken and worn engine in contrast with a new, smooth-running engine simply by listening to the sounds they make.

As infants, we have an innate ability for primitive stream segregation. As we experience the world we develop schemata for perceiving speech and other sound which enable us to understand the stimuli under many different and often adverse conditions. An example may help to further clarify the distinction: when listening to a foreign language for the first time we may be able to recognise the number of voices speaking but not the words being uttered (primitive stream segregation). To understand the words in a foreign language we must identify the contrastive speech sounds of that language (schema-based stream segregation) along with the combinations of these phonemes for the appropriate words which will help us build up a vocabulary.

By taking a more ecological approach to sound perception, auditory scene analysis enables us to partially bridge the gap between high-level and low-level auditory perception that was produced by a reductionist approach. It makes sense to posit that we are born with a certain level of perceptual ability which we build on as we *learn* to make sense out of the acoustic world. Such a view helps to explain skills such as those we all use for speech and those some of us develop for appreciating music to different levels of complexity; the potential to learn the difference between the call of a lesser spotted warbler and that of a greater blanched reed hen; or to tell if the engine in your 15-year-old car needs a new valve in cylinder number four.

The distinction between primitive stream segregation and schema-based segregation consequently forces us to make a distinction in the processes we use in speech perception. We must first have an ability to perceive sounds as speech, which infers an ability to ignore or segregate unwanted sounds occurring at the same time in the background. Second, we must also have the ability to understand and remember speech sounds as belonging to a language we are familiar with. To do this, we must be able to categorise acoustic variations of the same phoneme as equivalent. This second ability, of establishing and maintaining an internal representation of speech units, has been extensively researched for some time and will be discussed in the next section.

Categorical Perception

As we noted earlier, the same utterance can be perceived despite large variations in acoustic structure. We understand the word *cat*, for example, when uttered by a child or an adult male, by speakers with different regional accents, or by a speaker with a hoarse voice and blocked nose from a cold. Somehow we are able to get at the underlying information in speech despite the many varying ways in which the information can be communicated.

All of our perceptual systems (sight, hearing, touch etc.) share a similar attribute which enables us to cope with such complex situations, that of *perceptual constancy*. This refers to the constancy of a perception despite certain changes in the stimulus itself. For example, if you look at a TV screen from the side, the shape of the screen is not strictly a rectangle with 90° corners. The image on your retina reflects the slant of perspective and portrays a two-dimensional rhomboid, but you *perceive* the screen as being rectangular. Categorical perception in speech is a similar form of perceptual constancy. Usually, we perceive the word *cat* successfully because our auditory system deals with variation in the speech signal and enables us to perceive the phonemes giving meaning and understanding to the word spoken. It is important to remember, then, that phonemes are perceptual categories, not acoustic energy patterns.

An early example of the categorical perception of consonants was described by Liberman *et al.* (1957). They presented synthesised syllables of /bɑ/, /dɑ/ and /gɑ/ to their subjects and asked them to identify what they heard. The acoustic signals for these synthetic stimuli were very similar, with the only difference between them being the second formant transition (see Figure 4.3). The listeners identified the consonants fairly consistently, but the changeover from hearing /bɑ/ to /dɑ/ and from hearing /dɑ/ to /gɑ/ occurred very rapidly, taking roughly one or two steps in the formant transition. Later studies showed that subjects found it difficult to distinguish between variations within a category (e.g. /bɑ/[1] and /bɑ/[2]), and easy to distinguish across categories (e.g. /bɑ/[5] and /dɑ/[1]) even though the acoustic differences were the

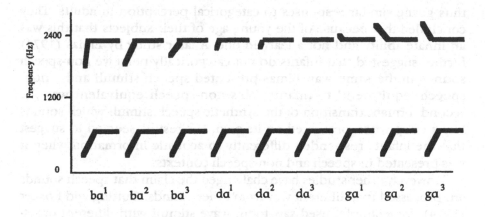

Figure 4.3: A schematic diagram of the synthetic consonants used by Liberman *et al.* (1957) of /bɑ/, /dɑ/, /gɑ/. Listeners hear these as distinct phonemes, find it difficult to discriminate differences within categories and change perceptions at roughly the same point.

same.

The explanation Liberman *et al.* gave was that the subjects processed the acoustic information to fit into the linguistic categories of either /b/, /d/ or /g/ in a way which was qualitatively different from the way we process other sounds. They suggested that humans had a specialised speech mechanism which allowed us to perceive speech sounds categorically and that this accounts for the ease with which we are able to cope with variations in the speech signal. The benefit of this is that we would only have to process the part of the acoustic signal relevant to the category (e.g. the second formant transition), thus making speech perception more robust and efficient. In defining speech perception as something special, the next question is: how do we get to treat speech in such a way? A simple and perhaps logical answer is that this special treatment of speech sounds is an innate ability. To test this hypothesis, it was necessary to investigate categorical perception in children. In the next section we discuss some of the important pieces of research which have helped to clarify this. For a more detailed review of categorical perception the reader is referred to Borden, Harris and Raphael (1994), Handel (1989) and Repp (1984).

Development of Categorical Perception

1. Is Speech Perception 'Special'?

One of the earliest attempts to see whether infants perceive speech categorically was a study by Eimas *et al.* (1971). They presented synthetic speech sounds to infants as young as 1 month old and found that they could distinguish across the categories but not within the categories, thus giving similar responses to categorical perception in adults. They concluded that because of the young age of their subjects that this was an innate ability and not a learned one. A later study by Eimas (1974) further suggested that infants do not categorically perceive non-speech sounds in the same way. Eimas presented speech stimuli and a non-speech 'equivalent' to infants. This non-speech equivalent was the second formant transition of the synthetic speech stimuli which sounds like a chirp when presented on its own. His results seemed to suggest that the infants responded differently to acoustic information when it was presented in speech and non-speech contexts.

However, other studies have challenged the claim that speech sounds are processed in a different way from other sounds. Cutting and Rosner (1974), for example, used saw-tooth wave stimuli with different onset-rise times which sound like musical instruments being either plucked (with a short onset rise time) or bowed (with a longer rise time). They found that their subjects perceived these sounds categorically and that their perception of the sound being plucked or bowed flipped from one to the other depending on the rise-time value (at around 35ms). The rise-times for these distinctions are comparable to those cues in certain speech contrasts (such as [tʃɑ] and [ʃɑ]) indicating that the same cue may be used categorically in both speech and non-speech contexts. Other research (e.g. Pastore, Li and Layer, 1990; and see also Handel, 1989; Bregman, 1990) has provided further evidence that speech perception is not as 'special' as previously thought but may involve general perceptual mechanisms.

The assertion that categorical perception is somehow unique to speech perception is further discredited by the fact that animals can do it (remember the budgies!: Dowling and Brown, 1990). Kuhl and Miller (1978) have even shown that chinchillas discriminate stop consonants in a way similar to human adults. This collection of evidence discredits the claim that speech may be processed in a 'special' way, but does not explain away the fact that infants perceive speech categorically at such young ages as one month after birth.

2. Is Speech Perception Innate?

The idea that speech perception is based on some innate characteristics of our perceptual system is supported by the observation that voice-onset time (VOT) seems to be a linguistically universal cue for categorical perception. VOT is the time difference between the release phase of a plosive and the start of the vibration of the vocal folds. Lisker and Abramson (1964, 1967) found that some phonemic categories for many languages can be divided up into one of three measures of VOT: long lead, short lag or long lag (see Figure 4.4). The fact that many different linguistic cultures use similar cues suggests that the cue may be the result of a characteristic of our perceptual system which makes it easy for us to detect this type of timing difference. This observation, together with the similarity between infant and adult performance on synthetic VOT stimuli, led Eimas (1975, 1978) to propose that infants are innately

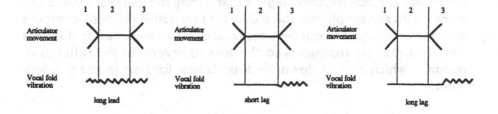

·**Figure 4.4**: Plosive sounds (e.g. [p t k b d g]) are produced in three stages: (1) the articulators are brought into firm contact (closure); (2) air pressure builds up in the vocal tract, behind the closure; (3) the articulators are quickly drawn apart (release) and the air in the vocal tract rushes out between them. In the case of long lead, vocal fold vibration occurs through all three stages; with short lag vocal fold vibration occurs immediately after release of the articulators; with long lag vocal fold vibration begins between 40 ms and 80 ms after release of the closure.

predisposed to detect certain features in speech.

Cross-linguistic research into categorical perception in the early 1970s established that infants can perceive categorical phonemic contrasts in non-native languages. For example, 6-month-old children born into Spanish and Kikuyu speaking cultures were found to discriminate English voiced–voiceless distinctions even though this is not prevalent in their linguistic environments (Lasky, Syrdal-Lasky and Klein, 1975; Streeter, 1976). Similarly, English infants have shown categorical perception of Hindi phonemic contrasts which are not used in English (e.g. Werker et al., 1981; Werker, 1989; Werker and Lalonde, 1988). These and other studies suggest that human infants are born with a linguistic-general ability to discriminate all possible phonetic contrasts.

It would appear, however, that we lose this sensitivity to certain phonetic contrasts if they are not reinforced by the linguistic environment. Whereas infant Japanese language-learners can discriminate English /l/–/r/ phonemes which are not used in Japanese, adult Japanese speakers have great difficulty in doing so. Research indicates that adult speakers are able to discriminate a few non-native phonetic contrasts but never as easily as native speakers (for a review of this area see Werker, 1992). The generally accepted view is that we lose the language-general ability in infancy as our speech perception becomes more efficient and effortless with regard to the important phonetic distinctions used in our native linguistic environments.

However, an alternative explanation may be offered. The study carried out by Lasky, Syrdal-Lasky and Klein (1975) found that their Guatamalan Spanish-learning infants could *not* discriminate some contrasts used by adult Spanish speakers. At first this would suggest that some phonetic distinctions are not immediately available to infants and have to be learnt (see Elliot, 1988). However, recent work reviewed by Werker and Polka (1993) suggests a more complex explanation. In a review of the literature, they suggest that during the first year of development we do not simply *lose* the ability for non-native phonetic contrasts but that we reorganise our perceptual abilities in a qualitively different way. This may be analogous to the loss of several of the reflexes in neonates which may lay down the foundations for later motor development.

3. The Link between Perception and Production

Consider what children have to accomplish before attempting to produce spoken language: they must be able to segregate the speech signal from other concurrent sounds; they must be able to categorise the sounds of speech (while taking variation into account); and they must have a robust method of remembering them; before finally equating these representations to production.

We have established above that categorical perception enables us to perceive phonemes regardless of some of the variation that may occur in the speech signal. This may help explain how a child comes to understand the link between perception and production. The vocal tract and fundamental frequency of adult speech along with the rate of articulation are widely different from those of a child. Consequently, the child cannot exactly reproduce the sounds of adult speech; instead we must think of the child as attempting to reproduce the articulations of adult speech. Whereas the speech imitated by mynah birds is almost an exact acoustic copy, infant speech differs in both temporal and spectral structure (Eguchi and Hirsh, 1969; Pentz, Gilbert and Zawadzki, 1979).

While learning to produce the most appropriate speech sounds, a child must be able to monitor its own articulations. This monitoring of their own sounds together with the responses from adult speakers helps to reinforce the learning process (see also 'Development of Feedback', Chapter 14). However, some problems may occur. Although it is generally considered that perception precedes production, this does not automatically mean that there is a one-to-one relationship between production and perception. Some studies have found that children can produce contrasts they are perceptually unaware of (Edwards, 1974). Other research indicates that children may be aware of perceptual distinctions in adult productions which they produce in their own speech but which we as adults do not class as phonemically noticeable (Macken and Barton, 1980; see also Chapter 14, this volume).

As a child's skill in articulation develops, dependence on auditory feedback may fade in favour of tactile and kinaesthetic feedback (see Kent, 1981). This may explain why certain 'functional' articulation errors, such as [w] for /r/ and [θ] for /s/, are often difficult to change even when the child's attention is drawn to the auditory distinction between error production and the correct production. For example, children who substitute [w] for /r/ can distinguish these sounds when spoken by an adult and hear their own recorded w–r productions as /w/ (Kent, 1981). In this case the child's internal representation of their own w–r productions may be more tactile and kinaesthetic than auditory.

In summary, we can say that speech perception is very complex and at present remains elusive of description or explanation. But there does seem to be some benefit in describing speech perception at two levels of explanation: basic auditory perception and internal representation. For a child with a noticeable problem in producing speech, we immediately have two potential explanations: (i) there may be a problem in basic auditory perception (for example, the child may not be able to perceive speech clearly in the presence of other sounds); (ii) there may be a problem in the categorisation of the speech sounds which help form and maintain a child's internal representation of speech units (this may or may not be caused by a lower-level problem). In the absence of identifiable problems at these two levels, we may infer that the production problem arises through motor coordination difficulties (see also Chapter 14, this volume).

This gives us some methodological direction with respect to the assessment of speech perception. Unfortunately, there are very few tests available which attempt to assess low-level auditory perceptual abilities, and the reader is directed towards the *Test of Basic Auditory Capabilities*, the *Staggered Spondaic Word Test* and the *Competing Environmental Sounds Test* (see Appendix for a short description of these tests). For the clinical assessment of speech perception we are restricted by research paradigms which have concentrated on the perception of isolated single words so that the natural environment of spoken communication has been ignored. Consequently, we may often be left with the unsatisfactory situation that when we have assessed a client in the 'ideal' situation of a quiet room, this does not necessarily rule out the possibility that the client may still have a problem in perceiving speech in the real world. Such a dilemma consequently limits the inferences which may be drawn from such tests.

As clinicians, we are concerned with an individual's current ability to categorise speech sounds into phonemes. The kind of question we are seeking to answer is 'Can children who consistently replace /k/ with [t] in the speech they produce perceive the distinction /k/ vs. /t/ in the speech of others?'. The next section evaluates assessment procedures which attempt to answer this question.

The Assessment of Speech Perception

It is perhaps natural to assume that speech production problems unaccountable for in terms of structural abnormality or neurological impairment are caused by faulty perception. In fact, research findings are conflicting. Bird and Bishop (1992) evaluated studies of auditory discrimination in phonologically impaired children and suggest a number of methodological factors which may have contributed to the apparent contradictions. These include the facts that severity and nature of impairment have been variable across studies, as have language status and age range; group data analysis may have masked individual differences; and tests used in the studies to assess perceptual skills were not as revealing as they have been assumed to be. This latter point is of particular relevance to this chapter.

The pertinent question to be addressed by any test of speech perception is: *'Does the child who produces X* (e.g. [ti]) for X (e.g. *tea*) and for Y (e.g. *key*) perceive X and Y as X?'. In a critique of speech perception assessments Locke (1980a) identified eight criteria which he considered essential to address this question. He stated that the assessment must:

1. *examine the child's perception of the replaced sound in relation to the replacing sound*. That is, the target phoneme versus its substitution phoneme, for example if the child produces [t] for /k/, /t/ versus /k/ should be tested. In the case of complete omission, target versus silence should be tested, for example *bow* versus *boat*;
2. *observe the same phonemes in identical phonetic environments in production and perception*. That is, if a child produces 'wabbit' for 'rabbit', it is not enough to extrapolate that [w] is substituted for /r/ and to test *wing* versus *ring*; 'wabbit' versus 'rabbit' should be tested;
3. *permit comparison of the child's performance on target and replacing sounds with his/her discrimination of target and perceptually similar control sounds*. If a child produces [w] for /r/, for example, then both the perception of /w/ versus /r/ and /r/ versus /l/ (a perceptually similar sound) should be tested. Successful discrimination between target and perceptually similar control sound (which is never substituted for the target by the child) indicates that the child is attending, cooperative and has understood the task;
4. *be based on a comparison of an adult's surface form and the child's own internal representation*. That is, the child has to decide whether what he or she has heard falls into their own potentially idiosyncratic phonemic categories. In order to do this the assessment should...
5. *present repeated opportunities for the child to reveal his or her perceptual decisions*. In other words, a single presentation of a test item is not enough on which to base a decision about perceptual ability;

6. *prevent non-perceptual errors from masquerading as perceptual errors*, for example, fatigue, distraction or guessing;
7. *require a response easily within a young child's conceptual capacities and repertoire of responses*. That is, use words likely to be in the child's vocabulary and tasks likely to be within the child's level of understanding;
8. *allow a determination of the direction of misperception*. For example, a child may think that /r/ could be realised either by [r] or [w] but that /w/ can only be realised as [w] (this last criterion is noted by Locke to be desirable rather than essential).

Locke went on to evaluate two auditory discrimination tests, the Wepman (1973) and the Templin (1957), and concluded that these tests met none of the eight criteria. He also evaluated picture-identification perception assessments; the Goldman–Fristoe–Woodcock (*Test of Auditory Discrimination*, 1970), the Templin (1957) and the Boston (Provonost and Dumbleton, 1953) and noted that these assessments met criteria 4 and 7 only. The Goldman–Fristoe–Woodcock addressed criterion 8 but with too few trials to be reliable. His main criticism of these assessments was that few of the test items were production-relevant. That is, contrasts such as /d/ vs /f/; /n/ vs /g/ which are never confused in children's production were included in the tests whilst contrasts which are confused were either excluded or had too few trials to be reliable.

Currently, the only readily available test of speech perception in the UK is *The Auditory Discrimination and Attention Test* (MorganBarry, 1988). This test assesses the child's ability to discriminate between seventeen pairs of words each of which has one 'feature distinction' between them and which are grouped on the basis of:

voicing differences	(for example, *coat–goat; pear–bear*);
place differences	(for example, *cap–cat; wing–ring*);
manner differences	(for example, *mat–bat; watch–wash*);
cluster differences	(for example, *crown–clown; grass–glass*).

Each test item presents a pair of pictures (for example, *seat* and *feet*). Prior to testing perception, the assessor goes through all pairs asking the child to produce each word and teaches the vocabulary where necessary. The child's productions are transcribed and note is made where items needed to be taught. For the perception task, the child is required to indicate which of the pair has been uttered by the assessor. Pre-school children are given three repetitions of each word in the pair, older children (5–12 years) are given six repetitions. The tester is required to observe the child's attention/concentration during the test and to note on the score sheet a *level of attention* using the Cooper, Moodley and

Reynell (1978) scale. Table 4.1 summarises our evaluation of this test in relation to the Locke criteria.

As can be seen from this table, MorganBarry's test meets more of Locke's criteria than the assessments evaluated by Locke in 1980, but still does not meet them all. In particular, although some of the items in *The Auditory Discrimination and Attention Test* reflect errors that the child is likely to make in production (for example, *coat–goat*; *key–tea*); other test items are not production relevant. For example, we suggest it would be more appropriate to test *glass* ([glas]) versus *gas* than *glass* versus *grass*; and *cup* versus *cuff* rather than *cat* versus *cap*. Thus we conclude that fourteen years on from the Locke paper there is still no published assessment which adequately evaluates speech perception abilities. So how may we assess speech perception? There are a number of procedures, discussed in detail by Locke (1980b), which do meet his criteria and may readily be employed by speech and language therapists. In the next section we will outline some of these procedures.

Table 4.1: Applying Locke's criteria to the Auditory Discrimination and Attention Test

Locke Criteria	The Auditory Discrimination and Attention Test MorganBarry (1988)
1. Examine the child's perception of the replaced sound in relation to the replacing sound	No
2. Observe the same phonemes in identical phonetic environments in production and perception	No
3. Permit comparison of the child's performance on target and replacing sounds with his/her discrimination of target and perceptually similar control sounds	No
4. Be based on a comparison of an adult's surface form and the child's own internal representation	Yes
5. Present repeated opportunities for the child to reveal his or her perceptual decisions	Yes
6. Prevent non-perceptual errors from masquerading as perceptual errors	Yes
7. Require a response easily within a young child's conceptual capacities and repertoire of responses	Yes
8. Allow a determination of the direction of misperception	Yes

Procedures for Speech Perception Assessment

When a child produces, for example, [ti] in response to pictures of both *tea* and *key*, there are two questions we may want to ask:

1. Is the child's internal representation of *key* [ti]?
2. Can the child perceive a distinction between the adult's productions of *tea* and *key*?

Answers to these two questions may be inferred from accessing two general types of perceptual processing identified by Locke (*op. cit.*) as Type I and Type II. Type I tasks use external referents, usually pictures and sometimes objects. The adult names the referent and the child is required either to point to the appropriate picture or to verify that the picture has been named correctly. Thus for Type I processing the child has to compare the adult's utterance (or surface form) with his or her own knowledge of words (or internal representations). Type I processing tasks therefore aim to address question 1.

Type II tasks aim to address question 2. They require the child to listen to two or more adult utterances and make a decision as to whether they are the same or different. It is possible for the child to make a same–different judgement about two adult surface forms without reference to his or her own internal representations. Nevertheless, when real words are used in Type II tasks, we cannot be certain that the child does not refer to his or her own internal knowledge. Auditory processing occurs very rapidly; a child may hear *tea*, associate it with an internal representation, then hear *key* and associate it with an internal representation and base his or her same–different response on a comparison of internal representations of *key* and *tea*. To attempt to ensure that the child is processing the adult utterances without reference to his or her own internal representations, non-words may be used. Stackhouse and Wells (1993) cite research which indicates that some children with impaired intelligibility perform better on real-word Type II processing tasks whereas others perform better on non-word Type II processing tasks. Thus they advocate that speech perception assessments should incorporate both real-word and non-word items so that a precise profile of auditory processing abilities and deficits may be identified.

Below we outline one Type I processing task, *The Speech Production–Perception Task*, and three Type II processing tasks, *The AX, ABX* and *4IAX Tasks*.

Speech Production–Perception Task (SP–PT)

There are no pre-determined stimuli for this task; test items are decided following a speech production assessment of the child. So, for example, if the production assessment reveals that a child produces [ti] for adult target /si/, then /si/ may be chosen as a test item. A picture of the sea serves as the stimulus and the adult asks a series of randomly ordered stimulus-questions: '*Is this* /si/?', correct articulation of the stimulus phoneme (SP); '*Is this* /ti/?', incorrect articulation using the child's response phoneme (RP); *'Is this /ʃi/?'*, incorrect articulation using a perceptually similar control phoneme (CP). The child is simply required to respond 'yes' or 'no'. Each stimulus type (SP, RP, CP) is presented six times. The random ordering of the stimuli is constrained to ensure that: no stimulus type occurs more than twice in succession; each block of six items includes two of each type of stimulus; and no more than two *yes* and three *no* responses occur consecutively. Table 4.2 shows the assessment format used by Locke. It is possible to determine the direction of misperception with this task by repeating the test items using a stimulus picture depicting the response phoneme (in the above example, *tea*).

Table 4.2: An example of the assessment format used by Locke (1980b). The first column has been completed using *sea* and *tea* to exemplify. With kind permission of John Locke.

Speech Production–Perception Task

Child's Name:
Date of Birth: Sex: M F

Production task		Production task		Production task	
Stimulus	Response	Stimulus	Response	Stimulus	Response
/si /	[ti]	/ /	[ ]	/ /	[ ]
SP / s /RP/ t /CP/ ʃ /		SP/ /RP/ /CP/ /		SP/ /RP/ /CP/ /	

Stimulus Class		Response		Stimulus Class		Response		Stimulus Class		Response	
1/ ʃ /CP	yes	NO		1/ /SP	YES	no		1/ /RP	yes	NO
2/ t /RP	yes	NO		2/ /CP	yes	NO		2/ /CP	yes	NO
3/ s /SP	YES	no		3/ /SP	YES	no		3/ /CP	yes	NO
4/ s /SP	YES	no		4/ /CP	yes	NO		4/ /SP	YES	no
5/ t /RP	yes	NO		5/ /RP	yes	NO		5/ /SP	YES	no
6/ ʃ /CP	yes	NO		6/ /RP	yes	NO		6/ /RP	yes	NO
7/ ʃ /CP	yes	NO		7/ /SP	YES	no		7/ /RP	yes	NO
8/ s /SP	YES	no		8/ /RP	yes	NO		8/ /SP	YES	no
9/ t /RP	YES	NO		9/ /SP	YES	no		9/ /CP	yes	NO
10/ s /SP	YES	no		10/ /CP	yes	NO		10/ /SP	YES	no
11/ t /RP	yes	NO		11/ /CP	yes	NO		11/ /CP	yes	NO
12/ ʃ /CP	yes	NO		12/ /RP	yes	NO		12/ /RP	yes	NO
13/ t /RP	YES	NO		13/ /SP	YES	no		13/ /SP	YES	no
14/ s /SP	YES	no		14/ /CP	yes	NO		14/ /RP	yes	NO
15/ ʃ /CP	yes	NO		15/ /RP	yes	NO		15/ /SP	YES	no
16/ t /RP	yes	NO		16/ /SP	YES	no		16/ /CP	yes	NO
17/ s /SP	YES	no		17/ /RP	yes	NO		17/ /CP	yes	NO
18/ ʃ /CP	YES	NO		18/ /CP	yes	NO		18/ /RP	yes	NO

Errors   Errors   Errors

RP _2_ CP _I_ SP _0_   RP ___ CP ___ SP ___   RP ___ CP ___ SP ___

AX Tasks

Traditionally, AX (or same–different) tasks present the child with a pair of words (e.g. *wing–ring; pin–bin; car–car*) and require the child to respond 'same' when the two words are the same and 'different' when the two words are different. A major criticism of such tests is that failure may be due to lack of understanding of the concepts *same* and *different* rather than due to inability to perceive differences between words. Bird and Bishop (1992) report on a procedure which appears to reduce the cognitive demands of the same–different judgement. They use two puppets, one of which is a 'copycat'. The first puppet says a word and the second puppet copies it. The child has to decide whether or not the second puppet is right or wrong. Task training includes asking the child to predict what the second puppet is going to say. For example, the tester holds up the first puppet, says 'horse' and asks the child what he or she thinks the copycat puppet is going to say. The child is encouraged to say 'horse'. The tester then holds up the second puppet and says 'vorse' and the child is asked whether or not the second puppet is right. As in the SP–PT test outlined above, test items for the Bird and Bishop task were specific to individual children and thus determined after a production assessment.

Locke (1980a) raises another concern with regard to AX tasks. He points out that children may fail on such tasks not because they do not perceive differences between items but because they ignore such differences as unimportant. That is, just as an adult may state that [kat^h] and [kat$^\cdot$] are the same because the variations in pronunciation of the word final /t/ are allophonic, a child may view [w] and [r] as allophones of the same phoneme and thus judge *ring* and *wing* to be the same. The ABX and 4IAX tasks outlined below go some way to addressing this problem.

ABX Task

In the ABX task the child has to decide which of two items a third item is most like. Two different items are presented (AB) and the third item (X) is either the same as A or the same as B. Locke used puppets for this task. The first puppet is held up and the tester says the word with the target phoneme (T), for example 'pear'; the second puppet is then held up and the tester says the word with the substitution phoneme (S) 'bear'; the child is asked 'Who said _____?' (either *pear* or *bear*). In this task it is given that the two puppets said different things and that the tester has repeated one puppet's word. Thus a child who is ignoring the /p/ versus /b/ difference as allophonic is forced to acknowledge the distinction and decide which of the two words is most like the third. As with the SP–PT test, Locke recommends that a perceptually similar control sound (C) is used and thus the task must have at least eight items:

TST	TCT
TSS	TCC
STT	CTT
STS	CTC

Locke notes that a sixteen-item test including two of each item can be administered in a few minutes.

4IAX Task

The 4IAX (or four-interval AX test) was developed by Pisoni (1971) to evaluate adults' ability to discriminate sub-phonemic differences. Pisoni and Lazarus (1974) compared the 4IAX and the ABX procedures and noted that the 4IAX yielded significantly more accurate discrimination decisions than the ABX. Locke adapted the 4IAX task for children, again using puppets. This time each puppet 'says' two words and the child is asked 'Who said "same sounds"?' For example the first puppet might 'say' *wing–ring* and the second puppet *ring–ring*; the child would be asked 'Who said *ring–ring*?' Locke used eight Target-Substitution items (e.g. w–r, r–r) and eight Target Control items (e.g. l–r, r–r). As with the ABX task, the child who perceives phonemic differences but ignores them as unimportant has to acknowledge the difference in the 4IAX task. Locke suggests that 'as in none of the other tasks, the 4IAX procedure appears to provide the subject with a clear perceptual reference for sameness' (1980b, p. 462).

It is worth noting here that on the ABX and 4IAX tests some children responded 'They both did' (in response to 'Who said _____?' (ABX) and 'Who said "same sounds"?' (4IAX)). Locke's solution to this problem was to add a TBD (they both did) category and to give the child half a point for a TBD response on the basis that if he or she had guessed, chance would render them accurate 50% of the time.

Prior to the advent of published phonological assessment procedures, many clinicians devised their own assessments based on phonological procedures. We suggest here that speech and language therapists adapt one or more of the above procedures to evaluate speech perception. Notwithstanding this, it should be noted that as speech perception is an internal process and cannot be directly observed, the results of assessment should be treated with caution. A correct response to test items may be inferred to indicate that a child has perceived a distinction 'accurately'. Yet it is possible that the child's discrimination decision is based on non-salient acoustic cues, imperceptible to the adult. For example a child may correctly discriminate *tea* versus *key* but may arrive at the discrimination decision on the basis of Voice Onset Time differences rather than F2 differences. Further, if we infer that the child perceives speech accurately, that is not to say that he or she has never had speech perception difficulties. It may be that earlier perception problems have resolved and production difficulties still exist owing to a lag between development of perception and development of production (Bird and Bishop, 1992; Locke, 1980a, 1980b). From incorrect responses we could infer that the child misperceives a contrast. Alternatively, it could be that the child perceives the acoustic differences but ignores them (Locke, 1980b).

We should also consider that the perceptual task in any of the above procedures is very different from speech perception in the real world. The first section of this chapter has given some indication of the complexities of the speech perception process. In the real world people normally use longer utterances than the one-word test items used in the tasks, against a background of competing auditory and other sensory stimuli. If a child fails a speech perception task under favourable conditions we may infer that he or she may have quite significant difficulties with perception of 'real world' speech. On the other hand, if a child succeeds at a speech perception task under favourable conditions, can we be sure that she or he experiences no difficulties with perception of real-world speech?

Summary

In this chapter we have attempted to convey the complex nature of speech perception and some of the inherent difficulties in researching processes of speech perception. We have concentrated on questions relating to the perception of speech by children but this should not be taken to imply that for adults with acquired speech and language impairments speech perception is not significant. Chapter 15 addresses some issues concerning the relation between speech production and speech perception in adults and we would suggest that the procedures outlined in the latter half of this chapter could be adapted to assess speech perception in adults with acquired disorders.

Perhaps in acknowledgement of the inadequacies of available assessment procedures, clinical assessment of speech perception declined in the latter half of the 1980s. Recent psycholinguistic research indicates a revival of interest in the relation between speech production and speech perception. We hope that this chapter will contribute to the extension of this interest into routine clinical work.

References

Arnst, D. and Katz, J. (Eds) (1982). *Central Auditory Assessment: The SSW Test.* San Diego, CA: College-Hill Press.

Bird, J. and Bishop, D. (1992). Perception and awareness of phonemes in phonologically impaired children. *European Journal of Disorders of Communication* 27, 289–311.

Bregman, A.S. (1990). *Auditory Scene Analysis*. Cambridge, MA: MIT Press.

Borden, G.J., Harris, K.S. and Raphael, L.J. (1994). *Speech Science Primer: Physiology, Acoustics and Perception of Speech* 3rd edn. Baltimore, MD: Williams & Wilkins.

Christopherson, L.A. and Humes, L.E. (1992). Some psychometric properties of the Test of Basic Auditory Capabilities (TBAC). *Journal of Speech and Hearing Research* 35, 929–935.

Cooper, J., Moodley, M. and Reynell, J. (1978). *Helping Language Development. A Developmental Programme for Children with Early Language Handicaps*. London: Edward Arnold.

Cutting, J.E. and Rosner, B.S. (1974). Categories and boundaries in speech and music. Perception and Psychophysics 16, 564–571.

Denes, P.B. and Pinson, E.N. (1993). *The Speech Chain: The Physics and Biology of Spoken Language*. New York: W.H. Freeman.

Dooling R.J. and Brown, S.D. (1990). Speech perception by budgerigars (*Melopsittacus undulatus*): Spoken vowels. *Perception and Psychophysics* 47(6), 568–574.

Edwards, M.L. (1974). Perception and production in child phonology: the testing of four hypotheses. *Journal of Child Language* 1, 205–219.

Eguchi, S. and Hirsh, I.J. (1969). Development of speech sounds in children. *Acta Otolaryngogica*, Supplement 257.

Eimas, P.D. (1974). Auditory and linguistic processing of cues for place of articulation by infants. *Perception and Psychophysics* 16, 513–521.

Eimas, P.D. (1975). Speech perception in early infancy. In: L.B. Cohen and P. Salapatek (Eds), *Infant Perception: From Sensation to Cognition*, Vol. 2. New York: Academic Press.

Eimas, P.D. (1978). Developmental aspects of speech perception. In: R. Held, H.W. Leibbowitz and H.-L. Teuber (Ed.), *Handbook of Sensory Physiology VIII: Perception*. Berlin: Springer-Verlag.

Eimas, P.D., Siqueland, E.R., Jusczyck, P. and Vigorito, J. (1971). Speech perception in infants. *Science* 71, 303–306.

Elliot, A.J. (1988). *Child Language*. Cambridge, UK: Cambridge University Press.

Gibson, J.J. (1966). *The Senses Considered as Perceptual Systems*. Boston: Houghton Mifflin.

Goldman, R., Fristoe, M. and Woodcock, R.W. (1970). *Goldman–Fristoe–Woodcock Test of Auditory Discrimination*. Circle Pines, MN: American Guidance Service.

Handel, S. (1989). *Listening: An Introduction to the Perception of Auditory Events*. Cambridge, MA: MIT Press.

Hammarberg, R. (1976). *The metaphysics of coarticulation*. Journal of Phonetics 4(4), 353–363.

Jenkins, J.J. (1985). Acoustic information for objects, places and events. In: W.H. Warren Jr and R.E. Shaw (Eds), *Persistence and Change: Proceedings of the 1st International Conference on Event Perception*. Hillsdale, NJ: Lawrence Earlbaum.

Johnson, D.W., Enfield, M.L. and Sherman, R.E. (1981). The use of the staggered spondaic word test and the competing environmental sounds test in the evaluation of central auditory function of learning disabled children. *Ear and Hearing* 2(2), 70–77.

Katz, J. (Ed.) (1994). *The Handbook of Clinical Audiology*. Baltimore and London: Williams & Wilkins.

Kent, R.D. (1981). Sensorimotor aspects of speech development. In: R.N. Aslin, J.R.

Alberts and M.R. Petersen (Eds), *Development of Perception: Psychobiological Perspectives*, Vol. 1. London: Academic Press.

Klatt, D.H. and Stefanski, R.A. (1974). How does a mynah bird imitate human speech? *Journal of the Acoustical Society of America* 55, 822–832.

Kuhl, P.K. and Miller, J.D. (1978). Speech perception in the chinchilla: identification functions for synthetic VOT stimuli. *Journal of the Acoustical Society of America* 63, 905–917.

Laksy, R.E., Syrdal-Lasky, A. and Klein, R.E. (1975). VOT discrimination by four and six-and-a-half-month-old infants from Spanish environments. *Journal of Experimental Child Psychology* 20, 215–225.

Liberman, A.M., Harris, K.S., Hoffman, H.S. and Griffith, B.C. (1957). The discrimination of speech sounds within and across phoneme boundaries. *Journal of Experimental Psychology* 54(5), 358–368.

Lisker, L. and Abramson, A.S. (1964). A cross language study of voicing in initial stops: acoustical measurements. *Word* 20, 384–422.

Lisker, L. and Abramson, A.S. (1967). The voicing dimension: some experiments in comparative phonetics. In: *Proceedings of the Sixth International Congress of Phonetic Sciences*. Prague: Academia (1970).

Locke, J. (1980a). The inference of speech perception in the phonologically disordered child, Part I: a rationale, some criteria, the conventional tests. *Journal of Speech and Hearing Disorders* 45, 431–444.

Locke, J. (1980b). The inference of speech perception in the phonologically disordered child, Part II: some clinically novel procedures, their use, some findings. *Journal of Speech and Hearing Disorders* 45, 445–468.

Macken, M.A. and Barton, D. (1980). The acquisition of voicing contrast in English: the study of voice onset time in word-initial stop consonants. *Journal of Child Language* 7, 41–47.

MorganBarry, R. (1988). *The Auditory Discrimination and Attention Test*. Windsor: NFER-Nelson.

Pastore, R.E., Li, X. and Layer, J.K. (1990). Categorical perception of nonspeech chirps and bleats. *Perception and Psychophysics* 48(2), 151–156.

Pentz, A., Gilbert, H.R. and Zawadzki, P. (1979). Spectral properties of fricative consonants in children. *Journal of the Acoustical Society of America* 66, 1891–1893.

Pisoni, D.B. (1971). On the nature of categorical perception of speech sounds. *Status Report on Speech Research (SR-27)*. New Haven, CT: Haskins Laboratories.

Pisoni, D.B. and Lazarus, J.H. (1974). Categorical and noncategorical modes of speech perception along the voicing continuum. *Journal of the Acoustical Society of America* 55, 328–333.

Provonost, W. and Dumbleton, C. (1953). A picture-type speech sound discrimination test. *Journal of Speech and Hearing Disorders* 18, 258–266.

Repp, B.H. (1981). On levels of description in speech research. *Journal of the Acoustical Society of America* 69(5), 1462–1464.

Repp, B.H. (1984). Categorical perception: issues, methods and findings. In: N. Lass (Ed.), *Speech and Language*, Vol. 10: *Advances in Basic Research and Practice*, pp. 244–335. Orlando, FL: Academic Press.

Samuel, A.G. (1981). Phonemic restoration: insights from a new methodology. *Journal of Experimental Psychology: General* 110(4), 474–494.

Stackhouse, J. and Wells, B. (1993). Psycholinguistic assessment of developmental speech disorders. *European Journal of Disorders of Communication* 28(4), 331–348.

Streeter, L.A. (1976). Language Perception of Two-month-old Infants shows Effects of both Innate Mechanisms and Experience. *Nature* 259, 39–41.

Templin, M.C. (1957). *Certain Language Skills in Children*, Institute of Child Welfare Monogram No. 26. Minneapolis: University of Minnesota.

Warren, R.M. (1970). Perceptual restoration of missing speech sounds.*Science* 167(3917), 392–393.

Wepman, J.M. (1973). *Auditory Discrimination Test*. Chicago: Language Research Associates.

Werker, J.F. (1989). Becoming a native listener. *American Scientist* 77, 54–59.

Werker, J.F. (1992). Cross language speech perception: developmental change does not involve loss. In: J. Goodman and H.C. Nusbaum (Eds), *Speech Perception and Word Recognition*. Cambridge, MA: MIT Press.

Werker, J.F., Gilbert, J.H.V., Humphrey, K. and Tees, R.C. (1981). Developmental aspects of cross-language speech perception. *Child Development* 52, 349–353.

Werker, J.F. and Lalonde, C.E. (1988). Cross language speech perception: initial capabilities and developmental change. *Developmental Psychology* 24, 672–683.

Werker, J.F. and Polka, L. (1993). Developmental changes in speech perception: new challenges and new directions.*Journal of Phonetics* 21, 83–101.

Appendix

Test of Basic Auditory Capabilities

Available on DAT or audio cassette (US$105 approx.)
CDT Inc., 205 South Walnut Avenue, Bloomington, IN 47404, USA.
The Test of Basic Auditory Capabilities consists of a battery of seven discriminatory subtests and one nonsense-syllable identification subtest. The seven discriminatory subtests require the subject to compare a standard sound to one of two following sounds and to indicate which of them differs from the standard sound. The trials are presented in groups of six. Within each set of six, the difficulty of the discrimination ranges from easy to difficult. The subtests consist of the following:

1. frequency discrimination;
2. intensity discrimination;
3. duration discrimination;
4. rhythm discrimination;
5. duration discrimination within tone sequences;
6. order discrimination within tone sequences;
7. order discrimination within syllable sequences;
8. identification of nonsense syllables.

The test has been standardised and several studies have recorded a high level of reliability (e.g. Christopherson and Humes, 1992). The authors of this test intended this to be a test which goes a little bit further to explain why two people with similar hearing loss may present different abilities to resolve speech.

Staggered Spondaic Word Test and Competing Environmental Sounds Test

Precision Acoustics, 411 NE 87th Avenue, Suite B, Vancouver, WA 98664, Canada.

The SSWT (see Arnst and Katz, 1982; Johnson, Enfield and Sherman, 1981; Katz, 1994) was developed in the 1960s as a tool for the study of both hearing ability and auditory processing ability and is one of the most widely used tests of central auditory dysfunction in the United States. The test is essentially constructed from pairs of two-syllable words which are presented with the syllables staggered and overlapping to each ear. The first word is presented to one ear so that its first syllable is heard clearly; the first syllable of the second word is presented to the other ear and is timed to be simultaneous with the second syllable of the first word. The subject is forced to interpret these dichotic and competing stimuli, which is carried out by the central nervous system.

The subject's response consists of him or her repeating the actual words in the correct order with each ear leading the presentation order.

There are extensive normative data for age populations (5–70) and for children with learning difficulties and specific reading disorders.

The CEST is a complementary test to the SSWT, aimed at assessing central auditory dysfunction. The SSWT is sensitive to verbal processing problems whilst the CEST uses non-speech sounds to test auditory processing, which in most cases is carried out in the right hemisphere of the cortex. The test's main aim is to assess whether there is any dysfunction in the pathways between the two hemispheres and is usually used in conjunction with the SSWT.

Chapter 5
Assessment of Phonology

PAMELA GRUNWELL

Introduction

As we have seen from the chapter by Evershed Martin and Hirson, approaches and techniques for the clinical assessment of speech production have recently developed a high level of sophistication. Notwithstanding these procedures for measuring articulatory skills and the increasing number of instrumental investigations of articulatory performance, the non-technological and less quantitative approach of linguistic analysis remains an essential tool in the speech and language therapist's range of assessment procedures for disordered speech. In assessing disorders of speech production it is of course important to describe in detail the articulatory characteristics of the disordered production process, but in most instances it is at least equally important to take into consideration also the *communicative* implications and outcomes of the disorder.

It is necessary to assess whether and to what extent the disordered pronunciation results in failures on the part of speakers to convey their intended messages adequately. Speech therapists routinely encounter clients who have virtually unintelligible speech resulting from 'multiple misarticulation' (that is, severe pronunciation problems) which may or may not be associated with identifiable disorders or disabilities affecting speech production processes, (see Chapters 14 and 15, this volume). In order to describe the characteristics of these pronunciation disorders from a communicative perspective a *phonological* framework of analysis and assessment is required. As already discussed in Section 1, phonology is concerned with describing the patterns in spoken language whereby sound differences function to signal meaning differences. Phonology is therefore complementary to phonetics in that it investigates how the phenomena of speech are used in spoken language. A phonological investigation therefore is dependent upon and is derived from phonetic investigation, as described in Section II, Chapter 3. For routine clinical purposes the phonetic investigation that is the appropriate basis for a phonological investigation is a narrow (i.e. detailed) phonetic auditory-articulatory transcription. A clinical phonological analysis and assessment of disordered speech therefore describes the functional consequences of the different pronunciation patterns of the disordered speaker. On the basis of such descriptions the speech and language therapist can assess the relative severity, in functional terms, of the disordered characteristics of an individual's pronunciation patterns and formulate a principled treatment programme designed to enhance a client's intelligibility, and hence communicative adequacy.

In this chapter we shall consider a range of different approaches and procedures for the phonological assessment of disordered speech. Both formalised assessment tools and informal techniques of analysis will be discussed as both approaches are currently employed in clinical investigations (cf. Harris and Cottam, 1985; Shriberg *et al.*, 1986). In considering the types of clinical procedures available for the assessment of phonology, it is important to appreciate that the term *phonology* has acquired different applications and interpretations when employed in clinical contexts. For some clinical linguists and speech and language therapists a phonological analysis of a transcribed data sample simply *describes* the patterns in the client's disordered pronunciation, with no cross-reference as to the nature of the disorders or disabilities in the speaker's speech mechanism and the production processes which may have created these patterns. For other analysts the phonological analysis provides an *explanation*, or at least contributes directly to an explanation, of the nature of the speech disorder/disability *per se*. This difference in interpretation has been termed (by Hewlett, 1985), the 'data-oriented' versus the 'speaker-oriented' approach. As Grunwell (1985a) has pointed out, both positions are tenable at present, and appropriate in clinical assessment *provided* the clinician is aware of their different implications. With a data-oriented approach, we assume that the phonological assessment is merely a description of the patterns in the transcribed speech sample. Clearly a richer interpretation that attempts to see beyond descriptive statements and to evaluate and understand the current state of a client's phonological knowledge, skills and potential for phonological change generates a more potent clinical approach. However, this explanatory approach to phonological analysis and assessment cannot be undertaken in a linguistic vacuum. Information from a wide variety of clinical observations and assessment procedures (auditory, perceptual, articulatory, medical, cognitive, social, etc.) needs to be brought to bear in arriving at clinical hypotheses about the psycho-physiological nature of pronunciation disorders. Such considerations are not within the remit of this chapter (but see further Section III).

Of more relevance to our present concerns are the differences in the applications and interpretations of the different phonological frameworks of analysis that have been employed in clinical assessment procedures. Whether we attempt a rich interpretation or not, the phonological analysis is at the least a descriptive statement of the *patterns* in the client's pronunciation. It has, however, been pointed out (e.g. Grunwell, 1987b), that it is essential for the clinician to appreciate the distinction between descriptive statements that present an analysis of the client's pronunciation patterns as an independent, self-contained phonological system, and statements that describe the systematic phonological relationships between the disordered speaker's pronunciation patterns and normal pronunciation patterns. This distinction will be discussed further in our consideration of different assessment procedures.

Clinical procedures for phonological analysis and assessment were originally devised primarily for use with children with developmental phonological disorders (see further Chapter 14, this volume). Indeed phonological analysis led to the discovery of the nature of these disorders (Ingram 1976; 1989; Grunwell 1981). Phonological assessment is also valuable in the investigation of other types of speech disorders where there is an apparent organic basis for the disorder, such as cleft palate. The phonological assessment reveals whether there are functional implications for any of the disordered speech patterns and indicates if there are any co-occurring characteristics of disordered phonological development (see Grunwell 1990; 1993).

It should be noted that this chapter is solely concerned with the phonological assessment of the segmental aspects of speech. Wells, Peppé and Vance (Chapter 10) address the issues concerned in the phonological assessment of the suprasegmental or prosodic aspects of speech. They similarly focus on the functional dimensions of prosody and highlight the distinction between phonetic and phonological phenomena.

Principles for Phonological Assessment

Before we proceed to an examination of assessment procedures we need to consider the basic clinical requirements that have to be satisfied by a phonological analysis of disordered speech. It is essential that clinical judgements about diagnosis and treatment of speech disorders are informed by reliable, appropriate and detailed phonological descriptions. Grunwell (1985b) has delineated the criteria for such descriptions. A clinical phonological assessment must satisfy three fundamental linguistic criteria. It must be:

1. *Exhaustive*: the framework for the analysis must be capable of describing and classifying all the data examined by the assessment procedure. If it cannot, then relevant data will either be excluded from the analysis or spuriously misclassified. The resultant assessment is potentially misleading as it is only a partial description of a client's pronunciation patterns.
2. *Replicable*: the procedures for analysing and classifying the data must

be explicitly and unambiguously stated, such that two analyses of the same data sample by two different analysts (or by the same analyst on two different occasions) will provide identical results. This criterion is thus equivalent to the requirement for inter-tester and intra-tester reliability in psychometric assessments. If the procedures for an assessment are not adequately presented then the users of the procedure may be forced to make *ad hoc* classifications on an unprincipled basis and the results of the analysis might thus be haphazard and unreliable.

3. *Predictive*: the analytical statements must be interpreted as descriptions of the speaker's habitual pronunciation patterns. In order to satisfy this criterion, the analysis should be based on a reliable, representative data sample that is known to be typical of the speaker and large enough to include, as far as possible, the full range of different types of target segments and sequences.

As well as these linguistic criteria, a further number of clinical requirements need to be fulfilled. Procedures must:

1. provide a description of the patterns in the speaker's pronunciation of the language;
2. identify the differences between the expected normal patterns and the patterns used by the disordered speaker; these differences are the aspects of the client's speech which render it unacceptable and/or unintelligible to the linguistic community of which the speaker is a member. It is therefore these aspects of the client's pronunciation patterns that will be the target of any intervention procedures;
3. indicate the communicative implications of the disordered pronunciation patterns; this is the essentially phonological dimension in an assessment procedure, in that it examines the functional consequences of the disordered speech and identifies the phonological contrasts that are absent. The results of this assessment provide an appropriate basis for the formulation of prioritised treatment aims.

In evaluating children's pronunciation patterns, we require a further assessment procedure which may suggest a different set of treatment priorities. Therefore:

4. when a clinical assessment of a child's pronunciation patterns is required, the procedure should also provide an indication of the developmental status of the child's speech. This assessment can thus provide a different set of guidelines for planning treatment, with priorities established by reference to the criteria of developmental normality and relative severity of delay.

As well as providing a basis for planning treatment, the communicative and developmental assessments can be used to identify and evaluate treatment outcomes and to assess any type of change in a client's pronunciation patterns. It is very important for clinical purposes that an assessment procedure is also an informative reassessment procedure. On reassessment, changes in pronunciation patterns must not only be identified; they must be evaluated as regards their involving developmental progress and improvement in communicative adequacy.

Finally, it should be a long-term aspiration of clinical linguists and speech and language therapists to formulate diagnostic classifications of different types of pronunciation disorders based on clearly stated descriptions of their phonological characteristics. The diagnostic characteristics of developmental phonological disorders have been delineated (see later in this chapter). As phonological assessments are used more routinely in the investigation of other disorders, further descriptive diagnoses will become formulated (see Grunwell 1988; 1990; 1993). These clinical linguistic descriptive diagnoses would then be cross-matched to speech pathological diagnostic categories (Grunwell, 1988). When such a situation is achieved the theoretical base of clinical speech–language pathology will have been considerably advanced.

Studies of the phonological disorders have described, almost exclusively, the consonantal characteristics of the disordered pronunciation patterns. The assessment procedures described below are therefore designed only to analyse consonantal aspects of pronunciation. There have been a small number of published studies of disordered vowel systems (Pollock & Keiser 1990; Reynolds, 1990; Stoel-Gammon and Herrington 1990; Pollock & Hall 1991; Gibbon, Shockey and Reid 1992; Penney, Fee and Dowdle 1994). These are primarily case studies. No phonological assessment procedure for vowel systems has been published as yet (*pace* Crystal, 1982; see below). As with prosody (see Chapter 10, this volume) accent and dialect variations are a major factor in the assessment of vowels. This, together with the apparent relative infrequency of disordered vowels, probably accounts for the lack of formalised assessment methods.

Procedures for Phonological Assessment

A number of approaches to the clinical assessment of phonology have been proposed over the last twenty years. These have reflected the waxing and waning influences of mainstream (linguistic) approaches to phonology on clinical practice (Grunwell, 1992a; cf. the relationship between theoretical linguistics and child phonology as portrayed by Menn, 1980). During this period both distinctive feature analysis and generative phonological analysis have been applied in clinical assessment (see McReynolds and Engmann, 1975; Compton and Hutton, 1978; for comprehensive reviews of these approaches see Edwards and

Schriberg, 1983; Grunwell, 1987a). In the 1980s one approach attained a pre-eminent position in clinical phonology: phonological process analysis. This is not to imply that other procedures are not available; several alternatives will be outlined below. It is also important to appreciate that phonological process analysis shares many descriptive similarities with other approaches which preceded it or indeed coexist with and complement it.

When employed in descriptive assessments phonological processes are relational statements about the systematic correspondences between the speaker's pronunciation patterns and the target (normal) pronunciation patterns. They describe:

1. the feature differences between natural classes of sounds in a replacement relationship; i.e. *substitutions*.
2. the rearrangements or deletions of natural classes of sounds in transpositions or omission-type relationships; i.e. *metatheses* and *omissions*.

Processes involving replacement relationships include:

1. *fronting* of target velar consonants to alveolar place of articulation, i.e.

$$k \rightarrow t$$
$$g \rightarrow d$$
$$\eta \rightarrow n$$

2. *stopping* of target fricative and affricate consonants to homorganic (with the same place of articulation) plosive realisations, e.g.

$$f \rightarrow p$$
$$s \rightarrow t$$
$$z \rightarrow d$$
$$\int \rightarrow t$$
$$t\int \rightarrow t$$
$$d\mathfrak{z} \rightarrow d$$

3. *gliding* of target 'liquids' /r l/ to 'glides' [w j].

Processes describing omission relationships include:

1. *weak syllable deletion*, i.e. omission of unstressed syllables either before or after the stressed syllable, e.g. *again* [gɛn] *telephone* ['tɛfon];
2. *final consonant deletion*, i.e. omission of the word final consonant, e.g. *horse* [hɔ] *bed* [bɛ];

3. *cluster reduction*, i.e. omission of one or more consonants from a target consonant cluster; the most comprehensively described patterns are those for target syllable-initial word-initial clusters, e.g.

    /s/ + plosives /p t k/ → plosive

    /s/ + nasals /m n/ → nasal

    plosives + approximants → plosives

    (for further details see Grunwell, 1987b).

There are also processes which involve an assimilative interaction between the affected target consonant and contextual factors or the features of other consonants in the target pronunciation of the word/phrase. These include:

1. *consonant harmony*, where one consonant is assimilated to (harmonised with) another consonant in the word; most commonly the place of articulation features interact, e.g. *dark* [gɑk] *neck* [ŋɛk];

2. *context-sensitive voicing* where all word-initial and within-word obstruents are voiced and all word-final obstruents are voiceless, the initial consonant being assimilated to the voicing feature of the following vowel, the final consonant being assimilated to the following potential silence, e.g. *bed, pet* [bɛt] *packet* [badɪt] *cupboard* [ˈgʊbət].

It will be evident from these descriptions and examples that phonological processes provide a systematic, linguistically defined set of descriptive categories which match the traditional pronunciation error categories of *substitutions, omissions, additions* and *transpositions*. It is also apparent that phonological processes employ similar concepts to those integral to other phonological frameworks of analysis, such as distinctive features, natural class, system and structure in pronunciation patterns. In regard to the last-named concepts, it must be emphasised that the processes decribe the relationships between two pronunciation systems: those of the disordered speaker and those used by the normal speakers of the same language. Furthermore, the processes only describe those aspects of pronunciation where the two pronunciation systems differ. As a consequence, there is no overall description of the relationship between the two systems; nor is there a complete description of the pronunciation system of the disordered speaker when a phonological process analysis is carried out. For example, in a phonological process analysis patterns such as fronting, stopping and cluster reduction would be identified, but the analytical framework does not *per se* lead to a statement of the phonological consequences of those patterns, namely:

$$/k/ \rightarrow [t]$$

$$\left.\begin{array}{l} /s/ \\ /\int/ \\ /t\int/ \end{array}\right\} \rightarrow [t]$$

$$\left.\begin{array}{l} /st/ \\ /tr/ \end{array}\right\} \rightarrow [t]$$

Nowhere is it stated that:

$$/t/ \rightarrow [t]$$

The processes imply losses of contrast without explicitly stating these consequences and the framework as such completely ignores the occurrence of matches between the two systems.

Notwithstanding this shortcoming, the theoretical definition of phonological processes accords them explanatory power, in that they are claimed to reflect an innate set of phonological tendencies towards simplification of the speech production processes:

> A phonological process is a mental operation that applies in speech to substitute for a class of sounds or sound sequences presenting a common difficulty to the speech capacity of the individual, an alternative class identical but lacking in the difficult property. (Stampe, 1979, p.1)

In order for this definition to be operationally valid, it has to be assumed that the disordered speaker (or child learning to pronounce) has stored knowledge of the correct form of the words and sounds at the least in perceptual terms. According to Stampe (the creator of phonological process analysis), this is so and the operation of the processes is entirely attributable to production (i.e. articulatory) constraints. Ingram (1976) on the other hand, in applying phonological process analysis to clinical data, hypothesises that processes may operate at any of three levels in the speech mechanism: perception, organisation or production. Ingram's viewpoint seems more plausible and potentially insightful, especially when processes are identified in children's speech. Leonard (1985) is one of the researchers to expound this view in explaining the nature of disordered patterns in children:

> The child stores for recognition some of the information available from the adult words spoken in the environment. This stored information does not necessarily preserve all the characteristics of the adult form. Differences between the child's stored form and the adult form may be the result of perceptual encoding rules or a failure to adequately store in memory less familiar though correctly perceived phonetic details. Output rules relate the child's stored form for a word to his or her produced form. Importantly, these rules are both motivated and restricted by severe output constraints. These constraints may be the result of the child's limited ability to hit particular articulatory targets or to plan sequences of articulatory gestures. Of

course, cases where accurately produced exceptions to a child's rule are
subsequently produced less accurately to conform to the rule...serve as examples that output rules can operate as organisational devices even in the
absence of articulatory limitations. (p. 8)

Leonard is therefore suggesting first that a child's knowledge of adult
words may be restricted by an inability to process auditorily all of the
information in the acoustic signal; this processing constraint may reflect
information overload or active restrictions on perceptual analysis, a kind
of perceptual avoidance strategy. Second, he suggests that a child has
production strategies that constrain articulatory output in terms of types
of targets or sequences attempted. Finally, he indicates that even when
there is evidence that a child can produce an articulatory target, in
certain contexts the child's phonological rules impose patterns that
prevent an accurate realisation.

Review of Phonological Assessment Procedures

Procedures Based on Phonological Process Analysis

There are currently six widely known informal phonological assessment
procedures based on phonological process analysis, all of which are
designed for the assessment of child speech. They are:

Weiner (1979): *Phonological Process Analysis (PPA)*;
Shriberg and Kwiatkowski (1980): *Natural Process Analysis (NPA)*;
Hodson (1980): *Assessment of Phonological Processes (APP)*;
Ingram (1981): *Procedures for the Phonological Analysis of Children's
     Language (PPACL)*;
Grunwell (1985b): *Phonological Assessment of Child Speech (PACS)*;
Dean *et al.* (1990) *Metaphon Resource Pack*.

In Ingram (1981) and Grunwell (1985b), the phonological process
analysis procedures are part of a set of procedures which involve a variety of different approaches to clinical phonological assessment (see
further below). The other four procedures focus virtually exclusively on
the process analysis as the main basis for the clinical assessment. Unfortunately, all six procedures employ ostensibly different sets of processes;
these are listed in Table 5.1. On closer inspection, however, the similarity between the analytical frameworks becomes apparent, the differences being largely attributable to different classification systems and
varying levels of detail in regard to the descriptive definition of each
process. For example, in PPA the processes are categorised into three
types:

Syllable Structure Processes;
Harmony Processes;
Feature Contrast Processes.

This classification reflects that originally proposed by Ingram (1976/1989) with minor changes in nomenclature; the original terms are Syllable Structure Processes; Assimilatory Processes; Substitution Processes. This classification is still in effect used by Ingram in PPACL, even though it is not specified, namely:

Syllable Structure Processes:
Deletion of Final Consonant;
Reduction of Consonant Clusters;
Syllable Deletion and Reduplication.

Substitution Processes:
Fronting;
Stopping;
Simplification of Liquids and Nasals;
Other substitution processes.

Assimilation Processes.

PACS employs a comparable classificatory framework, categorising processes according to whether they effect *structural* or *systemic simplifications* in children's speech by comparison with the adult pronunciation patterns. Metaphon follows this framework, based on Grunwell (1985b). APP's classification shares some of the principles evident in the three procedures already considered, for example in distinguishing *articulatory shifts* (i.e. phonetic maturational pronunciation differences) from the other processes which involve phonemic differences, and in identifying assimilations. The categorisation into *basic* versus *miscellaneous processes*, however, appears to be somewhat *ad hoc*, especially when stopping (a common developmental process) is classified as a 'miscellaneous process'.

Notwithstanding these classificatory and terminological differences, all six procedures operate with the same principles of analysis. Furthermore, the four procedures discussed so far consider the phonological processes in some detail and all are to a certain extent open-ended, in that they specifically allow for and encourage the analyst/clinician to identify other processes (see further below). In contrast, NPA is extremely limited in its range of processes, being restricted to eight, which, even though they are process categories rather than the detailed processes themselves, do not cover all the types of phonological simplifying relationships included in the other four procedures. *Voicing* is in fact specifically excluded by the authors of NPA, as they claim it cannot be reliably transcribed and identified in child speech. In addition, no

Table 5.1: Clinical assessment procedures using Phonological Process Anaylysis

Weiner (1979)	Shriberg and Kwiatkowski (1980)	Hodson (1980)
Syllable Structure Process		*Basic Phonological* Processes
Deletion of final cons.	1. Final consonant deletion	Syllable reduction
Cluster Reductions:	2. Velar fronting:	Cluster reduction
Initial stop + liquid	Initial	Prevocalic obstruent
Initial fric + liquid	Final	singleton omissions
Initial /s/ clusters	3. Stopping:	Postvocalic obstruent
Final /s/ + stop	Initial	singleton omissions
Final liquid + stop	Final	Stridency deletion
Final nasal + stop	4. Palatal fronting:	Velar deviations
Weak syllable deletion	Initial	
Glottal replacement	Final	
	5. Liquid simplification:	*Miscellaneous Phonological*
	Initial	*Processes*
	Final	
Harmony Processes	6. Assimilation:	Prevocalic voicing
	Progressive	Postvocalic devoicing
Labial assimilation	Regressive	Glottal replacement
Alveolar assimilation	7. Cluster reduction:	Backing
Velar assimilation	Initial	Stopping
Prevocalic voicing	Final	Affrication
Final cons. devoicing	8. Unstressed Syllable	Deaffrication
Syllable harmony	Deletion	Palatalisation
		Depalatalisation
		Coalescence
Feature Contrast Processes		Epenthesis
		Metathesis
Stopping		
Gliding of frics		*Sonorant Deviations*
Affrication		
Fronting		Liquid /l/
Denasalisation		Liquid /ɚ/
Gliding of liquids		Nasals
Vocalisation		Glides
		Vowels
		Assimilations
		Nasal
		Velar
		Labial
		Alveolar
		Articulatory Shifts
		Substitutions of
		/f v s z/ for /θ ð/
		Frontal lisp
		Dentalisation of /t d n l/
		Lateralisation
		Other Patterns

Table 5.1 Cont.

Ingram (1981)	Grunwell (1985)	Dean et al. (1990)
Deletion of Final Consonants	**Structural Simplifications**	**Systemic Processes**
1. Nasals	Weak syllable deletion:	Velar fronting
2. Voiced stops	pretonic	Palato alveolar fronting
3. Voiceless stops	posttonic	Stopping of fricatives
4. Voiced fricatives	Final consonant deletion:	Stopping of affricates
5. Voiceless fricatives	nasals	Word final devoicing
	plosives	Context Sensitive voicing
Reduction of Consonant	fricatives	(i.e. WI)
Clusters	affricates	Liquid gliding
	clusters – 1	Fricative simplifications
6. Liquids	– 2 +	($\theta \rightarrow$ f; $\delta \rightarrow$ v)
7. Nasals	Vocalisation:	Backing of alveolar stops
8. /s/ clusters	/l/	(unusual/atypical process)
	other C	
Syllable Deletion and	Reduplication:	**Structural Processes**
Reduplication	complete	
	partial	Final consonant deletion
9. Reduction of disyllables	Consonant harmony:	Initial cluster/reduction/deletion
10. Unstressed syllable deletion	velar	Initial consonant l:Seletion
11. Reduplication	alveolar	(Unusual/atypical process)
	labial	Final cluster reduction/deletion
Fronting	manner	(unusual/atypical process)
	other	
12. of palatals	S.I. cluster reduction:	
13. of velars	plosive + approx.	
	fricative + approx.	
Stopping	/s/ + plosive	
	/s/ + nasal	
14. of initial voiceless frics.	/s/ + approx.	
15. of initial voiced frics.	/s/ + plosive + approx.	
16. of initial affricates	**Systemic Simplifications**	
Simplification of Liquids and	Fronting:	
Nasals	velars	
	palato-alveolars	
17. Liquid Gliding	Stopping:	
18. Vocalisation	/f/ /v/	
19. Denasalisation	/θ/ /ð/	
	/s/ /z/	
Other Substitution Processes	/ʃ/	
	/tʃ/ /dʒ/	
20. Deaffrication	/l/ /r/	
21. Deletion of initial cons.	Gliding:	
22. Apicalisation	/r/	
23. Labialisation	/l/	
	fricatives	
Assimilation Processes	Context sensitive voicing:	
	WI and WF	
24. Velar assimilation	Voicing WI	
25, Labial assimilation	Voicing WW	
26. Prevocalic voicing	Devoicing WF	
27. Devoicing of final cons.	Glottal replacement:	
	WI	
	WW	
	WF	
	Glottal insertion	

combinations of processes are allowed in the interpretation of the child's pronunciations; thus /kl/ → [t] would be one process of *cluster reduction* rather than the more transparent combination of *cluster reduction* and *velar fronting*. For these and other facets of the detailed applications of the NPA procedures NPA is by far the least satisfactory of these six assessments (see further Grunwell, 1987b). *Metaphon* is also somewhat restricted though it explicitly includes atypical or unusual processes. These are: backing of alveolar stops; initial consonant deletion and, curiously, final cluster reduction/deletion. This last is of note as it is not in this author's view an atypical pattern. The processes included in this procedure are those processes 'which our clinical experience suggests occur most frequently in phonologically disordered speech' (Howell and Dean 1991, p.20).

These procedures, nevertheless, share the same principles of description which lead to the same primary treatment aims. They all describe the systematic phonological relationships between adult and child pronunciation patterns; where they differ from each other is in terms of natural 'simplifying' processes. The clinical aim of all the assessments is primarily to lead to the implementation of a systematically structured therapy programme designed to facilitate progressive change in those aspects of a child's pronunciation where the processes are operative.

Although phonological process analysis has achieved its current position as the dominant approach to clinical assessment of child speech because of its use in studies of the normal development of phonology in children, only PACS directly leads to a developmental assessment profile (see Table 5.2). There is, however, quite detailed discussion of normal developmental patterns in both Shriberg and Kwiatkowski (1980) and Ingram (1981); but these discussions constitute descriptive accounts rather than normative profiles. Metaphon provides an indication of the age range by which processes are expected to disappear in normal development. As indicated above, Metaphon also includes three processes identified by its authors as atypical/unusual. With regard to the clinical evaluation of a child's pronunciation patterns, NPA, APP, PPACL and PACS all consider the characteristics of disordered use of phonological processes.

NPA includes an appendix in which clinical case studies of children with speech disorders are presented in some detail. APP covers in its list of processes unusual patterns such as *glottal replacement, backing, nasal deviations*. Ingram, in the manual for PPACL, describes and discusses the characteristics of disordered child phonology. Grunwell, in the PACS manual, provides the most comprehensive framework for a clinical evaluation of a phonological process assessment. In the PACS procedures themselves *glottal realisations: replacement and insertions* are specifically included to cater for these commonly occurring patterns in the speech of children with disordered development. In addition, there is provision for the detailed analysis of 'other' systemic and structural

Table 5.2: Developmental assessment (PACS)

Stage	Type	Labial		Lingual		Protowords and First Words
Stage I (0;9 – 1;6)	Nasal					Show phonetic variability and all phon processes. *Examples*
	Plosive					
	Fricative					
	Approximant					
Stage II (1;6 – 2;0)		m		n		Reduplication · Consonant Harmony · FINAL CONS. DELETION · CLUSTER REDUCTION
		p b	t	d		FRONTING · STOPPING · GLIDING · C.S.VOICING
		w				
Stage III (2;0 – 2;6)		m		n	(ŋ)	Final Cons. Deletion · CLUSTER REDUCTION
		p b	t	d	(k g)	Fronting · STOPPING · GLIDING · C.S.VOICING
		w			(h)	
Stage IV (2;6 – 3;0)		m		n	ŋ	Final Cons. Deletion · CLUSTER REDUCTION
		p b	t	d	k g	STOPPING/v ð z tʃ dʒ/ · FRONTING/ʃ/→[s] · GLIDING · C.S.Voicing
		f	s			
		w	(l)	j	h	
Stage V (3;0 – 3;6)		m		n	ŋ	Clusters used: obs. + approx. /s/ + cons.
		p b	t	d (tʃ)	k g	STOPPING/v ð z/ · FRONTING/ʃ tʃ dʒ/ · GLIDING · /θ/→[f]
		f	s	(ʃ)		
		w	l	j	h	
Stage VI (3;6 – 4;6)		m		n	ŋ	Clusters used: obs. + approx. /s/ + cons.
		p b	t	d tʃ dʒ	k g	/ð/→[d] or [v] · PALATALIZATION/ʃ tʃ dʒ/ · GLIDING · /θ/→[f]
		f v	s	z ʃ		
		w	l (r)	j	h	
Stage VII (4;6 <)		m		n	ŋ	Clusters used: obs. + approx. /s/ + cons.
		p b	t	d tʃ dʒ	k g	/ð/→[d] or [v] · /r/→[w] or [ʋ] · /θ/→[f]
		f v	θ s	ð z	ʃ (ʒ)	
		w	l r	j	h	

Comments and Notes

Source: Grunwell (1985). Reproduced by permission of the author.

processes, which Grunwell indicates in the PACS manual (pp. 58–59) are apparently unusual in the normally developing child population, or idiosyncratic to an individual child in either the normal or clinical context. Examples of the other processes illustrated include:

initial consonant adjunction: the addition of a consonant before a word-initial vowel;
backing: the opposite of fronting; target alveolars pronounced as velars;
weakening (spirantisation):target plosives weakened to fricatives;
denasalisation: target nasals pronounced as non-nasals.

PACS also provides a checklist of the diagnostic characteristics of developmental phonological disorders, which are as follows (for further details see Grunwell, 1985b):

persisting normal processes: those normal processes which remain in the child's pronunciation patterns long after the age at which they would normally have disappeared; i.e. delayed development;
chronological mismatch: the co-occurrence of some of the earliest patterns with some patterns characteristic of later stages in phonological development, i.e. uneven development;
unusual/idiosyncratic processes: the occurrence of patterns rarely or never attested in normal speech development, suggesting abnormal development (see above for examples of 'other processes').
systematic sound preference: one type of consonant is used for a large range of different target types, usually consequent upon a conspiracy of processes; e.g. fronting, stopping, stopping of liquids and voicing all conspire to the realisation of targets /k g s ʃ tʃ dʒ d l/ → [d]. This phenomenon usually involves persisting normal processes and some unusual processes, and results in a massive loss of the ability to signal phonological contrasts.
variable use of processes: more than one simplifying process routinely operates with the same type of target segments or structures; given that during the developmental period children's speech patterns are necessarily variable, this variability can only be appraised as abnormal under two conditions:

1. where the variability is static and does not appear to be resolving itself into developmentally more progressive patterns;
2. where the variability *per se* is not progressive; i.e. where two processes are operating on the same targets and neither realisation represents a developmental advance upon the other.

There is not the space here to describe in detail each of the six procedures introduced in this section. Having established their shared similarities and significant differences in terms of the phonological process analysis, we shall now consider another important aspect of their construction: the elicitation procedures advocated by or required by the authors. NPA, PPACL and PACS are all intended for use with spontaneous speech samples. NPA is restricted in this regard as the analytical procedure fully analyses only monosyllabic words, and only the first occurrence of those, thus excluding any possibility of detecting word-based variability in a child's pronunciation patterns. The other two procedures are designed to analyse all facets of a spontaneous speech sample, which should be:

1. representative of the target phonology;
2. representative of the habitual patterns used by the speaker;
3. large enough to reveal variability (i.e. 200–250 words);
4. homogeneous in time and type;
5. glossed (see further Grunwell, 1985b; 1987a).

PPA, APP and Metaphon employ predetermined elicitation procedures designed to obtain a specified sample of one-word utterances. PPA is based on the presentation of pictures to elicit 136 words by cued naming and delayed imitation. APP uses a set of 20 words in a screening version and 55 in the full version, both sets being obtained largely through the naming of a collection of objects. Metaphon has a screening procedure consisting of 44 words. Analysis of the responses to this procedure allows the clinician to identify when a process occurs on 50% or more of possible targets. If this is the case then the appropriate Process-specific Probe should be carried out. Both procedures employ object- and picture-naming tasks.

   As might be anticipated, given the basic similarities of these procedures, assessments of children's speech are convergent when the procedures are compared. This has been demonstrated for NPA, APP and PPACL (Paden and Moss, 1985), and for selected processes from APP and PPACL (Benjamin and Greenwood, 1983). (For further detailed critical discussion of these procedures see Grunwell, 1987b.)

Other Approaches to Phonological Analysis

The *Profile of Phonology* (Crystal, 1982; 1992; hereafter PROPH) is a procedure for analysing spontaneous speech samples (of 100 words), for clinical assessment based on the traditional speech pathology framework of error analysis but related to a comprehensive description of the target English phonology. The disordered speaker's pronunciations of the target segments are classified into the traditional categories of correct, omitted, substituted, and these realisations of the target pronunciations are entered on to a comprehensive chart for the exhaustive analysis of the data into categories which represent the structural and systemic contrasts available in the language. To satisfy this criterion:

PROPH...is essentially a presentation of the English sound system on a 2-page chart. To facilitate the compilation of the Profile a transcriptional page is added. To facilitate the interpretation of the Profile a separate 3-page section provides various suggestions about ways of summarizing the main patterns in the data. (Crystal, 1982, p. 54)

The primary analytical procedure in PROPH, however, involves classifying the child's realisations of target phonemes according to the three traditional definitions, categorised also with reference to position in word and syllable structure and stress placement. PROPH analyses all target singleton consonant phonemes and all target consonant clusters and target vowels. The target vowel system employed is RP (received pronunciation), but Crystal emphasises that local accent norms must be taken into account when assessing vowels.

It is stated that 'Having completed the transcriptional page and the accompanying profile chart, and allowed for the existence of awkward cases, the PROPH procedure is in a sense complete'. It is suggested that principled therapy can be formulated on the basis of this assessment. The additional procedures are therefore supplementary rather than essential. They include:

1. *inventory of phones*: a phonetic classification of phones in the sample;
2. *target analysis*: an analysis into articulatory categories of both correct and substituted phones;
3. *feature and process analysis*: both of which are rather limited and vaguely defined outlines of these types of approaches to phonological assessment.

Thus PROPH is primarily an exhaustive error analysis. What it gains in comprehensiveness, it unfortunately forfeits in failing to identify patterns in disordered pronunciation, and in lacking an acquisitional dimension to the assessment procedure.

Elbert and Gierut (1986) present their approach to the phonological analysis of child speech as an assessment of productive phonological knowledge, i.e. the knowledge that children possess of the pronunciation of their spoken language, no account being taken of their perceptual knowledge or skills. Although the authors claim that their procedures are drawn from 'standard generative phonology', their analytical approach bears more resemblance to the classic phonemic analysis framework. The aim is to focus on the child's sound system as a 'unique phonology'; however, there is an ambivalence in the analysis which is strikingly different from the traditional framework of error analysis. The child's phonology is described in terms of *static rules* and *dynamic rules*. Static rules describe phonotactic constraints, i.e.:

1. *inventory constraints*: certain sounds do not occur in the child's inventory;
2. *positional constraints*: certain sounds only occur in certain positions;
3. *sequence constraints*: certain sound combinations do not occur.

Dynamic rules include: *allophonic rules* which describe allophonic variants determined using the concepts of free variation and complementary distribution; and *neutralisation rules* which describe the merging of two otherwise contrastive sounds at a certain position in word structure.

Thus far the analysis appears to be describing, as intended, the child's phonology. However, when the child's phonology is compared with the target system there is a perplexing and unfortunate restriction. The definitions of types of phonological knowledge (see Table 5.3) encapsulate this difficulty in carrying out the assessment. If the correct realisation of the target phoneme is achieved, the child is credited with having complete phonological knowledge of that phoneme (i.e. Type 1 knowledge). No account is taken of whether or not the child is also using that same phonetic segment for the realisation of other target phonemes. By adopting this method of evaluating the match between the adult and the child pronunciations, Elbert and Gierut are not describing an independent child phonological system. They concentrate upon the matches between the two systems, and do not provide a mechanism for identifying the pronunciations used for the target consonants of which the child does not have 'phonological knowledge'.

Table 5.3: Types of phonological knowledge which have been observed in phonologically disordered children (Gierut 1985a)

Knowledge Type	Lexical Representation	Breadth of Distribution		Rule Account
		Positions	Morphemes	
1	Adult-like	All	All	None
2	Adult-like	All	All	Opt./oblig. rules
3	Adult-like	All	Some	Fossilized forms
4	Adult-like	Some	All	Positional constraint
5	Adult-like	Some	Some	Combination of 3 and 4
6	Non–adult-like	All	All	Inventory constraint

Note: Type 5 represents a logical possibility, but this combination of adult-like lexical representations for some morphemes in most positions has yet not been documented in our studies of phonological knowledge.
Source: Reproduced from Elbert and Gierut (1986), *Handbook of Clinical Phonology*, by permission of College Hill Press, Boston, USA.

In the past ten years a new approach to clinical phonological analysis has begun to emerge. This approach is based on the theoretical framework of non-linear phonology (see Spencer, 1984; Bernhardt, 1992a; 1992b; Bernhardt and Stoel-Gammon, 1994). There is as yet no formalised assessment procedure associated with this approach and a very limited number of examples of its clinical applications. It uses a multi-tiered analysis of the feature content of segments which promotes the description of interactions between adjacent and even non-adjacent segments at different levels in the hierarchy of tiers, thus accounting, for example, for consonant harmony and consonant-vowel harmony (where the place of articulation of a consonant is determined by the height of the following vowel; see Grunwell, 1981). There is not the space to discuss this approach further here; interested readers are referred to the tutorial article by Bernhardt and Stoel-Gammon (1994). As an approach to phonological assessment it is unlikely to be used routinely unless and until a formalised procedure is developed based on its analytical techniques.

Multifaceted Phonological Assessment Procedures

As pointed out some years ago by Lund and Duchan (1978), clinical phonological assessment procedures based on one theoretical approach tend to be too constrained and inflexible for the analysis of the wide range of different types of disordered pronunciation patterns encountered in a routine clinical population. A comprehensive procedure with a number of different types of analysis is more applicable for clinical assessment, as it provides for the clinician the flexibility to select the most appropriate framework for investigating and evaluating the patterns used by each disordered speaker on an individual basis.

Ingram's (1981) *Procedures for the Phonological Analysis of Child Language* (PPACL) and Grunwell's (1985b) *Phonological Assessment of Child Speech* (PACS), both provide such an eclectic and comprehensive range of assessment procedures. As we have already seen they both include procedures based on phonological process analysis. PPACL in addition contains:

1. *phonetic analysis*: to establish a child's phonetic inventories for word initial, medial and final position, and the frequency of preferred syllable shapes;
2. *analysis of homonymy*: to determine the occurrence of homonyms in a child's speech sample and to conclude whether the child's speech is highly homonymous by comparison with the adult language;
3. *substitution analysis*: to determine the substitutions used in the child's production of the initial, final and ambisyllabic consonants and clusters of the adult language.

The Phonological Process Analysis in PPACL is based upon the Substitution Analysis, although it can be carried out without a prior analysis. It will be seen from this brief résumé that the PPACL procedures are capable in large part of meeting the criteria for clinical phonological assessments. Furthermore, because a number of numerical formulae are derived from the various procedures, reassessment can be a precise and relatively objective exercise, provided that closely comparable data samples are the basis for both assessments. This is especially necessary for the *analysis of homonymy*, as the identification of homonyms present in a child's speech is fortuitous, being entirely dependent upon what the child chooses to say on any one particular occasion. However, as has already been mentioned, PPACL lacks a developmental profile. Furthermore, Ingram does not specify how treatment goals can be derived from the assessment results. Notwithstanding these shortcomings, PPACL represents a significant advance in clinical phonological assessments by way of its eclecticism and comprehensiveness.

PACS was specifically designed to satisfy the criteria outlined above and therefore contains a large number of different types of analytical procedures. These are:

Phonetic Inventory and Distribution: an analysis of the phonetic types of consonants used by the child and their distribution in four positions in syllable and word structure and in clusters.

Contrastive Assessment: a comparative analysis and assessment of the child's systems of contrastive phones and clusters with the adult systems of consonants in order to identify the matches and mismatches between the two systems.

Phonotactic Analysis and Assessment: a comparative analysis and assessment of the child's range of types of syllable structures in monosyllabic, disyllabic and polysyllabic words with adult range of syllabic structures.

Phonological Process Analysis: this has already been described above.

Developmental Assessment (see Table 5.2): this is based partly on the phonological process analysis, but can also be derived from the contrastive assessment procedure.

These six procedures are the main assessments in PACS. There are however a number of additional approaches suggested, including Evaluations of Communicative Adequacy:

Feature Analysis;

Analysis of Homophony (i.e. Homonymy);

Analysis of Multiple Loss of Phonemic Contrasts (i.e. identification of occurrences where one child phone matches/mismatches many adult phonemes);

Analysis of Variability (i.e. identification of occurrences where many child phones match/mismatch one adult phoneme).

There are also procedures for examining the sequential constraints in the combinations and ordering of consonants, i.e. *Polysystemic Phonotactic Analysis*.

PACS thus presents the speech and language therapist with a wide range of different approaches. However, it is not intended that all of the procedures should always be used. The clinician should select those which are appropriate for each individual child. None of the procedures is crucially dependent upon another. Furthermore, reassessment is facilitated and PACS procedures are sensitive to change in children's pronunciation patterns (see Grunwell, 1985b; 1992b; 1992c; Grunwell and Russell, 1987; Grunwell and Dive, 1988; Grunwell *et al.*, 1988).

Treatment guidelines are directly derivable from the assessments in a principled way and are directly aimed at facilitating improvements in communicative adequacy. In these ways PACS is clearly a comprehensive and clinically applicable assessment tool.

Reassessment

As indicated above, it is essential that phonological assessments provide the basis for informative reassessments which enable clinicians to evaluate change. In the framework of phonological process analysis progress is indicated if a process which was present in a child's pronunciation patterns is no longer present, or if there is a reduction in the frequency of its occurrence. This is a straightforward measure but it is probably overly simplistic and unable to detect subtle ongoing developments and potentials for change that are important in the planning of therapy that is responsive to an individual child's needs. Recently devised measures based on PACS address this point.

PACS as originally published in 1985 contains two primary procedures for evaluating change. The first, which has already been discussed, is the Developmental Assessment which provides a profile of normal development against which to measure a child's pronunciation patterns and to chart their progress. The second is the Contrastive Assessment which identifies the matches and mismatches between the child and adult pronunciation patterns. Clearly an increase in the number of matches with adult targets is indicative of progressive change.

Grunwell (1992b) refined this measurement into a set of phonological performance indicators (PPIs). For each position in word structure the types of matches are calculated as follows:

1. number of targets attempted against number possible;
2. number of different consonants;
3. number of stable correct matches;
4. number of stable mismatches (i.e. consistent errors);
5. number of variable matches including mismatches (i.e. errors) and correct matches;
6. number of variable matches involving correct matches (a subset of 5).

For word final position the following measures are calculated in addition:

7. number of stable zero realisations (omissions);
8. number of variable zero realisations;
9. number of variable realisations including zero that also involve correct matches (a subset of 8).

These measures focus precisely upon the presence of variability in a child's pronunciation patterns. They identify progressive variability in the form of the occurrence of some correct matches alongside mismatches. They also involve an active comparison of the patterns of child realisations at different positions in word structures. These are all factors which are highly relevant to effective and responsive treatment planning. (see Grunwell, 1992a; 1992b; 1994). The purpose of PPIs is to compare two Contrastive Assessments in order to identify where changes have occurred so that treatment targets can be delineated that respond to incipient and ongoing progressive developments in the child's pronunciation patterns.

Screening Tests in Phonological Assessment

'Articulation Tests' (see preceding chapter), as their name implies, are designed on the premise that speech development, maintenance and disorders involve solely articulatory abilities and that remediation of disordered pronunciation patterns requires correction of faulty articulatory performance of individual consonant segments. As has been demonstrated here, and will be discussed further in Section III, for many speech disorders this is an inaccurate and clinically misleading characterisation of a speaker's disabilities. Nevertheless, an articulation test still has its place in clinical assessment of speech disorders, as a *screening procedure* to identify speakers with major pronunciation problems.

The *Edinburgh Articulation Test* (EAT; Anthony *et al.*, 1971) is probably one of the most commonly used published screening procedures in the UK (see Grunwell, 1993a for a review). It is a very useful clinical tool because it not only screens for the presence of problems in learning pronunciation patterns but also provides in its *Qualitative Assessment* a preliminary diagnosis of delayed development by comparison with atypical development. In addition it diagnoses different degrees of delay. The

EAT is an articulation test which does not conform to the traditional phonemic structure of testing every target consonant phoneme once in every word position. It has a highly sophisticated structure that ensures that the phonetic, phonological and developmental dimensions of the English consonant system are assessed in a clinically informative way. It is a clinical procedure that is under-valued and under-utilised. It is worthy of in-depth study in order for clinicians to appreciate its full potential.

As has already been mentioned, APP and Metaphon have screening and in-depth procedures. Recently a screening procedure based on PACS has been developed, known as PACS TOYS (Grunwell and Harding, 1995). As the name suggests, this is an elicitation procedure that uses objects/toys primarily, with a few pictures. More significantly in the context of this chapter, it is designed to elicit a limited representative sample of English consonants in all word postions, following the guidelines outlined above. The analytical procedures include a Contrastive Assessment as well as classifications of the child's realisations into developmentally typical and atypical targets. It is designed for use across an age range from 1;6 to 6;0; thus it is a procedure that extends down the age range to the first words stage. It is also a procedure that is constructed in such a way that it can be completed in one clinical session and provide information as to the next stage in clinical management.

Phonological Assessment of Adult Speech Disorders

Thus far the discussion in this chapter has been primarily orientated towards the phonological assessment of children's speech. Similar principles and procedures are applicable in the assessment of adult speech disorders, especially pronunciation difficulties associated with acquired aphasia and acquired apraxia of speech. As with child speech disorders, phonological process analysis has been one of the most recent and popular approaches employed (Klich, Ireland and Weidner, 1979; Crary and Fokes, 1980; Edwards and Shriberg, 1983). These studies have demonstrated the systematicity of some of the pronunciation errors in acquired speech disorders and supported the hypothesis that some of the patterns revealed lead to a systematic reduction in the complexity of the speech produced. Similar findings have been reported in studies employing the framework of distinctive feature analysis and the concept of naturalness in phonology. (These studies include Marquardt, Reinhart and Peterson, 1979; Wolk, 1986.) Both studies conclude that acquired speech disorders involve reduced markedness in the error pronunciations by comparison with the target pronunciations; they therefore suggest that simpler pronunciation patterns are used characteristically by adult speakers with acquired disorders. It has to be acknowledged that studies such as these, because of the characteristics of the analytic frameworks employed, only analyse phonemic substitution errors. As a result, a considerable amount of relevant data, such as, for example, *additions* and *metatheses*, are ignored. Space does not permit detailed discussion here of the phonological characteristics of these disorders.

In this volume, Miller and Docherty place the assessment of acquired neurogenic speech disorders in a neuropsychological model and consequently do not apply any particular theoretically based phonological analysis to the speech data. However, their treatment strategies are firmly founded on the key phonological concept: the need to facilitate the signalling of sound contrasts (phonemic distinctions) in order to improve a speaker's ability to communicate.

Conclusion

Over the past fifteen to twenty years phonological assessment has gradually become established as a routine clinical procedure. During this time it has been recognised that a range of eclectic and comprehensive analytical tools is required for flexible, clinically applicable phonological investigations and evaluations. It is now possible for clinical phonological descriptive assessments to: reliably inform treatment planning and implementation; and inform diagnoses and provide insights into possible explanations of the nature of different speech disorders.

References

Anthony, A., Bogle, D., Ingram, T.T.S. and McIsaac, M.W. (1971). *Edinburgh Articulation Test*. Edinburgh: Churchill Livingstone.

Benjamin, B. J. and Greenwood, J. (1983). A comparison of three phonological assessment procedures. *Journal of Childhood Communication Disorders* 7, 19–27.

Bernhardt, B. (1992a). Developmental implications of non-linear phonological theory. *Clinical Linguistics & Phonetics* 6, 259–281.

Bernhardt, B. (1992b). The application of non linear phonological theory to intervention with one phonologically disordered child. *Clinical Linguistics & Phonetics* 6, 283–316.

Bernhardt, B. and Stoel-Gammon, C. (1994). Non linear phonology: introduction and clinical application. *Journal of Speech and Hearing Research* 37, 123–143.

Compton, A. J. and Hutton, J. S. (1978). *Compton–Hutton Phonological Assessment*. San Francisco, CA: Carousel House.

Crary, M. A. and Fokes, J. (1980). Phonological processes in apraxia of speech: a systematic simplification of articulatory performance. *Aphasia, Apraxia and Agnosia* 4, 1–13.

Crystal, D. (1982). *Profiling Linguistic Disability*. London: Edward Arnold.

Crystal, D. (1992). *Profiling Linguistic Disability*, 2nd edn. London: Whurr Publishers.

Dean, E., Howell, J., Hill A. and Waters, D. (1990). *Metaphon Resource Pack*. Windsor: NFER-Nelson.

Edwards, M. L. and Shriberg, L. D. (1983). *Phonology: Applications in Communicative Disorders*. San Diego, CA: College Hill Press.

Elbert, M. and Gierut, J. (1986). *Handbook of Clinical Phonology*. London: Taylor & Francis.

Gibbon, F., Shockey, L. and Reid, J. (1992). Description and treatment of abnormal vowels. *Child Language Teaching & Therapy* 8, 30–59.

Grunwell, P. (1981). *The Nature of Phonological Disability in Children*. London: Academic Press.

Grunwell, P. (1985a). Comment on the terms 'phonetics' and 'phonology' as applied in the investigation of speech disorders. *British Journal of Disorders of Communication* 20, 165–170.

Grunwell, P. (1985b). *Phonological Assessment of Child Speech (PACS)*. Windsor: NFER-Nelson.

Grunwell, P. (1987a). *Clinical Phonology*, 2nd edn. London: Croom Helm.

Grunwell, P. (1987b). *PACS Pictures*. Windsor: NFER-Nelson.

Grunwell, P. (1988). Phonological assessment, evaluation and explanation of speech disorders in children. *Clinical Linguistics & Phonetics* 2, 221–252.

Grunwell, P. (Ed.) (1990). *Developmental Speech Disorders*. Edinburgh: Churchill Livingstone/London: Whurr Publishers.

Grunwell, P. (1992a). Assessment of child phonology in the clinical context. In: C.A. Ferguson, L. Menn and C. Stoel-Gammon (Eds.), *Phonological Development, Models, Research, Implications*. Timonium, MD: York Press.

Grunwell, P. (1992b). Processes of change in developmental speech disorders.*Clinical Linguistics & Phonetics* 6, 101–122.

Grunwell, P. (1992c). Principled decision-making in the remediation of children with phonological disorders. In: P. Fletcher and D. Hall (Eds.), *Specific Speech and Language Disorders in Children*. London: Whurr Publishers.

Grunwell, P. (Ed.) (1993a). *Analysing Cleft Palate Speech*. London: Whurr Publishers.

Grunwell, P. (1993b). Assessment of articulation and phonology. In: J.R. Beech and L. Harding, with D. Hilton-Jones (Eds.), *Assessment in Speech and Language Therapy*. London: Routledge.

Grunwell, P. (1994). Phonological therapy: the linguistic challenge to facilitate change. Keynote Lecture at the 3rd International Congress of the International Clinical Phonetics & Linguistics Association, Helsinki, 1993. (Published in the Proceedings, University of Helsinki, 1994.)

Grunwell, P. and Dive, D. (1988). Phonological factors in the evaluation and treatment of cleft palate speech. *Child Language Teaching and Therapy* 4, 193–210.

Grunwell, P. and Harding, A. (1995). *PACS TOYS*. Windsor: NFER-Nelson

Grunwell, P. and Russell, J. (1987). Phonological development in children with cleft lip and palate. Paper given at Fourth International Congress for the Study of Child Language, University of Lund, July 1987.

Grunwell, P., Yavas, M., Russell, J. and Lemaistre, H. (1988). Developing a phonological system – a case study. *Child Language Teaching and Therapy* 4, 142–153.

Harris, J. and Cottam, P. (1985). Phonetic features and phonological features in speech assessment. *British Journal of Disorders of Communication* 20, 61–74.

Hewlett, N. (1985). Phonological versus phonetic disorders: some suggested modifications to the current use of the distinction. *British Journal of Disorders of Communication* 20, 155–164.

Hodson, B. W. (1980). *The Assessment of Phonological Processes*. Danville, IL: Interstate.

Hodson, B. W. and Paden, E. P. (1983). *Targeting Intelligible Speech*. San Diego, CA: College Hill Press.

Howell, J. and Dean, E. (1991). *Treating Phonological Disorders in Children: Metaphon – Theory to Practice*. London: Whurr Publishers.

Ingram, D. (1976). *Phonological Disability in Children*. London: Edward Arnold.

Ingram, D. (1981). *Procedures for the Phonological Analysis of Children's Language*. Baltimore, MD: University Park Press.

Ingram, D. (1989). *Phonological Disability in Children*, 2nd edn. London: Whurr Publishers.

Klich, R. J., Ireland, J. V. and Weidner, W. E. (1979). Articulatory and phonological aspects of consonant substitutions in apraxia of speech. *Cortex* 15, 451–470.

Leonard, L. B. (1985). Unusual and subtle phonological behavior in the speech of phonologically disordered children. *Journal of Speech and Hearing Disorders* 50, 4–13.

Lund, N. L. and Duchan, J. F. (1978). Phonological analysis; a multi-faceted approach. *British Journal of Disorders of Communication* 13, 119–126.

Marquardt, T. P., Reinhart, J. B. and Peterson, H. A. (1979). Markedness analysis of phonemic substitution errors in apraxia of speech. *Journal of Communication Disorders* 12, 481–494.

McReynolds, L. V. and Engmann, D. (1975). *Distinctive Feature Analysis of Misarticulations*. Baltimore, MD: University Park Press.

Menn, L. (1980). Phonological theory and child phonology. In: G.H. Yeni-Komshian, J.F. Kavanagh and C.A. Ferguson (Eds), *Child Phonology*, Vol. I: *Production*. New York: Academic Press.

Paden, E. P. and Moss, S. A. (1985). Comparison of three phonological analysis procedures. *Language Speech and Hearing Services in Schools* 16, 103–109.

Penney, G., Fee, E.J. and Dowdle, C. (1994). Vowel assessment and remediation: a case study. *Child Language Teaching & Therapy* 10, 47–66.

Pollock, K.E. and Hall, P.K. (1991). An analysis of the vowel misarticulations of five children with developmental apraxia of speech. *Clinical Linguistics & Phonetics* 5, 207–224.

Pollock, K.E. and Keiser, N.J. (1990). An examination of vowel errors in phonologically disordered children. *Clinical Linguistics & Phonetics* 4, 161–178.

Reynolds, J. (1990). Abnormal vowel pattern : some data and a hypothesis. *British Journal of Disorders of Communication* 25, 115–148.

Shriberg, L. D. and Kwiatkowski, J. (1980). *Natural Process Analysis (NPA)*. New York: Wiley.

Shriberg, L. D., Kwiatkowski, J., Best, S., Hengst, J. and Terselic-Webber, B. (1986). Characteristics of children with phonological disorders of unknown origin. *Journal of Speech and Hearing Disorders* 51, 140–161.

Spencer, A. (1984). A nonlinear analysis of phonological disability. *Journal of Communication Disorders* 17, 325–348.

Stoel-Gammon, C. and Herrington, P.B. (1990). Vowel systems of normally developing and phonologically disordered children. *Clinical Linguistics & Phonetics* 4, 145–160.

Stampe, D. (1979). *A Dissertation on Natural Phonology*. New York: Garland.

Weiner, F.F. (1979). *Phonological Process Analysis (PPA)*. Baltimore, MD: University Park Press.

Wolk, L. (1986). Markedness analysis of consonant error productions in apraxia of Speech. *Journal of Communication Disorders* 19, 133–160.

Chapter 6
Syntactic Assessment of Expressive Language

MICHAEL GARMAN AND SUSAN EDWARDS

Introduction

This chapter attempts to provide a clinician's guide to some issues in the syntactic assessment of samples of expressive language data. We make a distinction here between research studies and clinical practice. Research studies are aimed at pushing back the frontier of knowledge concerning language impairment and may use groups or individuals for study in certain ways. Clinical practice should be informed by research but necessarily is distinct from it in various ways. Whilst for research studies it may be essential to select and focus on certain types of client, an important requirement of clinical practice is that it deals with clients who present with language impairment in a range of contexts (including the presence of more or fewer other individual handicapping conditions). The result is that the clinician is routinely dealing with individuals whose language abilities are a complex function of intact and impaired elements, and it may be difficult to know where the boundary between the two lies. In acquired language impairment, a previously intact language system may continue to function *gracefully*, as a system, under the pressure of the impairment; and, even in the case of impaired development, this response characteristic of the language system as a whole may be just as important. The clinician is dealing with a range of symptoms of which some ultimately derive from whatever might be the underlying deficit(s), others reflect intact abilities more or less directly (the perceived strengths of the client), and still others represent the response of the language system to the underlying deficit. These are all aspects of the impaired resources that the client has to draw on; and it is these aspects that linguistic assessment must address, in our case at the level of syntax.

'Syntax' is understood here to form an important part of 'internal organisation of multi-word utterances'. Clinically, difficulties in this sort of language ability are encountered as a wide range of identifiable phenomena, as reflected in case-note remarks that range from 'cannot put his ideas together' (which may refer to difficulties involving word selection and message structure), to more specific descriptions such as 'confuses pronouns' (or prepositions, etc.), or 'has few auxiliary verbs' (or determiners, etc.), 'doesn't put endings on verbs', or 'cannot construct complete sentences'.

Because of this wide-ranging clinical symptomatology, it is as well to recognise at the outset that it may be difficult in practice, and not clinically desirable, to insist on delimiting one's field of enquiry by too rigid a separation of such descriptive levels as *morphology, syntax* and *semantics/pragmatics*; or on a division of hierarchies between elements within the domain of the sentence (*syntax*) versus those in the domain of the word (*lexis*). It is rarely the case that a disorder will respect a linguistic boundary such as that between morphology and syntax; or syntax and lexis; or that disorders affecting these areas and the wider area of meaning will be independent of each other. We may refer to the range of relevant clinical phenomena, quite generally, as reflecting some language impairment, and recognise that morpho-syntax is a good place to start one's enquiry into any example of this type of complex disorder. We shall, however, try to indicate ways forward from syntax into vocabulary assessment of expressive speech samples, and into semantics/pragmatics.

The other term in the title of this chapter is 'assessment'. We shall take this to refer to a treatment of the expressive language data that is systematic in terms of *elicitation, transcription, analysis* and *interpretation*. This simply means that there must be a determinate set of ways of collecting the data, and representing them; also a set of categories to which the transcribed data can be assigned; and there must be a framework within which these categories are set, in order that an interpretation may be arrived at. This leads us to the important issue of comparisons, which we should say something about at the outset.

Comparisons

Ultimately, we need normative information in our interpretive framework: What do normal children, or adults, speak like in such-and-such a situation? But these are not the only comparisons we may work with, nor are they always the most obvious. Frequently clinicians work with comparisons between language-impaired individuals and groups. For convenience, we will use the abbreviations N, I (for normal and impaired groups) and n, i (for individuals).

In these terms, there may be scope for simple i–n comparisons, between a language-impaired individual and another who is language normal (Edwards and Garman, 1989). Obviously, such comparisons can be placed on a surer normative footing by collecting group-normative information, because the range of what is 'normal' may be surprisingly large (i–N). But this is not always possible: a special case of i–n is where the comparison is with the same individual, either following attainment of language normality after intervention, or where there are data on pre-morbid language behaviour. Likewise, there may be just one individual in an i–i comparison – as in a single-case study type of investigation (Coltheart, 1983). Other types of comparison involve what we might refer to as repeated i–i: where a clinician measures an individual up to a number of other individuals, which is not the same as doing a comparison with a group, i–I. This latter is more like trying to assess how well an individual seems to fit the characteristics of a defined syndrome.

Group studies were the order of the day in the older literature: most of the typology of aphasic syndromes, tentatively established on the basis of exploratory i-studies, are of the I–I sort (e.g. Goodglass and Kaplan, 1983; Kertesz, 1982). Hence we learn that, for example, Broca's aphasics (one I group) are distinct from, for example, Wernicke's aphasics (another I group) in respect of the symptoms of fluency and comprehension, but not repetition, and are distinct again from other groups on other symptoms, and so on. The same sort of typology was attempted, in this older tradition, for disorders observed in childhood, but the typology never carried much conviction, in the face of the acknowledged differences between emergent, or developmental, as opposed to acquired language impairment (Mejia and Eslava-Cobos, 1989). More effective group studies involved comparing I children with N under the influence of Brown's grammar-writing approach to child language acquisition (CLA) (Brown, 1973); studies such as Menyuk (1964) attempted to show qualitative distinctions between I and N grammars for children of the same age. But here an important consideration emerges which is peculiar to the developmental field of study (perhaps we should say it has been finessed, or never addressed, in the field of acquired adult disorders): on what measure do we establish which groups are comparable? For children, an obvious early answer was age. This led Menyuk to find qualitative differences between I groups and their N peer groups – a major plank in the 'deviance' interpretation of child language impairment. Morehead and Ingram (1973) suggested that a better answer might be Mean Length of Utterance (MLU), and on this basis I–N group comparisons revealed a different picture: that the I children were following essentially the same developmental path as their N peers, only at an older chronological age – considerable support for the 'delay' interpretation. Age comparisons are still useful, however, e.g. where mental age (MA) is to be distinguished from chronological age (CA) (Miller, 1992), and may be carried out alongside those based on MLU (Leonard, 1992).

More recent work has tended to highlight certain problems arising from dealing in group data. Aphasiologists have been concerned about the lack of predictive ability of the major syndromes, and their failure to highlight cross-cutting symptoms. Studies pursuing the 'delay' aspects of childhood language impairment have come under the influence, from mainstream CLA studies, of a concern to focus on individual differences in development. For instance, researchers have emphasised the existence of distinct sub-groups of children within a diagnostic category such as Specifically Language-Impaired (SLI) (Miller, 1987; Fletcher, 1992). But there is a continuing need for I–N studies that look for the common characteristics of such categories, founded on more refined linguistic analyses and statistical procedures. Gavin, Klee and Membrino (1993) identify two types of such study, one involving comparisons of the groups by linguistic feature, using univariate statistical analysis, the other analysing linguistic group profiles in terms of multivariate statistical analyses.

Let us bring our discussion back to the clinician in routine working conditions. He or she will naturally assess a child or adult client in terms of individual strengths and weaknesses, in relation to two sets of knowledge: (i) the pattern of strengths and weaknesses seen in other language-impaired individuals; and (ii) assumptions about the linguistic behaviour of normal individuals. The two sets of knowledge are both complex, and interlinked to a degree: on some measure, say morphological marking, one language-impaired individual may be 'normal' whilst another is not, but the situation may be reversed on another measure, such as proportion of complex clauses.

The most obvious embodiment of assessment measures is in the form of published, or widely available, assessment procedures, in which the measures are pre-selected, and are intended to be applied to data that are elicited, transcribed and selected in approved ways. As far as childhood language impairment is concerned, it is the purpose of such procedures (e.g. Developmental Sentence Analysis (DSA); Lee, 1974) to allow clinicians to carry out i–N comparisons, whereas, for the clinician using a typical procedure with adult clients (e.g. the Western Aphasia Battery; Kertesz, 1982), the comparison will be of the type i–I (the normative information being backgrounded in the assumption that normal speakers would score 100%, less some fraction for ordinary human frailty).

Clinically, such procedures have two main disadvantages. First, most clinicians actually have to use these standardised procedures in nonstandard ways, because the client they are assessing is not drawn from a comparable population, or the data cannot be elicited from a comparable situation, to those used in the relevant standardisation exercises. Second, the measures used may not be appropriate (usually, are not refined enough), in the clinician's view, to capture the nature of the individual client's difficulties. In this sense, progress in assessment is to be measured in terms of improvement of the measures used.

In our own experience, attempting to establish a normative reference base for interpreting the data from language-impaired individuals is not an easy matter. There must be some assumption of what range of measures should be incorporated. This in turn involves looking at both the language impaired and normal data, and making a selection that will be revealing of both. But how many possible measures are 'out there' in the complex nature of language? In this chapter we shall concentrate on three main areas where currently proposed syntactic measures seem to us to be in need of refinement: one is in definition of the unit of syntactic organisation; another is in the relation of phrasal syntax to clausal syntax; and the third is to be found in the conception of the relationships that syntactic units enter into, to form complex units of discourse. But first we shall consider the framework within which these measures must be set.

Naturally Displayed Evidence

The term used as the heading for this section comes from Garrett's (1982) review of research directed towards understanding the nature of normal, adult, everyday expression of language. The idea that is central to this term is that observable performance, particularly if it is representative of naturalistic functions, is a worthwhile source of evidence on the underlying abilities that we may wish to enquire into. This is just as true of child data as it is of adult, and of impaired as well as normal data.

Now let us consider briefly what sort of evidence is potentially available as soon as one starts considering expressive speech data. Setting aside here the evidence that reflects the participants and the situation (as these are part of discourse analysis and pragmatics), we have to consider the following categories (see Figure 6.1). In these terms, most research, in the normal as well as impaired processing of language, has focused on the following categories:

1. *Non-verbal*: possibly a surprising category to start with, but there are

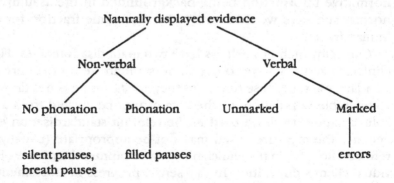

Figure 6.1: Simplified taxonomy of naturally displayed sources of evidence in spoken-language production.

typically pauses, and other non-verbal phenomena such as symbolic noises, to consider. Pauses may be filled (*um, er*) or empty, and reflect aspects of linguistic planning and execution (Goldman-Eisler, 1968; Butterworth, 1980; Butcher, 1981; Beattie, 1983), including grammatical structure (Gee and Grosjean, 1983). Symbolic noises may be integrated quite closely into grammatical structure, e.g. *it went (growling sound)*.

2. *Verbal, marked*:
(a) here we include a range of 'hesitation phenomena' (Butterworth, 1980) including false starts, backtrackings and structural mazes; these often accompany pauses, and may lead to incompletion of utterances;
(b) verbal behaviour may also reveal errors of one sort or another, and some (not all) of these may be associated with pausing and hesitation phenomena. A brief summary would include the following:

(i)   non-occurrence:
(a)   of response, e.g.:
      T: what happened to her/
      P: - - -
(b)   of grammatical categories, e.g.:
      P: can't open it/ (full form: *I can't open it*)
      P: bed/ (full form: *a bed*)
      P: this bath/ (full form: *this is a/the bath*)
      P: sit down there (full form: *he/the man's sitting down there*)

Note that certain utterances illustrate more than one non-occurrence.

(ii) substitution:
      P: other one again (appropriate form: *another one again*)
      P: I didn't know I had a stree (appropriate form: *a stroke*)

Without going into too much detail at this stage, we may observe:

(a) that some instances of non-occurrence may be attested in normal child and adult speech. For example, the subject-dropping observed in *can't* open it (above) may be best interpreted as conditioned by pragmatic factors such as the likelihood that, in context, the first person (speaker) may be understood to be the subject, unless the subject is otherwise specified;
(b) in other cases, structural factors may be operating, as in the example above where we have specified the 'full form' as *a bed*, in response to the query *what have you got there?* But this can only be considered a 'full' form if we assume the operation of normal processes of structural ellipsis;

(c) in many cases, the identification of missing elements may be uncertain (e.g. *a* versus *the* in *this (a/the?) bath*).

Now, although hesitation phenomena and error analysis have provided essential ways into the underlying processes of language production, it is rather striking that a large body of evidence has thus far gone relatively untapped, at least as far as adult performance is concerned (child data have been better served in this respect); the category of:

3. *Verbal, unmarked*: by which we refer to the structural and functional aspects of non-errorful, fluent utterances. The characterisation of these involves, potentially, all levels of linguistic description, from message structure to articulatory performance. As far as syntax is concerned, we need to take account of the following aspects of speech texts:

- those that are *major*, built on the traditional 'parts of speech' represented in classes of words such as nouns, verbs, prepositions, etc., versus those elements that are *minor*, standing outside this system, such as the so-called 'sentence particles' *yes* and *no*, 'interjections' such as *oh*, and stereotypic routines such as *how d'you do*;
- utterances that consist of 'one word at a time', versus those that exhibit constructional abilities;
- among the constructional types, some are patterned as clauses, some as phrases and some as both simultaneously.

There are word structure (morphological) patterns to consider also:

- *closed class* elements, typically drawn from small, systematically organised sets of terms (such as determiners, personal pronouns and auxiliary verbs), and whose function is to modify or mark grammatical relationships, versus *open class* elements, typically drawn from large sets of semantically representative terms, constituting the lexicon;
- elements that are building blocks of grammatical organisation (the choice really lies between words or morphemes here) versus elements that constitute the domain of grammatical organisation (usually assumed to be the 'sentence', though 'clause' and 'utterance' may also be used in this sense; as noted below, we shall use the concept of *text units*);
- elements of the *intra*-grammatical domain, forming part of the internal grammatical organisation of utterances (noun phrase, subject, main verb, determiner, adverbial, etc.) versus elements of the *inter*-grammatical domain, forging links between utterances within a text, either closely or at a distance (such as conjunctions, backward-referring pronouns, ellipsis, and thematic ordering of items).

Regarding the elements of the intra-grammatical domain, we should note that a basic distinction that has been usefully brought to the fore in recent years is that of *complement* versus *adjunct* (see Radford, 1988). Like many basic distinctions, it has a number of problems of detail, but it can be quite simply stated and illustrated by clear cases. Words within clauses are grouped into phrases, as we have seen, but not all phrases have the same status within the clause. We can illustrate with a single phrase in two different clauses: the prepositional phrase (PP) *in the garden* is a complement in

John is in the garden

but it is an adjunct in

John was reading a book in the garden.

The usual account of this distinction is that the verb *be* (*is* in the first clause above) requires a specification of location, which the PP supplies, and without which the clause would be incomplete; whilst the verb *read* (*was reading* in the second clause), requires an object NP, which *a book* supplies, but not a location. So an adjunct is an extra item, over and above what is actually demanded by the syntactic requirements of (in this case) the verb. (Other constituents than verbs also make specifiable syntactic demands, in analogous fashion.) We can say that any constituent that is demanded within the domain of another is a *complement*; anything else is an *adjunct*. Extending this argument slightly, we can say that all verbs in English demand that they should have a subject NP; so *John* is part of the complement-structure of both above examples.

Now, it is of the essence of adjuncts that they are 'optional extras'; but it would be a mistake to assume that, by contrast, all complements are obligatory. Taking the second example above, we could imagine a version like

John was reading in the garden

where what we want to call the same verb, *was reading*, appears without its object NP complement, but with its adjunct. This is where the discussion of complements and adjuncts starts to get tricky; we may well take the view that real-world, pragmatic factors such as focus and emphasis, as well as what the listener may reasonably be expected to work out for him- or herself, are influencing the syntactic form of the sentence. This is not to deny the fundamental importance of the grammatical distinction between the processes that attach complements to their demanding constituents, yielding what we may call *clause-complement structures* (CCSs); and those processes that, more loosely, attach adjuncts to these CCSs. An obvious question arises at this point: are there cases of language impairment where these processes are differentially affected?

Further Issues in Word and Sentence

At this point we should note that there are two, quite basic, issues to be addressed. One relates to misgivings that many students of unplanned discourse have, that speakers, whether normal or impaired, don't actually speak in 'sentences', as these are traditionally exemplified in the linguists' textbooks. Speech seems to be executed in units that are often smaller, and sometimes bigger, than sentences, and it is not clear that sentences form a natural 'half-way' unit at all. An open-minded approach would use a term such as *utterance*, and leave it open as to what sorts of grammatical domains are exemplified within such units. But, of course, that means that such units have to be defined, prior to assessment.

To illustrate, let us consider an extract from the transcript of a normal 5-year-old child (C) engaging with an adult (E) in placing stickers of objects and animals on a farm picture. The child utterances are presented here as turns in the dialogue:

C: Is that the mother one?
E: Do you know what I think?
C: What?
E: I think that's a turkey.
C: I do, because what's that thing sticking out?
E: Don't know.
E: Do you think it's his ear?
C: Yeah, oh this is a tiny one.
E: What do you think that is?
C: What's that one?
E: It's a chicken.
C: No, look it's got this thing.

Without going into too much detail at this stage, it is clear that we have to consider how far we can establish segmentation of the data within the child's turn contributions. Do elements such as *yeah, no, oh* belong with their neighbouring elements in such segments? Does *look* represent a distinguishable element? How do we handle the instances of tags and complex clause sequences? If we attempt to identify such constituents of turns, and set each out on its own line, then how many lines will there be in the extract above?

Such issues are important for the basic measure of Mean Length of Utterance (MLU), of course, but they also affect a number of other measures which more specifically relate to grammatical structuring ability, e.g. the proportion of complex utterances, the proportion of utterances with adverbial modification, and so on.

Another issue concerns words: no one doubts that speakers use them, but again they need to be defined for the purpose of assessment. Different analysts, for example, may take the pronoun forms *I* and *me* as two instances (tokens) of the same abstract lexeme (type), or as two distinct types, each with their own tokens. Consider also how the word *one* may appear, as a numeral (*one, two, three...*), or as a noun-substitute (*try these ones* – rather like *thing*), or as a pro-NP element (*one fell down*): are these different words, or different functions of the same word? Whilst we shall not consider vocabulary assessment as such in this chapter, we should simply note here that a basic measure such as Type Token Ratio (TTR) will be affected by such differences, and it is incumbent on assessment procedures to make such decisions explicit.

We shall now illustrate our own response to the need for explicitness in respect of both utterance and word, as found in our discussion of adult and child data samples in the later sections. Obviously, other positions are possible and defensible; but we believe the issues we highlight here need to be explicitly addressed in any assessment procedure dealing with grammatical assessment.

Units in Utterances

We said above that speakers may not speak in sentences. What sort of units do they use, then?

We start with the consideration that texts may be organised in a number of ways simultaneously. The units of organisation include speaker–listener turns, which may be as short as a single word, but are frequently much longer and may contain what we want to call a number of utterances whose sequencing calls for analysis. Within these, speech is prosodically structured also, in *tone groups* and other constituent units that relate to, but are not identical to, units of syntax (Crystal, 1979). This means that we have to do our syntax without any dependence on prosodic criteria for defining 'utterance'. This, however, does not mean that prosodic criteria play no role in providing for the syntactic analysis. As the transcriber works from the taped record, prosodic factors will often help to mark the status of a word or phrase in a way that is relevant for syntactic analysis: e.g. minor and stereotypic elements such as *well*, *don't know*, etc. may be distinguished from their analytical counterparts at this stage. This is no more than the traditional role of intonation in transcription, helping to disambiguate, say, a verbless structure such as *that boat* as either a noun phrase (Determiner + Noun) or a clause (Subject + Complement). But it does mean that, as such identifications are made as part of the transcription process, no prosodic marking is required in the transcription format that is the basis for syntactic analysis. (See also Perkins, 1994 for further issues in the determination of elements that speakers tend to use repetitively.)

Unclear:

Next, we recognise that not all parts of a text are intelligible, or clear in their analysis. Those stretches of speech that are unintelligible (marked X for each apparent syllable, up to XXX) may appear to be distinct utterances (wholly unintelligible); or they may appear as part of what on other grounds appear to be distinct utterances (partially unintelligible). Utterances that are incomplete by virtue of being abandoned, or interrupted, and never picked up again are also unclear, as they could potentially have been completed in indefinitely long and diverse ways. Stereotypic expressions are also unclear, because it is often difficult to know how much the structure they are apparently composed of is attributable to the speaker. Finally, errorful (including paraphasic) utterances are unclear, at least on a first analysis, as they are by definition deviations from whatever target might be hypothesised to account for them.

Minor:

Not all parts of a text have grammatical structure: e.g. Minors (see above), and these are segmented off on to separate distinct lines of the transcript (but see comments under 'linearisation', below). These constitute the first clear type of what we shall refer to as Text Units (TUs: Garman 1989b; 1990).

Clausal:

At the other extreme of grammatical sophistication, we find parts of the text exhibiting clause structure, possibly with phrase structure also represented within its constituents (see above). Here, we define a clause as having just one main verb, and at least one other element of clause structure: Subject (S), Object (O), Complement (C) or Adverbial (A). In addition, each consists only of complements of that verb.[1] For those used to working with Larsp (and a number of other surface-syntax procedures) this has two important consequences. First, many clause patterns of the type SVA, SVOA, SVAA, and so on will be segmented as SV/A, SVO/A, SVA/A, or SV/A/A, depending on whether the V in these structures takes the A as a complement, or not. Second, because each clausal TU has just one V, there is clearly a need for specifying the linkages

[1] Note here the distinction between the Quirk grammar/LARSP use of 'Complement' ('Complement with a big C'), and 'complement' (with a small 'c') which is in contrast with adjunct (see above). Huddleston (1984) makes it clear that it makes perfect sense to talk of 'Subject complements' and 'Object complements': these are rather cumbersome terms, but they make it clear that verbs in English *require* subjects, and those that take objects *require* those objects. We could also speak of 'Complement complements', for verbs like *be* which *require* an NP or AdjP Complement. It is when we get to Adverbials that, depending on the verb requirements, we may find either 'Adverbial complements' or 'Adverbial adjuncts'.

between multi-clausal sequences (as in Larsp Stage V). We shall come to each of these issues in a moment.

Phrasal/Lexical:

Between these two extremes we find portions of text that map on to multi- or single-word units (see above). The distinction between the two types may be somewhat artificial (because a single-word Adverbial Phrase such as here may have the same syntactic distribution as its multi-word counterparts), but it may prove clinically useful. The phrasal and lexical elements referred to here, it should be emphasised, are those which occur outside the clause structures recognised above. It is this that gives them the status of TUs. They may constitute portions of the text which stand alone, or which form part of a longer sequence. They may arise in a number of ways: through ellipsis, addition, or as the 'residue' of the segmentation procedures established above.

One of the virtues of this approach is that it focuses attention on the size of the units involved in discourse production: respecting the linguistic features of the designated units above seems to yield units that are considerably smaller than the sentence. At the same time, a number of them are clearly linked to each other, along grammatical dimensions, to form higher-order sequences that are considerably longer than the sentence.

Another virtue of the approach is that it makes an issue of the linearity (the left–right dimension) in language. This was long ago seen (Bolinger, 1952) as a neglected aspect of syntactic organisation (in comparison with hierarchy, the vertical dimension). The basic insight is that one and the same modifier (e.g. *slowly*) may be regarded as more closely integrated in the Text Unit (TU) if it occurs within it (*I slowly ate my breakfast*), and as more loosely linked if it occurs at the end (*I ate my breakfast slowly*). In processing terms, this makes sense: elements that are planned ahead are more closely integrated than those which are afterthoughts. So linearity is used as a defining feature of TUs: specifically, *slowly* would be taken as part of the TU in the first case above, but would be segmented off as a distinct TU in its own right in the second case. In similar fashion, Minors occurring within other TUs (e.g. *they were eating oh something really nice*) are regarded as belonging to them, by the principle of linearity.

Relations in Utterances

Specifying TUs presupposes that they are capable of linking up in various ways to form larger units of discourse. In the procedure illustrated in this chapter, we tap that subset of inter-TU relations that hold between immediately adjacent TUs: we refer to these as Immediate Grammatical Relations (IGRs). Effectively, these build utterances into higher-order units, many of which are considerably longer than traditional sentences. We shall introduce them in the following sections, in illustration of child and adult data.

Thus far, we have introduced (a) the potential sources of evidence contained in a sample of expressive speech, and (b) some of the ways in which unmarked as well as marked sources can be tapped for syntactic assessment. In the remainder of this chapter we shall illustrate with reference to child and adult data. We shall end with a brief summary and conclusions.

Child assessment

Assessment Procedures

In the first edition of this book, our chapter (Garman 1989a) compared the *Language Assessment and Screening Procedure* (LARSP) and *Developmental Sentence Analysis* (DSA), on a sample transcript, to highlight certain important features of these procedures. We noted the obvious differences: DSA is divided into two distinct procedures, *Developmental Sentence Types* (DST) and *Developmental Sentence Scoring* (DSS), whereas LARSP is unified; DSS is selective in its treatment of structures (only subject–predicate types are recognised), whereas LARSP is comprehensive; DSS is limited in the scoring categories it targets, whereas LARSP is exhaustive; DSS makes no principled distinction between morphology, phrase syntax and clause syntax, whereas LARSP does; DSS is standardised whereas LARSP is not. We also noted that some differences were more apparent than fundamental: e.g. whilst DSS delivers a score, it also provides a profile, at least implicitly. We went on to review a major research initiative for standardising an expressive language procedure on LARSP principles (Fletcher *et al,* 1986), using an improved transcription format, a more explicit procedure for segmentation of utterances, the provision of further categories of analysis, particularly for adverbials (Fletcher, 1987) and lexical items (Fletcher and Garman, 1988; French, 1988); and systematisation of the method of scoring complex constructions. A further development in this research initiative was the extension of the age range covered, up to normal 7-year-olds.

BLADES

As well as proposed developments to LARSP, of course, other procedures have been developed. The *Bristol Language Development Scales*

(BLADES) (Gutfreund, Harrison and Wells, 1989), coincidentally published in the same year as our chapter , is founded on the normative information provided by the *Bristol Child Language Project* (Wells, 1985). In this project, each child utterance is classified by conversational purpose, semantic and syntactic features, and BLADES aims to use this knowledge base to provide a sensitive assessment across the whole range of language use, at the same time using less technical means of general assessment. In the Bristol research data, Level I is up to 15 months; thereafter, Levels II to X represent nine further intervals up to age 5;0.

BLADES is organised into two scales: the Main Scale has items selected by the clearest evidence of order of emergence, greatest frequency and ease of definition, in pragmatics, semantics and syntax. The Therapy Planning form lists all of the items of language used in the original research project, by order of appearance, and is used for filling gaps in assessing a patchy sample, and for developing a comprehensive programme of therapy.

In terms of syntactic assessment, BLADES offers one of the three main subsystems on the Main Scale, entitled 'Syntactics' (the other subsystems are 'Pragmatics' and 'Semantics'). 'Syntactics' consists of three columns, headed 'Conjunctions', 'NP structure' and 'Sentence/clause'. There is also a central column, headed 'Noun Phrase Elements', which straddles the semantic and syntactic areas, containing items drawn from both systems. In spite of its title, this column is also used to include expressions of time and place, such as *here, now, in the garden, never* etc.

A sample is assigned a BLADES level by noting the number of items recorded on the Main Scale form for each subsystem, totalling these for each level and checking the result against the criterion score for that level. Getting a criterial score for Level V assigns the child to that level, even if the criterial score for Level IV is not attained.

BLADES is intended for use on a child's conversation, drawn from a naturalistic setting, of about 30 minutes' duration, ideally sampled through the day. At least 100 utterances are needed, particularly for the higher levels of development. Regarding the definition of this unit, BLADES notes:

> For our purposes, an utterance starts:
>
> (1) each time there is a change of speaker;
> (2) within one speaker's turn after a pause or change of intonation.

But it is made clear that there are exceptions to these rules of thumb. It does not recognise the distinction between complements and adjuncts, or provide for morphological analysis.

Comparative analyses

As well as such new developments, however, standard LARSP has continued to be used both in routine clinical work and in research. In the latter area, it is most often used for comparative analyses, either of other measures (e.g. Blake, Quartaro and Onorati, 1993), or of characteristics of specific groups of language-impaired children (e.g. Gavin, Klee and Membrino, 1993).

Blake *et al.* (1993) used LARSP as a frame of reference for assessing the relation between MLU and certain indices of syntactic complexity across the age range 1;6 to 4;9. From the first five stages of LARSP, they derived 10 LARSP scores for each child, including (unlike earlier studies) weighted mean stage scores for both clausal and phrasal levels. They also calculated their own syntactic complexity measure by totalling the LARSP categories S, V, O, C, A. They found that some LARSP measures were less valid than others, but found significant changes across MLU groups for almost all LARSP measures. They conclude that MLU is a valid measure of clausal constructions at LARSP stages I–II, and V, and in terms of average clausal complexity, and that their own syntactic complexity measure was also promising in this respect. In contrast, neither measure was sensitive to phrasal syntax beyond the lowest group.

In the context of such recent work, it seems to us that fundamental issues concerning the definition of utterance, and analytic decisions regarding adjunct vs complement, clausal vs phrasal syntax, etc. remain to be addressed. We shall now present some results of the analysis of child data within a framework of syntactic assessment that represents a further development of LARSP principles, in an effort to meet the desiderata that we have outlined in the earlier section. In particular, we shall use Text Units and Immediate Grammatical Relations, and explicitly distinguish between phrasal utterances vs phrasal expansions in clausal utterances.

Data Illustration and the Profile Chart

First, we shall introduce some data and analysis categories from a 6-year-old language-impaired child whom we shall refer to as 'B', and who will be reported on more fully below. An illustrative sample worksheet for data analysis is presented in simplified form in Table 6.1.

The first column, **Unc**(lear), corresponds to LARSP Section A, i.e. it is where structures are logged if they are unclear in terms of how or whether they are to be analysed: Codes are U(nintelligible), $ (stereotypic), A(mbiguous), I(ncomplete), etc.

The next column, **Min**(ors), will be familiar from LARSP, as will the division into those minors that are R(esponses) vs O(thers).

Table 6.1: Sample worksheet, Child B

Child B	Age 6;0		Text Unit categories					
No.	Text	Unc	Min	Lex	Phr	Cla	IGR	
1	put the girl in seesaw					VOA		
2	girl's got	I						
3	the girl on the bike	A						
4	this			P				
5	look			V				
6	don't know		$					
7	what			P				
8	it's got a jacket on					SVOA		
9	yeah		R					
10	yea		R					
11	back bike	A						
12	riding the bike					VO		
13	put mummy in the seesaw					VOA		
14	and the boy watch mummy					a Cl		
15	girl			N				
16	got black hair					VO		
17	no		R					
18	in the slide				PDN			
19	yeah		R					
20	'cos watch this					s Cl		
		4	4	4	1	7	0	

The middle column, **Lex**(ical), corresponds to LARSP Stage I Major, but has a fuller notation for parts of speech, to unpack the LARSP Other category, e.g. **J** = Adjective, **B** = Adverb, **P** = Pronoun, beside **V** = Verb and **N** = Noun. But the category **O**(ther) remains, for a restricted set of items. (We use an **Amb**(iguous) category here to capture those items which LARSP calls Problematic, falling between two or more categories, e.g. *run*, noun or verb?).

The next two columns bring us into multi-word syntax. **Phr**(asal) has, despite its familiar label, no exact parallel in LARSP: it records the number of TUs that are constructed as phrases, i.e. have phrase structure as their highest level of organisation. It thus captures independent utterances such as *at home*, e.g. in response to a question stimulus; but also as adverbial adjuncts which extend a basic clausal text unit, such as *at home* in *I got one of those/at home*. LARSP makes no distinction, under its 'Phrase' column, between such phrases and those that occur as expansions of clause-elements such as A in clause units. However, LARSP does provide a subsidiary categorisation of 'expansions', and points out that this is a potentially important feature of grammatical organisation. The present profile thus implements this LARSP distinction in a clearer way. Symbols are as in LARSP, supplemented by **J, B, R** as above and (slightly modified) **A**(uxiliary verb), **P**(reposition). So PDN above represents LARSP PrDN.

The **Cla**(usal) column will appear straightforwardly LARSP-based, though it should be recalled that these are clause-complement sequences, with adverbial adjuncts hived off to distinct text-units, so the proportion of A-modified sequences is lower than would be the case in standard LARSP. Connectives (LARSP and, c, s) are represented as **a**, **c**, **s**. The clauses that they connect to are not further specified as particular patterns of elements, but are simply represented as **Cl**; so **aCl** above represents a clause introduced by *and*. This accords with the principle of marking each utterance just once, for its most advanced feature (which is the connectivity marker).

Finally, the **IGR** column collects the inter-TU relations referred to earlier; there are none in this sample extract, and we shall in any case not go into the subtypes of IGRs in detail in this chapter. It is worth noting, however, that the mere occurrence of connectives does not guarantee the presence of an IGR; this distinction reflects the LARSP practice of marking connectives separately from instances of true coordination and subordination, at Stage V.

The Profile Chart

From the layout of the worksheet above, it is a short step to the construction of a profile chart. The one shown in Table 6.2 represents the full sample consisting of 100 utterances, from which the extract above was taken. The data in the profile chart are organised in the same columns as the worksheet, but frequency ordered, with the most frequent items at the top.

From this display, we may see clearly enough that child B has a low number of IGRs, and high numbers of Minors and Lexicals. However, it is difficult to go further unless one has other profile charts to compare: what constitutes a 'low' or 'high' number of Phrasal and Clausal utterances, for samples of particular types of elicited/free conversational data?

Table 6.2: B's TUs and IGRs (profile display)

Unclear	Minor	Lexical	Phrase	Clause	IGRs
Amb 4	R 31	N 10	PDN 2	SVO 6	A 1
$ 3		R 4	PR 1	a Cl 5	P 1
		O 4	JN 1	VOA 5	C 1
		Amb 2	PB 1	VO 5	O 1
		Q 1	VV 1	SVC 4	
		V 1		SVOA 3	
				s Cl 2	
				QVS 2	
				SVA 1	
				XA 1	

We may start to point up some of these interpretive issues by providing the profile of a 100-utterance sample from another language-impaired child, G (aged 7;1). G's profile (Table 6.3) clearly illustrates a more fully developed system of structured TUs (Phrasal and Clausal types), and IGRs, than we found in B.

Table 6.3: G's TUs and IGRs (profile display)

Unclear	Minor	Lexical	Phrase	Clause	IGRs
Amb 3	R 17	N 4	PDN 4	AX 15	A 14
		B 4	PN 3	s Cl 10	S 3
		J 1	PR 3	a Cl 6	R 3
		O 1	DN 1	SVA 6	C 2
			PDJN 1	SVC 5	P 2
			ODN 1	SV 4	T 1
			PJO 1	c Cl 2	W 1
			BJ 1	SC 1	
			cB 1	AAXY 1	
			cN 1	SVCA 1	
			cDN 1	VSV 1	

But we really need to put a range of children into the picture, in order to see what sorts of variation may occur, over the analysis categories that have been presented so far. In effect, this will involve us in making a number of i–i comparisons, in terms of the first section. For this purpose, we have taken a number of children of different ages, but all having some grammatical involvement in their pattern of language impairment. Our purpose is to ensure that we have a reasonably mixed, typical cross-section of the sort of children that clinicians frequently see, among which the different levels of syntax may be more or less compromised, in the context of individual differences of strengths and weakness.

We shall consider 10 samples, each sized at 100 Complete & Intelligible (C&I) utterances (by the SALT program, Miller and Chapman, 1985) except for three: one falls slightly short, at 94 C&I, whilst the other two are considerably shorter, at 73 and 64. We shall report on proportioned data for these samples. As well as TU analysis, each sample has been analysed for the presence of bound morphemes, providing an analogue of the LARSP Word-level count.

General Characteristics

Some general characteristics of these samples are given in Table 6.4 (from SALT standard summary information). The MLU(m) values given here are used to rank the samples, and the labels A–J reflect this ordering (note that the labels B and G for the children illustrated above derive from this ordering, and the same samples appear in this table as B and

G). This ordering gives some idea of the 'language age' range the children represent. It is clearly distinct from their chronological age, as we would expect in such a mixed group. However, we should note that the MLU(m) values are lower than those that are standardly cited in the research literature, because 'utterances' here are defined as text units, which tend to be shorter than the usual notion of 'utterance' in such sample analyses. Unfortunately, it is not possible to say precisely what the more usual MLU values for these samples would be, because the standard definitions of 'utterance' are, unlike 'text unit', inexplicit.

Table 6.4: The 10 language-impaired samples

Child	A	B	C	D	E	F	G	H	I	J	Range
Age	3;7	6;0	5;0	3;10	5;11	6;5	7;1	5;8	10;5	4;4	3;7–10;5
Total utts	100	100	100	94	100	73	100	100	100	64	64–100
MLU(m)	1.67	2.3	2.7	2.76*	2.85	2.89*	2.94	3.07	3.34	3.84*	1.67–3.84

Note: MLU(m) = mean length of utterance, counting morphemes; * = proportioned to take account of varying sample size).

Basic Text Unit Measures

Table 6.5 provides the proportioned number of tokens of each of the categories we introduced above, from the profile charts for each of the 10 children. Clearly, we have considerable variation on the four main categories of text-units (we leave unclear units out of this account), IGRs and bound morphemes. But certain stable features emerge. First, Clausal TUs show both a relatively narrow range, and a marked preponderance over other types of TUs, accounting for nearly half of the utterances, on average: in this respect, sample A is marked as unusually low, and sample J as high. Minors are next most frequent, overall, at around a fifth of the data on average: samples H and F represent the extremes. Next, we may note that Phrasal and Lexical TUs have similar dominance in the samples, at around 15% on average: we can now say that B turns out to be particularly low on Phrasals. Finally, we can note that IGRs average out at just over 10 per 100 TUs in these data: in this respect, sample G is indeed high, at 26.

Pursuing this approach, we can illustrate five main patterns of grammatical impairment in our data, by taking those samples that represent the more extreme points on two or more of these measures, as in Table 6.6. These patterns are quite complex, although relationships and similarities are discernible (e.g. between A and B). The dimensions of syntax that are represented in these measures appear to be quite independent of each other. We shall now provide some further discussion and illustration of these children's syntactic abilities, on the more refined measures below.

Table 6.5: 100 C&I utterances for the group: basic TU tokens (proportioned)

Child	A	B	C	D	E	F	G	H	I	J	Range
TUs											
Tokens											
CL	20	34	49	39	43	41	52	47	46	64	20–64
PH	8	6	14	15	21	12	18	27	25	11	6–27
LE	37	22	6	19	12	5	10	21	11	8	5–37
MI	26	31	30	22	24	37	17	5	16	11	5–37
IGRs											
Tokens	0	4	15	8	17	3	26	11	20	8	0–26
Bound morphemes											
Tokens	6	14	29	23	27	26	32	36	26	39	6–39

Table 6.6: Five main patterns of grammatical impairment in the data samples

Child	Text units				IGR	BM
	Min	Lex	Phr	Cla		
A		High	Low	Low		Low	Low
B	High		Low			Low	Low
F	High	Low				Low	
H	High		High				High
J				High			High

Further Details, Phrasal Syntax

We may go back to consider B in more detail. We argued above that the phrasal syntax involved in expansions of clausal elements should be considered independently of Phrasal TUs. We have already noted that B is low on the latter category, in comparison with the other nine child samples. Table 6.7 gives the data relating to B's phrasal expansions. This reveals a restricted range of types and tokens in each position, consistent with the picture of low use of phrasal syntax at TU level. The proportion of elements expanded is highest for those elements that tend to occupy post-V positions, as we would expect; the proportion of V expansions is, strikingly, lowest of all.

Table 6.7: B's clause elements and phrasal expansions (profile display)

Clause elements					
Type, number	S 20	V 34	O 23	C 5	A 14
Expansions					
Type, number	DN 5	AV 3	DN 7	DN 1	PDN 6
		ANV 1	JN 1	IJ 1	PN 1
Proportion	0.25	0.12	0.35	0.4	0.5

We could compare this with the data from G, or H, to show how a child with more obvious phrasal structuring abilities handles expansions: but we may bring F in here for a more revealing comparison. F is in the lower range for Phrasal TUs (12 out of 100) but, in spite of this, we can see from Table 6.8 that F's phrasal syntax in expansions is proportionately much more developed than B's.

Table 6.8: F's clause elements and phrasal expansions (profile display)

Clause elements Type, number	S 29	V 30	O 13	C 11	A 14
Expansions Type, number	DN 3	AV 7	JN 3	DN 2	PR 2
			DN 2	JN 2	PDN 2
			DJN 2	NPDN 1	PN 2
			NN 1		PNN 1
					PB 1
Proportion	0.10	0.23	0.61	0.45	0.57

There are proportionately many more O-expansions than B has, and rather more V-expansions too (though they are still fairly low). Just as striking is the range of phrasal types used: among the post-V elements B has 6 to F's 12.

Bound Morphemes

To complete the picture regarding B's low grammatical structuring ability, consider the bound morphemes measure (Table 6.9). B shows the lowest number of types and tokens in the group. Only one instance marks a noun inflection (-*s*, plural); of the 13 verb inflections, nine are contracted forms, which may not be representative of fully productive knowledge. Among these, seven are instances of the form '*s*, of which one occurs in the context of the contracted auxiliary *have*, whilst the other six are contracted copulas. The single instance of *3s* represents one of three obligatory contexts for this morpheme, the other two contexts showing omission.

Table 6.9: B's bound morphemes

Stem category:	Verb		Noun	
	's	7	pl	1
	ing	3		
	'll	2		
	3s	1		

To point a contrast, we do not need to go to the 'High' bound morpheme users, but may consider sample G's use of bound morphemes (Table 6.10), which is in the upper range for tokens (32) but actually has more types than any other child in the group. These are mainly verbal (26), and include a number of contracted forms, but the bulk of these morphemes (14) mark person, tense and aspect on lexical verb stems.

Table 6.10: G's bound morphemes

Stem category:	Verb		Noun	
	'll	1	pl	5
	'm	3	gen	1
	're	2		
	's	4		
	've	2		
	3s	2		
	ed	7		
	en	1		
	ing	4		

There is only one example of a bound morpheme ('m) failing to occur in an obligatory context.

Summary

In summary of these profiles and comparisons, we may say that B is constructing his discourse out of those elements that require least structuring in terms of morphological and phrasal organisation, on the one hand, and clause linkage on the other. Between these two, as it were, his clause syntax appears to be relatively well developed, in the range of types used, although the overall Clausal TU incidence is the lowest in the group by virtue of his reliance on the Minor and Lexical TUs. This would appear to be a case where the profile of types is crucial to interpretation.

Finally, in illustration of how vocabulary analysis may integrate with syntactic profiling, we may consider the verbs that stand in the Clausal TUs that B uses. Consistent with what we have seen thus far, B uses a relatively large number of different main verbs, at 18 (Group range: 10–21). However, when we look at the closed class of auxiliary verbs, we may not be surprised to find that the picture is very different: B is the lowest in the group, with just three types (Group range 3–10).

Adult assessment

Most carers and non-language specialists associated with aphasic speakers judge language impairment and reduction of that impairment by the aphasic person's spoken output. However, it is recognised that whilst the description of connected speech is an important part of aphasia assessment, both deciding what the components of that description should be and how the data should be quantified are problematic (Menn, Ramsberger and Helm-Estabrooks, 1994). The investigator may undertake to investigate every aspect of connected (or spontaneous) spoken language, pragmatic, grammatical, semantic, lexical and phonemic or, for reasons of clinical expediency or research focus, decide to undertake a detailed investigation of one aspect of language functioning. In this chapter, although we are focusing on the grammatical assessment, it will be seen that it is not really possible to look at one aspect of language in isolation and we will consider how, for example, deployment of lexical elements affects the distribution of grammatical structures.

Assessment Procedures

Most existing aphasia assessments consist of a series of tasks which test various language abilities such as the naming and selection of single words, as in the *Boston Diagnostic Aphasia Examination* (BDAE; Goodglass and Kaplan, 1983), or the *Psycholinguistic Assessment of Language Processing in Aphasia* (PALPA; Kay, Lesser and Coltheart, 1992). Such procedures either do not provide means of assessing continuous speech (PALPA specifically excludes this feature), or, if they do (as in the BDAE), they provide a mixture of semantic, prosodic, pragmatic and grammatical criteria and thus offer some index of expressive ability, but fail to produce a fine-grained grammatical analysis. *The Shewan Spontaneous Language Analysis* (SSLA; Shewan, 1988) which was developed to describe and quantify aphasic speakers' connected language, computes twelve aspects which include: *Number of Utterances* (where Utterance is defined as a complete thought marked by content, intonation and/or pause); *Time* (length of sample); *Length* (the number of utterances of five or fewer words divided by total number of utterances multiplied by 100); *Melody* (which is judged to be absent, normal but limited to short phrases, or normal); *Articulation* (which also has a three-category rating); *Rate; Errors* (which may involve omission of bound or free grammatical morphemes, subject omission, mazes); *Content Units* (based on information conveyed); *Complex Sentences*. Complexity is defined as a sentence which contains at least one independent clause and one or more dependent clause (p. 127). Non-finite clauses as in *the boy wants to get his knife* and conjoined clauses such as *the boy is trying to get a kite and rescue it* are not counted as independent clauses. Although this procedure can capture some varied aspects of spoken output it is not without some problems. First, the criteria for segmenting the data depend on semantic and prosodic criteria which may not correspond with grammatical boundaries in aphasic speakers and may, for example, result in the under-estimation of grammatical structures used by aphasic speakers who frequently pause. Second, categorising features such as subject omission under Errors is problematic if we are dealing with spontaneous speech where subject omission is permissible in certain situations. These observations should not detract, however, from the overall strength of this system but investigators who wish to obtain a more detailed analysis of grammatical features in spontaneous speech may wish to consider other procedures which focus on grammar.

Some grammatical profiles of aphasic speakers have been produced. Penn and Berhmann (1986) used LARSP (Crystal *et al.*, 1976), a procedure originally developed to quantify child language, with a group of aphasic people. More recently, procedures specifically designed for the quantification of grammatical aspects of adult aphasic speech have been developed. There are two recently published procedures which we will consider before moving on to describe our procedure. Saffran, Berndt and Schwartz (1989) produced the *Quantitative Production Analysis* (QPA) which offers quantification of lexical and syntactic features of output. Menn *et al.* (1994) published the *Linguistic Communicative Measure* which provides a measure of lexical output and the use of obligatory grammatical morphemes. The development of these procedures reflects the need to have some reliable way of quantifying grammatical aspects of aphasic speech. Saffran *et al.* provide a detailed method for producing a fine-grained analysis of certain lexical and grammatical aspects of a continuous narrative. They recommend a sample of minimally 150 words which are selected from the aphasic individual's retelling of a well-known fairy story. The corpus consists of 'narrative' words: all other lexical and phrasal items such as repetitions, comments, discourse markers, interruptions, are excluded. The profile obtained, therefore, is based on different material from that used in our profile which has been devised to describe all aspects of spontaneous speech and can therefore be used for conversational data as well as narrative.

The procedure published by Menn *et al.* (1994) was developed to measure change over time also in an aphasic speaker's ability to produce oral narratives. There are some similarities with the SSLA in that it aims to measure the aphasic speaker's grammatical ability as well as the ability to convey information by quantifying 'amount of information conveyed, emptiness of speech and grammatical acceptability' (p. 343). It yields two indices: *Lexical Efficiency*, which is computed by dividing the total number of words used by the content units produced, and the index of *Grammatical Support*, which is computed by adding the correct number of 'endings' (bound grammatical morphemes), to total number of correct words and dividing the summed result by the number of content words. In the example given by the authors, the determiner *the* and the auxiliary verb *is* are termed 'supporting words': *ing* and plural *s* are segmented as 'endings'. The authors claim that this procedure is a 'quick and dirty' indicator of syntactic ability and can be used by those with 'minimal clinical experience' and no linguistic training (p. 344). It is not surprising, therefore, that, as far as a grammatical analysis is concerned, this procedure offers a limited grammatical analysis focusing on the use of bound morphemes. It does not identify omission of bound morphemes in obligatory contexts, examine the speaker's use of verb phrases, agreement, argument structures or the speaker's ability to use phrasal and clausal constructions. Investigators who wish to examine these aspects of grammar need to turn elsewhere. The development of these and other procedures reflects the interest in quantifying spontaneous speech output and especially in providing ways for examining grammatical features of speech that aphasic speakers use when unrestrained by clinical elicitation tasks. We can also see that the quantification of output, even quantification of one aspect, in our case, grammatical, is by no means straightforward.

Our protocol, which is described below, is intended to be part of the assessment process but, in common with the procedures already discussed, does not provide a full aphasic assessment. It will be seen that the protocol has been developed from that used by researchers at Reading University to investigate child language. However, it has become apparent that LARSP, which is widely used to quantify child language, is only partly successful when applied to adult data. Saffran *et al.* (1989) have rightly observed that the unit for analysis, based on prosodic features, is not suitable for adult data and we have tried to address this point. In developing procedures for quantifying adult aphasic speech, we have addressed a number of issues. First, the analysis has to be comprehensive enough to capture the complexity of adult speech; second, we wish to establish a reliable unit of analysis based on grammatical criteria; third, we are concerned that the analyses should reveal not only the grammatical units used by a speaker but also the lexico-syntactic devices used to connect those units; and finally, we considered it desirable to provide some control data whereby we could judge aphasic performance. Reliable units of analysis are essential if we are to quantify total output, produce meaningful proportions or compare performance across subjects or over time. Identifying the grammatical relationships between units gives some measure of grammatical complexity in that, for example, it can separate those speakers who, although able to use clausal constructions, are less able to use subordinate clauses. However, such differences may only be apparent when aphasic performance is compared with normal performance. Equally, if we wish to measure severity of aphasia in terms of comparisons with unimpaired performance rather than in comparison with other aphasic performance, then we need to know what normal speakers do. There is, however, little information on normal grammatical performance, in comparison with what is available for child language, and although our normative data are limited, they give the clinician some kind of yardstick. We hope to increase our normative data and we are aware that we may have to adjust our norms in the light of this.

Building a Grammatical Profile

We will now describe the method, giving examples from our database. The examples are mainly from spontaneous speech data of one of our ten aphasic subjects, G, a 62-year-old male aphasic who had made a good recovery and had an Aphasia Quotient (Kertesz, 1982) of 0.83 at the time of recording. Despite this relatively good score it can be seen from the examples and the analyses below that he continued to have difficulty with connected speech although, on the whole, he communicated his message well. Controls were generally spouses of aphasic subjects, or people otherwise well acquainted with, and involved in, their aphasic condition.

Data Illustration

In our research, we have collected recordings of both conversational and monologic speech, each under two conditions. In this section we shall illustrate from conversational speech on the topic of the onset of aphasia, which, in the data collected to date, seems to be most productive, from aphasic and control subjects alike. We have based the analyses on samples sized at 100 Text Units (TUs, see Section 2), which is larger than those usually recommended in the field, and therefore likely to be more representative.

We will now look at a brief example of text which is formatted according to the considerations outlined in Section 2. It is taken from part of his description of events just prior to his stroke. As with the child data, each TU is given a separate line and coded for the type and subtype, as in Table 6.11. Various features are revealed by this short example which will now be discussed. We will start by examining the types of TUs which G uses.

Clausal TUs can be seen at lines 2, 9, 11, 13, 14. Two clauses (at lines 11 and 13) have the same internal structure, that is, two elements, the verb plus adverbial. In both these clauses, the omission of the subject is permissible but we note that the subject is present in the other three examples (lines 2, 9 and 14). Adverbial complements occur as part of the clause structure in lines 9 (*away*), 11 (*up the road*) 13 (*to bed*) and 14 (*down*). Line 2 is tagged as a clausal TU although it contains a paraphasic element, because, in this case, the structure of the TU is not put in doubt by the paraphasia. Where it is impossible to judge grammatical status the TU would be marked as *unintelligible* (see below).

Table 6.11: Sample worksheet, aphasic adult G

Adult G Age 62		Text unit categories					
No.	Text	Unc	Min	Lex	Phr	Cla	IGR
1	well		O				
2	it *was* a bit (F) merkary					SVC	
3	no		O				
4	(F) it was as	I					
5	oh dear		O				
6	it was a bit (F)	I					
7	driving	Amb					
8	'nthat		O				
9	and of course I put me car away					a Cl	
10	like		O				
11	and walked up the road					a Cl	
12	'nthat		O				
13	and went to bed					a Cl	
14	and when I come down					a Cl	
15	in the morning				PDN		A
16	I was going to take (F) pota-	I					
17	no		O				
18	(F) onions			N			
19	'nthat		O				
20	up to me brother-in-law				PDN		
		4	8	1	2	5	1

Note: (F) = filled pause.

Phrasal TUs are found just at lines 15 and 20. The first is an example of an adjunct to the immediately preceding clause (the temporal phrase *in the morning* not being required by the verb of the preceding clause), and as such is indented here to indicate that it is linked by the IGR of type A. Not all phrasal TUs have a close relationship with the previous clause. In line 20, there is another phrasal construction *up to me brother-in-law*, but it is not immediately linked to its clause (in line 16). The distinction here is one of linearisation: the speaker's grammatical planning is interrupted by intervening TUs, in which he corrects *pota-* to *onions* and inserts two Minor elements *no* and *'nthat*.

Lexical TUs occur just at line 18, which can unequivocally be designated *noun*, and at line 7, which is more problematic. Such words receive grammatical status from context which is missing here. The previous text units suggest that the speaker is still looking for a descriptor to complete *it was* having tried to self-correct at lines 3 to 6, but there are other possible explanations. The item *driving* is therefore tagged as ambiguous, within the *unclear* category.

Minor TUs, even in this short example, are found on eight of the 20 lines. Intuitively, this would seem to be a high proportion although it is obviously important to consider a larger sample in order to see how representative this frequency is. The Minors used are all what LARSP would call Other (non-Response), and seem to have two functions: *no* and *oh dear* follow incomplete TUs or lexical errors (lines 2/3 and 4/5) and mark self-corrections; *well, like* and *'nthat* are more typical of fluent discoursal markers. Both these types of Minors might have been used by G before he was aphasic but, as we will see below, our analysis suggests a significant frequency of Minors and correspondingly low use of grammatically productive TUs in G compared with our normal controls.

Incomplete TUs are syntactically the most abnormal type, occurring here in lines 4, 6 and 16. However, such TUs also occur in the control data when, for example, the speaker backtracks or inserts a discoursal comment. In the following example the speaker (normal control, retelling the Noah's Ark story) breaks off at line 22 to check a word:

		TUs
21	and he saved all the animals	C
22	male and female of (each) (F) each	I
23	you can't say variety	C
24	can you	C

Or the speaker may self-correct, as at line 27 in the following example:

		TUs
25	(F) and I said	C
26	I'll get you a drink of water	C
27	what's	I
28	try and tell me	C
29	what's happened	C

However, as with the Minor TUs, Incompletes may be much more frequent in certain types of aphasic speech.

IGRs between adjacent TUs are infrequent in the G data (there is just the one, type A, referred to already in the above excerpt) although others did occur in the full transcript, e.g. the *that*-clause (Type T) in lines 32/33 below:

		TUs	IGRs
30	and (F) then (F)	I	
31	(and she said) and she said (F)	I	
32	she was saying	C	
33	that I was Garry	C	T
34	like	M	

G's infrequent use and restricted range of IGRs can be seen as an index of syntactic difficulty. Such difficulty is clearly present in non-fluent aphasic speech, but fluent aphasic speech may also exhibit similar characteristics.

Frequency and Normal Controls

If we now make some i-N comparisons (see first section, this chapter), we shall be in a position to firm up some of our impressionistic judgements about G's speech. In Table 6.12 we compare 100 Text Units from G with similar-sized samples collected from 10 control subjects on the same topic. In this comparison we have chosen to compare G's total scores with the range exhibited by the controls rather than the means. This is because, first, the range gives an indication of normal variation and, second, we want to see whether G's performance falls within that range rather than whether his score matches the mean.

Table 6.12: Aphasic (G)'s TU types in relation to control group range

	Unclear	Minor	Lexical	Phrasal	Clausal
G	15	37	8	12	28
Control range	1–7	3–21	4–15	10–31	41–84

A number of features are highlighted by this comparison. Unclear and Minor TUs are considerably more frequent in G's speech than in any of the control subjects; the proportions of Lexical and Phrasal TUs fall within the normal range; the proportion of clausal TUs falls well below the normal range. We now need to compare G's IGRs with those used by the normal controls and we can see from Table 6.13 that, overall, G uses fewer IGRs than any of our control subjects.

Table 6.13: Aphasic (G)'s IGR types in relation to control group range

	Type A	Other IGRs	Total IGRs
G	10	6	21
Control range	10–34	10–29	27–25

More significantly, G's low use of IGRs seems to be based on the types other than A. These are phrasal extensions of clausal constructions, and their incidence in G's speech just falls within normal limits, whilst the types that mark clause–clause links fall below the normal range, and may reflect a syntactic impairment that is reflected also in the low incidence of clausal TUs.

At this point, we may recall that some potential IGRs were 'lost' by G's frequent use of Minor and Incomplete TUs. The increase in Minors might be a conversational strategy used by the speaker or, more likely, a feature not within the speaker's conscious control but one that arises as a consequence of the aphasia and is specifically related to his reduced lexical access and/or his reduced ability to construct clauses and deploy grammatical linking devices between these clauses. It would be interesting to investigate whether G can link TU without the intrusion of Minor TUs. At this point a clinician might choose to devise a series of tasks to test this skill. Alternatively, or in addition to further exploration of G's grammatical abilities via specially designed tasks, the investigator may turn the focus of the assessment to G's lexicon: as clausal construction seems to be compromised it would also be important to examine the distribution of verbs.

Distribution of Main Verbs

For this analysis we will examine the distribution of main verbs which carry meaning, are usually designated as 'open' class, and which might be implicated if the speaker has problems of lexical access. Auxiliaries and catenative verbs which have a different function have been excluded, as has the copular form of *to be* in this illustrative analysis.

In the same 100 TU sample as used before, G had 15 different main verb types, and 30 tokens, just below the normal range (and so also with the Type–Token Ratio, TTR; see Table 6.14).

We already know, from the TU analysis and the low number of clausal constructions found, that G has most difficulty with clausal syntax, and we may now see that this may need to be interpreted in the light of the verb data. Although G is not far below the normal range, this might be an area to explore further in therapy; improved verb retrieval may result in continuous speech which has a greater proportion of clausally organised and linked TUs.

Table 6.14: Aphasic (G)'s verb types and tokens in relation to control group range

	Types	Tokens	TTR
G	15	30	0.50
Controls range	20–44	35–60	0.57–0.78

Conclusion

The approach we have outlined in this chapter has started from consideration of certain linguistic features that we think ought to be reflected in syntactic assessment. We have argued that error analysis is appropriate as long as it is part of a broader assessment of language abilities. Specifically, we have called attention to the distinction between phrase and clause syntax, as well as morphology; the distinction between adjuncts and complements; the different roles of hierarchical and linear organisation of constituents in syntax; the determination of units of syntactic organisation as actually observed in unplanned speech; and the many and varied relations that these units enter into, to build up into discourse.

We have illustrated a framework of assessment that addresses all these issues, in a way that allows decisions to be made (the analyst is free to 'set the switches' as seems appropriate), but ensures that they do not go by default. Explicitness establishes the conditions under which comparisons can be made more effectively, or not at all. We have considered what sorts of comparisons are useful in clinical assessment, and we have illustrated how such an approach may accommodate both child and adult data.

Finally, what can we say about the nature of language impairment, in these terms? Clearly, this has not been our main focus, but the question is fundamental. Our view derives from what we take to be the most pressing issue for linguistics in clinical practice: the provision of highly motivated, well-articulated assessment procedures for the purpose of intervention. This is at the heart of the profile (as distinct from the global score), which should deliver an outcome in terms of remedial goals. At any stage in clinical assessment, a particular client's profile will reflect a complex function of factors deriving from that client's individual language abilities as well as the impairment that may be present. In the remedial history of a particular client, it may never be clear exactly what the nature of the impairment is, or where the boundary is between impaired and intact abilities. It is for research to improve our knowledge of language impairment as such, to establish norms of language variation, and to identify reliable indices of language impairment. Meanwhile, clinical practice cannot, and should not, wait upon the determination of such issues. Assessment of the client's particular and complex needs will always require the skills of linguistically trained clinicians who are aware of the limitations of standard assessments, and who can supplement them with specific investigative procedures of their own devising.

References

Beattie, G. (1983). *Talk: An Analysis of Speech and Nonverbal Behaviour in Conversation.* Milton Keynes: Open University Press.

Blake, J., Quartaro, G. and Onorati, S. (1993). Evaluating quantitative measures of grammatical complexity in spontaneous speech samples. *Journal of Child Language* 20, 139–152.

Bolinger, D.L. (1952). Linear modification. *Publications of the Modern Language Association* 67, 1117–1144.

Brown, R. (1973). *A First Language: The Early Stages*. Cambridge, MA: Harvard University Press.

Butcher, A. (1981). Aspects of the speech pause: phonetic correlates and communicative functions. *Arbeitsberichte* 15, Institut fur Phonetik, Universitat Kiel.

Butterworth, B. (1980). Evidence from pauses in speech. In: Butterworth, B. (Ed.), *Language Production: Speech and Talk*. London: Academic Press.

Coltheart, M. (1983). Aphasia therapy research: a single-case study approach. In: Code, C. and Muller, D.J. (Eds.), *Aphasia Therapy*. London: Edward Arnold.

Crystal, D. (1979). Neglected grammatical factors in conversational English. In: Greenbaum, S., Leech, G. and Svartvik, J. (Eds.), *Studies in English Linguistics: For Randolph Quirk*. London: Longman.

Crystal, D., Fletcher, P. and Garman, M. (1976). *The Grammatical Analysis of Language Disability*. London: Edward Arnold. (2nd edn, 1981).

Edwards, S. and Garman, M. (1989). Case study of an adult. In: Grunwell, P. and James, A. (Eds.), *The Functional Evaluation of Language Disorders*. Beckenham: Croom Helm.

Fletcher, P. (1987). Tense and time adverbials in normal and language-impaired children. Paper presented to the Philological Society, March.

Fletcher, P. (1992). Sub-groups in school-age language-impaired children. In: Fletcher, P. and Hall, D. (Eds.), *Specific Speech and Language Disorders in Children: Correlates, Characteristics and Outcomes*. London: Whurr Publishers.

Fletcher, P. and Garman, M. (1988). LARSPing by numbers: a response to French. *British Journal of Disorders of Communication* 23, 309–322.

Fletcher, P., Garman, M., Johnson, M., Schelletter, C. and Stodel, L. (1986). Characterizing language impairment in terms of normal language development: advantages and limitations. In: *Proceedings of the Seventh Annual Wisconsin Symposium on Research in Child Language Disorders*. Madison: University of Wisconsin-Madison.

French, A. (1988). The LARSP profile of the normal 5 year old, with special reference to phrase structure. *British Journal of Disorders of Communication* 23, 293–308.

Garman, M. (1989a). Syntactic assessment of expressive language. In: Grundy, K. (Ed.), *Linguistics in Clinical Practice*, Ist edn. London: Taylor & Francis.

Garman, M. (1989b). The role of linguistics in speech therapy: assessment and interpretation. In: Grunwell, P. and James, A. (Eds.), *The Functional Evaluation of Language Disorders*. Beckenham: Croom Helm.

Garman, M. (1990). *Psycholinguistics*. Cambridge: Cambridge University Press.

Garrett, M.F. (1982). Production of speech: observations from normal and pathological language use. In: Ellis, A. W. (Ed.), *Normality and Pathology in Cognitive Functions*. London: Academic Press.

Gavin, W.J., Klee, T. and Membrino, I. (1993). Differentiating specific language impairment from normal language development using grammatical analysis. *Clinical Linguistics and Phonetics* 7, 191–206.

Gee, P. and Grosjean, F. (1983). Performance structures: a psycholinguistic and linguistic appraisal. *Cognitive Psychology* 15, 411–458.

Goldman-Eisler, F. (1968). *Psycholinguistics: Experiments in Spontaneous Speech*. London: Academic Press.

Goodglass, H. and Kaplan, E. (1983). *Boston Diagnostic Aphasia Examination (BDAE)*. Philadelphia: Lea & Febiger.

Gutfreund, M., Harrison, and Wells, G. (1989). *Bristol Language Development Scales (BLADES)*. Windsor: NFER-Nelson.

Huddleston, R. (1984). *Introduction to the Grammar of English*. Cambridge: Cambridge University Press.

Kay, J. Lesser, R. And Coltheart, M. (1992). *Psycholinguistic Assessment of Language Processing in Aphasia (PALPA)*. London: Erlbaum.

Kertesz, A. (1982). *Western Aphasia Battery (WAB)*. London: Grune & Stratton.

Klee, T. and Paul, R. (1981). A comparison of six structural analysis procedures: a case study. In: Miller, J. (Ed.), *Assessing Language Production in Children: Experimental Procedures*. Baltimore, MD: University Park Press.

Lee, L. L. (1974). *Developmental Sentence Analysis (DSA:DST DSS)*. Evanston, IL: Northwestern University.

Leonard, L. (1992). The use of morphology by children with specific language impairment: evidence from three languages. In: Chapman, R.S. (Ed.), *Processes in Language Acquisition and Disorders*. St. Louis: Mosby.

Mejia, L. and Eslava-Cobos, J. (1989). Disorders in language acquisition and cerebral maturation: a neurophysiological perspective. In: Ardila, A. and Ostosky-Solis, F. (Eds.), *Brain Organization of Language and Cognitive Processes*. New York: Plenum.

Menn, L., Ramsberger, G. and Helm-Estabrooks, N. (1994). A linguistic communication measure for aphasic narratives. *Aphasiology* 8, 343–359.

Menyuk, P. (1964). Comparison of grammar of children with functionally deviant and normal speech. *Journal of Speech and Hearing Research* 7, 109–121.

Miller, J. (1987). A grammatical characterization of language disorder. In: Martin, J.A.M., Fletcher, P., Grunwell, P. and Hall, D. (Eds.), *Proceedings of the First International Symposium on Specific Speech and Language Disorders in Children*. London: AFASIC.

Miller, J. (1992). Lexical development in young children with Down Syndrome. In: Chapman, R.S. (Ed.), *Processes in Language Acquisition and Disorders*. St. Louis: Mosby.

Miller, J. and Chapman, R. (1985). *SALT: Systematic Analysis of Language Transcripts*. Madison: Language Analysis Laboratory, Waisman Centre on Mental Retardation and Human Development, University of Wisconsin-Madison.

Morehead, D. and Ingram, D. (1973). The development of base syntax in normal and linguistically deviant children. *Journal of Speech and Hearing Research* 16, 330–352.

Penn, C. and Behrmann, M. (1986). Towards a classification scheme for aphasic syntax. *British Journal of Disorders of Communication* 21, 21–23.

Perkins, M. (1994). Repetitiveness in language disorders: a new analytical procedure. *Clinical Linguistics and Phonetics* 8, 321–336.

Quirk, R., Greenbaum, S., Leech, G. and Svartvik, J. (1985). *A Comprehensive Grammar of the English Language*. London: Longman.

Radford, A. (1988). *Transformational Syntax*. Cambridge: Cambridge University Press.

Saffran, E., Berndt, R. and Schwartz, M. (1989). The quantitative analysis of agrammatic production: procedure & data. *Brain & Language* 37, 440–479.

Shewan, C. (1988). The Shewan Spontaneous Language Analysis (SSLA) system for aphasic adults: description, reliability and validity. *Journal of Communication Disorders* 21, 103–138.

Wells, G. (1985). *Language Development in the Pre-School Years*. Cambridge: Cambridge University Press.

Chapter 7
Investigating
Comprehension of Syntax

M. HAZEL DEWART

Introduction

An adult is reading a story to a young child. Is the child understanding what is being said and following the story? How can the adult tell? Perhaps the child looks interested, nods occasionally, asks a relevant question, laughs at an appropriate point. If the child is not giving these clear signals, it is quite difficult to tell the extent of the child's understanding. This is because the process of understanding is essentially an internal, covert activity that is not directly observable.

In investigating a person's understanding of language we are trying to find ways of making this internal process open to scrutiny. We have to find subtle ways of determining whether a person understands what is said, perhaps by giving instructions and asking the person to carry them out, by asking him or her to match words, phrases or sentences with real or pictorial referents, by posing questions to determine how appropriately they are answered or by carefully observing instances where the person seems spontaneously to have misunderstood what has been said.

In the psycholinguistic literature a considerable amount of creativity has been expended in devising ways of investigating people's understanding of a wide range of aspects of syntax. In this chapter, I argue that clinicians can make use of methods and approaches from psycholinguistic research and that to do so will enrich their clinical work in this area.

It must be acknowledged that clinical applications are often difficult to draw from research, which typically takes the form of group studies devised to test particular psycholinguistic hypotheses. The clinician is faced with an individual client and has to assess the extent of that person's abilities and difficulties in understanding language. Some judgement as to the explanation for any difficulties that may be found has also to be made. In an attempt to bridge this gap between research and clinicians' needs, I will approach this chapter from the context of clinical work: a client's comprehension of syntax is to be investigated.

How can we go about it? What factors have to be taken into account in considering an individual's performance?

The chapter will focus on the comprehension of syntactic aspects of language, though it will be argued that comprehension of syntax can never be studied to the exclusion of other aspects of language and of other factors that influence how people behave. The chapter will be mainly concerned with comprehension of the spoken as opposed to the written word.

Why Assess Syntactic Understanding?

The answer to this question is that a person's knowledge of syntax is not necessarily reflected in their speech. This disparity can operate in two directions. Sometimes, one may suspect that an individual has more knowledge of syntax than is evident from his or her output. Some children with physical disability have little or no ability to produce spoken language but show clear evidence of some comprehension. On the other hand, instances can be found of syntactic structures being produced without full understanding of what they mean. The developmental relationship between production and comprehension of language is a complex one and does not necessarily conform to the notion that comprehension always and necessarily precedes production (Bloom and Lahey, 1978). Some autistic children may produce well-formed phrases or sentences but in situations to which they are inappropriate. A particularly dramatic example of the possible disparity between comprehension and production is presented by Curtiss (1982). She describes a boy with such severe cognitive impairment that he was virtually untestable on most assessments. He often misunderstood what was said to him and produced utterances that were semantically inappropriate. Nevertheless, the utterances were well formed syntactically. For example, when told to 'Draw a picture of Vivian', he said 'No it's not Vivian's, it's mine'. A person's level of syntactic understanding cannot, therefore, necessarily be predicted from their level of spoken language.

How is Language Comprehension Investigated?

Approaches to the investigation of language comprehension range from observation of a person's spontaneous comprehension in natural or slightly contrived communicative situations, to tightly controlled experimental tasks. Most studies have used one of a small number of techniques. Many have used the *picture choice* technique where the person has to choose a picture to match a phrase or sentence spoken by the investigator. The other most commonly employed technique is the *acting-out* task where the person has to carry out the actions involved in the sentence using a set of small objects or toys. Other techniques involve judgements, for example judgements of whether a sentence is grammatical or not, of which of two versions of a sentence sounds better or of whether or not a particular sentence is a correct description of a picture. Sometimes the person has to answer a series of questions devised to investigate how well a story or other piece of connected discourse has been understood. Sometimes the person is observed in a more natural setting where particular types of question or instruction are slipped into the conversation, an approach closer to everyday use of language but more difficult to control systematically.

In the widely used picture choice task, a match has to be made between a phrase or sentence and a picture that represents it. The appropriate picture is chosen from a number of other pictures, or distractors, which have been carefully selected to contrast with the correct picture in ways which help determine whether the response was based on the particular grammatical feature being investigated. For example, if the test sentence is 'The boy is being pushed by the girl', then an array of pictures might show the following:

| Girl pushing boy | Man pushing boy |
| Man pushing girl | Boy pushing girl |

Here the 'boy pushing girl' picture is the critical distractor for determining whether someone understands the word order distinction between active and passive sentences. The other pictures are lexical distractors, pictures that correspond to the test sentence except for one content word. Inclusion of these means that the person is less likely to choose the correct picture merely on the basis of recognising one of the content words.

Performance on the picture choice task will be influenced by the person's ability to interpret pictorial representations and it cannot always be assumed that a child, or an adult with brain injury, will interpret a picture in the same way as the investigator. Performance will also be influenced by the ability to attend one by one to a series of pictures and to discriminate between them. In addition, the range of possible errors is determined by the set of alternative pictures provided by the investigator.

In the acting-out task the person must act out a sentence spoken by the investigator, either by carrying out an action or by manipulating objects or small toys. For example, the investigator may say 'Before moving the book, pick up the comb' or 'The lorry is pushed by the car', and the task is to move the objects appropriately. Sometimes the investigator selects the relevant objects from an array, whereas in other studies the person being tested has to choose the relevant objects from the array before beginning to act out the sentence.

Although the acting-out task gets round the problems associated with picture identification and the need to be able to attend one by one to a series of pictures, performance is very susceptible to the nature of the objects to be manipulated. For example, faced with a doll and a toy bed, young children will tend to put the doll in the bed, regardless of whether the instruction is to put the doll in, on, under or beside the bed. Several studies have demonstrated how the child's understanding of prepositions can be influenced by the conventional (or *canonical*) relationship between the objects chosen for acting out (Clark, 1973; Wilcox and Palermo, 1975). Another drawback is that some aspects of syntax do not lend themselves to the acting-out format. For example, number, tense and aspect of the verb are difficult to investigate in this mode.

In the clinical setting, performance may be influenced by familiarity with the objects concerned. In the case of some young children and people with severe cognitive impairment, recognition of miniature objects may be a problem.

Factors Influencing Comprehension of Syntax

Drawing conclusions as to whether or not a person understands a particular syntactic construction is not a straightforward matter. This is because understanding of language cannot take place in the absence of a shared social and situational context (Bransford and Nitsch, 1977). In everyday life a number of other linguistic and non-linguistic factors interact in the comprehension of language and these can never be totally excluded in any testing situation.

If, for example, someone makes no response at all to something that is said, this need not mean that the person failed to understand. He or she may have understood but regarded the message as uninteresting, a routine statement to be taken for granted, or even as something worthy of contempt.

If the person does make a response that seems to imply understanding, this response could have been based on other sources of inspiration, with little understanding of the language and no understanding of the syntax at all. A speaker's intentions can often be guessed on the basis of tone of voice, gesture or facial expression. Knowledge of familiar routines for saying the same thing in the same situation may also assist. Interpretation of what is said can be based largely on the linguistic or conversational *context*.

Semantic information also comes into play (see Landells, this volume). Any sentence involves semantic as well as syntactic information, and sentence comprehension tasks really involve syntactic/semantic mapping rather than syntactic comprehension *per se*. Many statements can be interpreted simply by knowing the meanings of some of the words and working out their most likely relationship with one another. Some sentences are strongly biased towards a particular interpretation. For example, whilst syntactically complex, it does not take much knowledge of syntax to work out who did the biting and who was bitten in a sentence like 'It was a dog that the postman was bitten by'. In psycholinguistic research such sentences are termed 'non-reversible' in contrast to 'reversible' sentences which could have their meaning reversed without rendering the sentence implausible. An example of such a reversible sentence would be, 'The politician criticised the journalist'.

Sometimes a statement may be interpreted on the basis of cues from the situation in which it is expressed; children find it easier to act out 'The red car is pushed by the blue car' if they are holding the blue car rather than the red car (Huttenlocher, Eisenberg and Strauss, 1968). If both cars are in a 'car park' in front of them, they will often select the car parked nearer to their dominant hand as the one to do the pushing (Bridges, 1980). Older children and adults are less likely to be misled by implausible sentences or statements that violate situational expectations but they can still be influenced by them and this may show up in a longer response time. Thus, in investigating someone's understanding of syntax, semantic and situational influences must always be taken into consideration.

Anyone attempting to devise a task to investigate syntactic comprehension should be aware that it is never possible to eliminate these other factors totally. Comprehension cannot be investigated in a vacuum and whatever situation is chosen to carry out the investigation will carry with it its own set of expectations (Bridges, 1985). Nouns may be equated for animacy, toys and testing materials may be equated for size, conventional relationships between objects may be avoided and care may be taken not to stress one or other of the words in presenting a test sentence. These measures have their value in keeping context consistent from one test item to the next. However, despite all these measures, given a difficult or unfamiliar utterance to interpret, the person is unlikely just to give up. Instead, he or she will use some aspect of the linguistic input or some aspect of the non-linguistic, interpersonal situation as a basis for an interpretation. People can create their own context for an utterance, however hard an investigator tries to prevent them doing so.

Rather than attempting to exclude these factors, it is more realistic to acknowledge their role in the process of language comprehension and in the testing situation. Thus, a person's use of linguistic and non-linguistic context is an aspect which can be investigated in studying language comprehension.

Explaining Language Comprehension Difficulties

We have considered briefly the situations where a person fails to make a response, or makes an inappropriate response to language input. What can we conclude when a person gives incorrect responses? In clinical investigations, it is sometimes easy to jump to the conclusion that difficulty on tasks devised to test some aspect of understanding of language reflects a lack of linguistic knowledge. Thus, difficulty with sentences designed to test knowledge of relative clause constructions might be taken to imply that a person has incomplete knowledge of that syntactic construction. However, the difficulties may be caused not by a lack of linguistic knowledge so much as by problems associated with psychological processes involved in sentence comprehension. Such processes as auditory perception, selective attention and memory are all involved in language comprehension tasks and may be at the root of the difficulties displayed. In the clinical setting, it is important, though not easy, to determine the extent to which someone's problems with language comprehension tasks are caused by these more general psychological factors as opposed to linguistic factors or, alternatively, to a combination of the two.

When a client's comprehension of syntax is to be investigated, there is a series of questions to ask:

1. How does the client compare with others of the same age or status on comprehension of syntax?
2. Which syntactic constructions does the person understand and which give difficulty?
3. Why is the person having the difficulties that may be found? What processes underlie someone's comprehension of syntax?

These questions will be examined one by one and possible approaches to answering them presented.

How Does the Person Compare With Others of the Same Age or Status on Comprehension of Syntax?

This will often be the first question in the clinician's mind but, although this information is important, it is merely a first step. The usual way of approaching this question is by the use of standardised tests. In the development of these tests, a set of items is devised and presented to a number of people (usually representing a range of age-groups) using the same instructions and under similar conditions. Their performance can then be used to compare the level of performance of individual clients.

A number of standardised tests of language include items designed to test syntactic comprehension and some tests have been devised expressly for this purpose. Tests of both types are listed in Table 7.1.

Table 7.1: Tests of syntactic comprehension

Tests for children:
Northwestern Syntax Screening Test (Lee, 1969)
Test for Reception of Grammar (TROG) (Bishop, 1983)
Test for Auditory Comprehension of Language (Carrow, 1973)
Sentence Comprehension Test – Revised Version (Wheldall, Mittler and Hobsbaum, 1987)
Derbyshire Language Scheme (Revised): Detailed Test of Comprehension (Knowles and Masidlover, 1987)
Reynell Developmental Language Scales: Verbal Comprehension Scale (Reynell, 1977)
Clinical Evaluation of Language Function (CELF) (Semel and Wiig, 1980)

Tests for adults:
Token Test (De Renzi and Vignolo, 1962)
Boston Diagnostic Aphasia Examination (Goodglass and Kaplan, 1972)
Test for Reception of Grammar (TROG) (Bishop, 1983) – designed for children but centiles for 12-year-olds can be used for adults passing up to 18 blocks

Most of these tests involve a series of sentences providing a range of syntactic constructions. Whilst some of the tests (e.g. the Reynell test and the Token Test) use the acting-out technique, most use a picture-choice task.

Each of these tests has its strengths and weaknesses as an assessment tool and there is not space to review them individually here. The reader is referred to Darley (1979), Byng, Kay, Edmundson and Scott (1990) and Kersner (1992) for reviews of a number of the tests. There are, however, several points which should be taken into account in evaluating the available tests and selecting from them.

Like any psychometric assessment, a test of comprehension of syntax should be reliable and valid and provide evidence that it is so in the test manual. Not all the tests listed in Table 7.1 provide such information. The test should cover a range of syntactic structures and the rationale for the choice of structures should be discussed. Some structures may have been excluded from tests for reasons to do with test construction rather than because the structures themselves are not of interest. For example, structures may be excluded because they are difficult to represent pictorially or, as in the case of Wh-questions, because they are difficult to fit into either the picture-choice or acting-out format.

The rationale for the proposed order of difficulty of items should also be clear. Order of difficulty should not be confounded with sentence length so that the more complex sentences are also longer and thus make more demands on memory.

Another major consideration is the number of items included of each syntactic construction. The *Test for Auditory Comprehension of Language* (Carrow, 1973), for example, has only one sentence of each syntactic construction. On one item the guessing rate is 0.33 because one of the three pictures is correct. Even with tests where there are more items for each construction, one cannot draw conclusions about whether a person understands a particular structure unless there is a clear criterion set out for doing so. The *TROG* (Bishop, 1983) has four items of each construction and four pictures to choose from for each. The chances of getting all four correct on the basis of chance is 0.004. The test can, therefore, be used to determine a client's level of performance on individual constructions.

It is clearly important that the client is familiar with the vocabulary used in the test sentences, otherwise errors could be due to failure to understand the vocabulary rather than the syntax. Some tests pay little attention to this factor, whereas others encourage pre-testing in cases where there is doubt. *TROG*, for example, provides cards for pre-testing vocabulary.

Standardised tests that allow an individual to be compared with others of the same age or status on language comprehension certainly are of value to the clinician. They can help in determining whether someone's understanding of language is in line with their cognitive abilities or whether syntactic understanding is an area of particular difficulty for them. It can also be of interest to compare performance on a language comprehension test with performance on some assessment of production of language (though direct comparisons cannot be made unless both assessments were standardised on the same population). The score may be valuable as a baseline measure against which future progress should be monitored. It is also one way of communicating about some aspects of a child's abilities to other professionals.

It should be stressed, however, that such tests provide only a preliminary estimate of general comprehension ability and these estimates are subject to the same limitations as all language scores derived from psychometric tests (see Muller, 1985). For example, they are based on assumptions that language behaviour is normally distributed and that language can be assessed in one particular context without taking into account a range of natural contexts of use. In addition, scores for children and adults with particular types of disability have to be compared with norms for people without such disabilities (see further Chapters 6 and 9, this volume).

It is important to be aware that some people have specific language comprehension difficulties which may not be evident from scores on the sorts of tests described in this section. So, for example, on tests such as the *Boston Diagnostic Aphasia Examination*, people with Broca's aphasia will tend to show relatively intact comprehension compared with limited spoken output. However, on more specific testing a comprehension deficit may become apparent (Schwartz, Saffran and Marin, 1980).

In order to explore a person's language comprehension more fully so that remediation can be planned, it is necessary to investigate further. Multiple presentations of particular linguistic constructions should be carried out with such factors as context, semantic variables, sentence length and modality (written/spoken/signed) being systematically varied. The following sections will address these issues.

Which Syntactic Constructions Does the Person Understand and Which Give Difficulty?

In order to draw up a profile of someone's command of syntax, we need to know whether there are constructions which give that person particular difficulty, and others which are well understood. Most standardised tests have too few of each construction type and/or too narrow a range of constructions for this information to be gained satisfactorily.

We have, then, to devise a way of investigating an individual's understanding of particular syntactic constructions. Curtiss and her colleagues were faced with just this sort of task in the early stages of their psycholinguistic study of Genie (Curtiss, 1977). Genie was a young girl who had been brought up in virtual isolation from her early years until puberty. When she was discovered at the age of 13;9 with barely any communicative behaviour, she became the subject of an intensive study and remediation project. Curtiss wanted to measure Genie's performance and to monitor her progress on a range of syntactic constructions that went beyond the scope of the available standardised tests. She therefore devised a range of tests which are described in detail in the appendix to her book (Curtiss, 1977).

The tests involved multiple presentations of each linguistic structure and attempted as far as possible to eliminate semantic and pragmatic cues as a basis for interpretation. For instance, to test Genie's comprehension of the personal possessive pronoun, a picture of a boy and girl standing together was used, as well as Genie's and the investigator's own bodies. Genie's understanding of the vocabulary used in the test having been checked, she was then given a series of fourteen instructions asking her to point to, for example, 'their mouths', 'my chin', 'our noses'. To test comprehension of elements of the tense/aspect system Genie was shown sets of three pictures showing, for example, a girl about to open an umbrella, a girl in the act of opening an umbrella and a girl with a fully opened umbrella. She heard Curtiss talk a little about each picture and was instructed, 'Show me "The girl opened the umbrella"' or 'Show me "She is opening the umbrella"'. Apart from its intrinsic fascination, this study is of interest here for the systematic way in which these comprehension tests were planned.

There is scope for creativity in devising tests of this nature. A set of sentences of a particular structure or structures is presented under controlled conditions and the number and type of errors recorded. There must be a sufficient number of sentences of each construction to allow conclusions to be drawn and a clear criterion set in advance as to what level of performance will be taken to mean that the person does understand that construction.

It is important to remember that people may well be influenced by aspects of the test materials and the interpersonal situation in dealing with such comprehension tasks, and to be alert to this possibility in designing tests, and during testing and in analysing test scores, as will be discussed in the next section.

What Processes Underlie the Person's Comprehension of Syntax?

Ideally, we would approach this question from the viewpoint of a particular model of the cognitive processes involved in language comprehension and of the way these processes can be impaired. The consequences of different types of impairment on a range of comprehension tasks would be understood, allowing inferences to be drawn from performances on these tasks to underlying impairment. In an even more idealised world, knowledge of the nature of the processing impairment would have clear implications for our choice of a set of remediation strategies for the client. Although this general approach is the one actively being employed by cognitive neuropsychologists concerned with language processing (for a review see Ellis and Young, 1988), the psycholinguistic processes underlying language comprehension and its impairment are still far from being well understood (Howard, 1985).

We can, nevertheless, begin to gain some impression of the way people are going about language comprehension by studying their pattern of performance across construction types, across contexts and across comprehension tasks. We can observe whether their error pattern is random or systematic. Errors may be more likely to occur on sentences that extend beyond a certain length, that involve syntactic rules or representations of a particular type, that do not conform to the typical subject–verb–object word order, or that violate the usual semantic expectations. This type of investigation cannot be done without going beyond the available standardised tests, although *TROG* (Bishop, 1983) does give guidelines for beginning to look at some of these questions.

The cognitive neuropsychologists have pointed to the value of carefully designed and documented single case studies of people with comprehension difficulties in exploring these issues. It is interesting to take as an example a study carried out by Butterworth, Campbell and Howard (1986). They studied a subject, R.E., who had been found to have a severely reduced digit span and impaired phonological processing. Despite this fact, she had passed 'O' and 'A' level examinations and had a BA honours degree in Psychology. It might be predicted that a person with short-term memory limitations would show deficits in the comprehension of lengthy complex sentences. Intriguingly, Butterworth *et al.* found that, although R.E. showed impaired performance on sentence repetition, her performance was unimpaired on syntactic analysis and comprehension of long and complex material. What is of interest here is how Butterworth *et al.* approached the task of studying R.E.'s comprehension.

They began by testing R.E. on the *Token Test* (De Renzi and Vignolo, 1962) which required her to follow complicated instructions by manipulating cardboard tokens. The materials were presented under three conditions: aurally, in written form for reading silently, and in written form for reading aloud.

R.E. was also tested on *TROG* (Bishop, 1983) which was presented in both spoken and written form. This test has not been standardised with adults but is sometimes used in assessing adult clients whose scores can be compared with the 12-year-olds in the standardisation sample.

A more demanding sentence comprehension task was then devised, this time a verification task. On this task R.E. had to decide whether each of a set of syntactically complex reversible sentences such as 'The train is preceded by the horse which is above the square' was an accurate description of a picture. The picture either correctly depicted the sentence or involved a mismatch for one of the nouns, one of the verbs, or one of the prepositions in the sentence. As the sentences are reversible, correct performance on this task involves knowledge of syntactic structure.

R.E. was then tested on her ability to make difficult grammatical judgements, a task similar to that employed by Linebarger, Schwartz and Saffran (1983). She therefore had to judge whether sentences such as 'The backs of chairs were never designed to be suitable places *OF hanging fur coats' were grammatical or not.

This study provides an example of the way a single case study can proceed, with the use of standardised tests being supplemented by tasks devised to test out hypotheses about specific aspects of comprehension processing. Where tasks were not standardised, Butterworth *et al.* (1986) compared R.E.'s performance with that of ten matched control subjects.

The value of detailed psycholinguistic testing of language comprehension has become particularly apparent in relation to Broca's (or 'agrammatic') aphasia (see Chapter 11, this volume). As mentioned above, people with this type of brain damage have limited spoken output of language, but their comprehension was traditionally thought to be relatively unimpaired as on some tests and in everyday conversations they seem to understand what is said to them without difficulty. More detailed testing, however, has shown that they *do* have difficulties with language comprehension. These difficulties arise where they have to rely on grammatical information from sentence structure to determine relational meanings. So they often make errors on sentences that are semantically reversible, e.g. 'The man that the woman is hugging is happy' but not on 'The bicycle that the boy is holding is broken' (Caramazza and Zurif, 1976). They may well interpret a simple active declarative sentence such as 'The policeman shot the robber' as meaning that the robber did the shooting (Schwartz *et al.*, 1980). Further evidence suggests that even this generalisation may not apply to all people with aphasia of Broca's type, some individuals, for example, having impairment on speech production without comprehension deficits (Berndt, 1987; Howard, 1985). Detailed testing of comprehension of syntax has therefore contributed to the cognitive neuropsychologists' questioning of the adequacy of traditional diagnostic categories such as Broca's and Wernicke's aphasia (Ellis and Young, 1988).

It is important, therefore, to investigate each client's ability to use syntactic information in sentence comprehension. A useful tool for this and many other aspects of psycholinguistic functioning is the *Psycholinguistic Assessments of Language Processing in Aphasia* (PALPA) developed by Kay, Lesser and Coltheart (1992). *PALPA* consists of a set of carefully designed and controlled tasks for investigating aspects of language processing and was developed as a resource for speech and language therapists and cognitive neuropsychologists. It is not a fully standardised test battery but a collection of tasks that can be drawn upon for use in single-case study and clinical work. Sentence processing is investigated by sentence picture-matching tasks which systematically vary syntactic structure and semantic variables. The *PALPA* tasks provide excellent examples of the way methods used in psycholinguistic research can be adapted for clinical investigations.

When we move from the study of adults to the study of children, we discover a considerable interest in finding out what language comprehension processes children employ in circumstances where the linguistic input is rather difficult for them. It seems that children strive to make sense of what they have heard and seen, and do so by drawing on what they know of the situation as a whole. Consequently, children's performances on tests devised to assess their comprehension of language may be influenced by such factors as their knowledge of the usual (or 'canonical') relationship between two objects (for example, boats usually go under rather than over bridges) or the physical characteristics of test materials such as their relative sizes or orientations, or the layout of the test materials in front of the child (Bridges, 1985).

Eventually children come to be able to ignore contextual cues and interpret correctly sentences that do not conform to situational constraints. Studies of children's language comprehension can look at how situational information is used in going about making sense of language and the extent to which it is relied upon. Much of the research on children's comprehension of language has been aimed at identifying the use of what have come to be termed 'sentence comprehension strategies' (Bever, 1970).

A comprehension strategy has been defined by Chapman (1977) as a short cut for arriving at sentence meaning without full marshalling of the information in the sentence and one's linguistic knowledge. The child may often appear to understand because the strategy yields the correct interpretation but occasionally the strategy will lead to an incorrect interpretation. By using sentences that violate expected strategies, we can observe whether children interpret them correctly or systematically misinterpret them and thus we can infer whether a strategy has been employed. One such strategy, often ascribed to 3-year-olds, is the 'probable event' strategy (Bever, 1970; Strohner and Nelson, 1974) by which children rely heavily on their knowledge of events in the world to help them interpret sentences. They may interpret sentences that are biased semantically by ignoring word order and going for the interpretation that seems to them to be most probable. They might, therefore, interpret both 'The girl holds the baby' and 'The baby holds the girl' as meaning that the girl was doing the holding.

Another example is the word order strategy first described by Bever (1970) which interprets a noun–verb–noun sequence as agent–action–object. Use of this strategy would lead a child to interpret reversible active sentences such as 'The boy pushes the girl' correctly but to reverse the correct interpretation of reversible passive sentences such as 'The girl is pushed by the boy'.

Another strategy appears to follow the minimal distance principle (Chomsky, 1969) by which the noun preceding a complement is taken to be the agent for that complement. A sentence such as 'John told Mary to go away' conforms to this principle and would be interpreted correctly by a child following such a strategy. However, sentences such as 'John promised Mary to go away' are exceptions to the principle and would be misinterpreted by a child who was following the strategy.

By the *order-of-mention strategy* (Clark, 1971), the order of clauses is taken to correspond to the order in which the events described occur. 'After the boy played football, he went to the shop' conforms to this principle whereas 'The boy played football after he went to the shop' does not conform and would be misinterpreted by someone using the strategy.

There is not space here to go into all the strategies that have been proposed (see Chapman, 1977), or some of the controversies in the area (Cromer, 1976; Bridges, 1980). It should be pointed out, however, that most of the research on such strategies has taken the form of group studies. Where individual children's patterns of response have been analysed (e.g. Dewart, 1975; 1991; Bridges, 1980; Tager-Flusberg, 1981), developmental trends have not emerged so clearly, and evidence of considerable individual differences in strategy usage have been found.

A number of fascinating case-studies have been published that raise the possibility that syntactic abilities may be acquired relatively independently of non-linguistic cognitive abilities. Cromer (1991) discussed the language of D.H., a girl with spina bifida whose speech was fluent and syntactically complex, despite a severely impaired level of functioning on general cognitive tests. Smith and Tsimpli (1991) described 'Christopher', a 'savant' who, despite limited intellectual ability, possesses a prodigious talent for learning foreign languages that allows him to translate on sight passages from some 15 or 16 different languages.

The syntactic processing of children with specific language impairment appears to provide an interesting counterpoint to such cases. A series of experiments by van der Lely has investigated in depth the syntactic processing abilities of a group of such children (e.g. van der Lely and Dewart, 1986; van der Lely and Harris, 1990; van der Lely, 1994). Like the individuals with Broca's aphasia described above, these children have been found to have difficulties with semantically reversible sentences and these difficulties have been demonstrated across a range of sentence types (van der Lely and Harris, 1990). In interpreting passive sentences such as 'The fish is eaten' the children were found to opt for an adjectival rather than a transitive verbal interpretation, so choosing a picture of an already eaten fish on a plate rather than a man eating a fish (van der Lely, 1993). Van der Lely and Stollwerck (1993) argue that at least some children with specific language impairment can be shown to have impairments in syntactic processing that are independent of lexical, pragmatic or general world knowledge and that these impairments are particular to aspects of syntax that involve dependent structural relationships between constituents. They describe these aspects as those involving 'government and binding principles' in the sense of Chomsky (1981). They propose that these findings provide further evidence for the potential autonomy of syntax from general cognitive processing; in the case of these children, general cognitive functioning being at a normal level but syntactic abilities being severely impaired.

Future Directions

In this chapter I have strayed beyond the confines of a focus on syntax alone. This is because comprehension of syntax has to be considered in the broader context of the way the person uses semantic, pragmatic and contextual information, as well as knowledge of syntax, in order to impose meaning on language. I have tried to encourage the use of techniques and approaches derived from psycholinguistic research in the clinical investigation of language comprehension with individual clients. If we adopt a creative, problem-solving approach, we can readily go beyond the information available from most psychometric tests of language comprehension.

Extending the range of methods described so far is an approach that allows comprehension processes to be investigated 'on-line', that is, while word-by-word processing is actually taking place (Tyler and Warren, 1987; Tyler, 1992). These contrast with typical 'off-line' tasks, such as sentence–picture matching, where the response is made only after the message is completed and the person has time and opportunity to reflect on the response. In most everyday situations, comprehension is an ongoing process which allows little time to think about alternative meanings. Tyler (1992) reports on the successful use of on-line processing tasks for the investigation of language comprehension disorders in aphasia. This approach would appear to have great potential for furthering our knowledge in this area, although at present it is technically sophisticated for routine clinical applications.

Two other recent approaches hold promise for future developments. In one of these, 'the preferential looking paradigm' developed by Golinkoff and Hirsh-Pasek (1995), young children are presented with two video displays of events and a simultaneous auditory stimulus that matches one of the events, e.g. 'Big Bird is hugging Cookie Monster'. Children's preference for looking at the display that matches the linguistic input is taken as an indication of their understanding. Unfortunately, although this technique works for group comparisons, it has not yet proved possible to adapt it for the reliable investigation of individual children (Bates, 1993). The other new technique involves the use of electrophysiological recording of cortical event-related potentials. Electrodes are placed on subjects' scalps and the electrical activity of different regions of the brain is measured while specific stimuli are presented (Molfese, 1990). The application of this method to investigate sentence comprehension (Holcomb, Coffey and Neville, 1992) is still in its infancy but holds out exciting prospects. As it requires neither speech nor action on the part of the subject, it could be invaluable where people with cognitive or physical disability are being assessed.

Another way in which the approaches I have described can be extended is by going beyond the focus on sentence level to study the comprehension of connected discourse (Lund and Duchan, 1983). This can be investigated by, for instance, presenting short stories for recall and judging whether what has been omitted or altered reflects lack of understanding of the original story. Alternatively, the stories can be followed by inference questions to see if the person can draw inferences from statements they hear (as in *The Test of Language Competence*: *Making Inferences Subtest*, Wiig and Secord, 1985). The person can be asked to explain jokes and riddles to see if they have understood the shift from the expected meaning that is often involved.

The situations in which comprehension is usually investigated are undoubtedly somewhat unnatural: they involve repeated presentations of single sentences in contexts that are fairly remote from the child's or adult's own communicative needs. Whilst there are good reasons for testing comprehension in a controlled situation, a person's comprehension in this setting needs to be compared with comprehension in more naturalistic settings. How does someone cope with understanding what is said in more noisy situations; for example, the child in a busy classroom or the adult in a talkative family group? It is important to mention in this regard that some children may perform relatively well on sentence comprehension tasks but in everyday communicative interactions make responses that seem unusual, inappropriate or even bizarre. Children who have been described as having a 'pragmatic disability', for example, may often fit this description. Comprehension processes in these children are still far from being understood.

In conclusion, we are only beginning to find out how language comprehension processes in children and adults with communication problems can be impaired or remain intact. We have some of the tools for carrying out such investigations and it is to be hoped that more in-depth case studies of both adults' and children's language comprehension processing will emerge in the near future.

References

Bates, E. (1993). Commentary on 'Language and comprehension in ape and child'. *Monographs of the Society for Research in Child Development* 58(3–4), 222–242.

Berndt, R.S.(1987). Symptom co-occurrence and dissociation in the interpretation of agrammatism. In: M. Coltheart, G. Sartori and R. Job (Eds.), *The Cognitive Neuropsychology of Language*. Hillsdale, NJ: Lawrence Erlbaum.

Bever, T.G. (1970). The cognitive basis for linguistic structures. In: J.R. Hayes (Ed.), *Cognition and The Development of Language*. New York: Wiley.

Bishop, D.M.V. (1983). *Test for Reception of Grammar*. Available from the author at MRC Applied Psychology Unit, The University of Cambridge.

Bloom, L. and Lahey, M. (1978). *Language Development and Language Disorders*. New York: Wiley.

Bransford, J.D. and Nitsch, K.E. (1977). Coming to understand things we could not previously understand. In: J.F. Kavanaugh and W. Strange (Eds.), *Speech and Language in the Laboratory, School and Clinic*. Cambridge, MA: MIT Press.

Bridges, A. (1980). S.V.O. strategies reconsidered: the evidence of individual patterns of response. *Journal of Child Language* 7, 89–104.

Bridges, A. (1985). Ask a silly question...: some of what goes on in language comprehension tests. *Child Language Teaching and Therapy* 1, 135–148.

Butterworth, B., Campbell, R. and Howard, D. (1986). The uses of short-term memory: a case study. *Quarterly Journal of Experimental Psychology* 38A, 705–737.

Byng, S. (1988). Sentence processing deficits: theory and therapy. *Cognitive Neuropsychology* 5, 629–676.

Byng, S., Kay, J., Edmundson, A. and Scott, C.(1990). Aphasia tests reconsidered. *Aphasiology* 4(1), 67–91.

Carramazza, A. and Zurif, E.B. (1976). Dissociation of algorithmic and heuristic processes in language comprehension: evidence from aphasia. *Brain and Language* 3, 41–46.

Carrow, E. (1973). *Test for Auditory Comprehension of Language*. Teaching Resources Corporation.

Chapman, R. (1977). Comprehension strategies in children. In: J.F. Kavanaugh and W. Strange (Eds.), *Speech and Language in the Laboratory, School and Clinic*. Cambridge, MA: MIT Press.

Chomsky, C. (1969). *The Acquisition of Syntax in Children from 5 to 10*. Cambridge, MA: MIT Press.

Chomsky, N. (1981). *Lectures on Government and Binding*. Dordrecht: Foris.

Clark, E.V. (1971). On the acquisition of meaning of 'before' and 'after'. *Journal of Verbal Learning and Verbal Behavior* 10, 266–275.

Clark, E.V. (1973). Non-linguistic strategies and the acquisition of word meaning. *Cognition* 2, 161–182.

Cromer, R. (1976). Developmental strategies for language. In: V. Hamilton, and M.D. Vernon, *The Development of Cognitive Processes*. New York: Academic Press.

Cromer, R.F. (1991). The cognition hypothesis of language acquisition? In: R.F. Cromer, *Language and Thought in Normal and Handicapped Children*. Oxford: Blackwell.

Curtiss, S. (1977). *Genie: A Psycholinguistic Study of a Modern-day 'Wild Child'*. New York: Academic Press.

Curtiss, S. (1982). Developmental dissociations of language and cognition. In L.K. Obler and L. Menn (Eds.), *Exceptional Language and Linguistics*. New York: Academic Press.

Darley, F. L. (1979). *Evaluation of Appraisal Techniques in Speech and Language Pathology*. Reading, MA: Addison-Wesley.

De Renzi, E. and Vignolo, L.A. (1962). The Token Test: a sensitive test to detect receptive disturbances in aphasics. *Brain* 85, 665–678.

Dewart, M. H. (1975). A psychological investigation of sentence comprehension by children. Unpublished PhD Thesis, University of London.

Dewart, M.H. (1991). Age changes in language comprehension: a longitudinal study. Paper presented at Symposium in honour of Richard Cromer, The British Psychological Society Developmental Section Conference, Oxford.

Ellis, A.W. and Young, A.W. (1988). *Human Cognitive Neuropsychology*. Hove: Lawrence Erlbaum.

Golinkoff, R.M. and Hirsh-Pasek, K. (1995). Reinterpreting children's sentence comprehension: towards a new framework. In P. Fletcher and B. MacWhinney, *Handbook of Child Language*, pp. 430–461. Oxford: Blackwell.

Goodglass, H. and Kaplan, E. (1972). *Boston Diagnostic Aphasia Examination*. Philadelphia, PA: Lea & Febiger.

Holcomb, P.J., Coffey, S.A. and Neville, H. (1992). Visual and auditory sentence processing: a developmental analysis using event-related potentials. *Developmental Neuropsychology* 8, 203–241.

Howard, D. (1985). Agrammatism. In: S. Newman and R. Epstein (Eds.), *Current Perspectives in Dysphasia*. Edinburgh: Churchill Livingstone.

Huttenlocher, J., Eisenberg, K. and Strauss, S. (1968). Comprehension: relation between perceived actor and logical subject. *Journal of Verbal Learning and Verbal Behavior* 7, 527–530.

Kay, J., Lesser, R. and Coltheart, M. (1992). *Psycholinguistic Assessments of Language Processing in Aphasia*. Hove: Lawrence Erlbaum.

Kersner, M. (1992). *Tests in Speech, Voice and Language*. London: Whurr Publishers.

Knowles, W. and Masidlover, M. (1987). *The Derbyshire Language Scheme (Revised)*. Derbyshire: Educational Psychology Service.

Lee, L. (1969). *Northwestern Syntax Screening Test*. Evanston, Il: Northwestern University Press.

Linebarger, M.C., Schwartz, M. F. and Saffran, E. M. (1983). Sensitivity to grammatical structure in so-called agrammatic aphasics. *Cognition* 13, 361–392.

Lund, N.J. and Duchan, J. F. (1983). *Assessing Children's Language in Naturalistic Contexts*. Englewood Cliffs, NJ: Prentice-Hall.

Molfese, D. (1990). Auditory evoked responses recorded from 16-month-old human infants to words they did and did not know. *Brain and Language* 38, 345–363.

Muller, D. J. (1985). What does a language score really mean? *Child Language Teaching and Therapy* 1, 38–45.

Reynell, J. K. (1977). *Reynell Developmental Language Scales*, rev. edn. Windsor: NFER-Nelson.

Schwartz, M.F., Saffran, E.M. and Marin, O.M. (1980). The word order problem in agrammatism, I: Comprehension. *Brain and Language* 10, 249–262.

Semel, E. and Wiig, E. (1980). *Clinical Evaluation of Language Function (CELF)*. Columbus, OH: Charles E. Merrill.

Smith, N. and Tsimpli, I.M. (1991). Linguistic modularity? A case study of a 'savant' linguist. *Lingua*, 84, 315–351.

Strohner, H. and Nelson, K. (1974). The young child's development of sentence comprehension: influence of event probability, non-verbal context, syntactic form and strategies. *Child Development* 45, 567–576.

Tager-Flusberg, H. (1981). Sentence comprehension in autistic children. *Applied Psycholinguistics* 2, 5–24.

Tyler, L.K. (1992). *Spoken Language Comprehension: an Experimental Approach to Disordered and Normal Processing*. Cambridge, MA: MIT Press.

Tyler, L.K. and Warren, P. (1987). Local and global structure in spoken language comprehension. *Journal of Memory and Language* 26, 638–657.

Van der Lely, H.K.J. (1993). Specifically language impaired and normally developing children: verbal passive vs adjectival passive sentence interpretation. In: J. Clibbens and B. Pendleton (Eds.) *Proceedings of the Child Language Seminar*, pp. 59–80. Plymouth: University of Plymouth.

Van der Lely, H.K.J. (1994). Canonical linking rules: forward versus reverse linking in normally developing and specifically language impaired children. *Cognition* 51, 29–72.

Van der Lely, H.K.J. and Dewart, H. (1986). Sentence comprehension strategies in specifically language impaired children. *British Journal of Disorders of Communication* 21, 291–306.

Van der Lely, H.K.J. and Harris, M. (1990). Comprehension of reversible sentences in specifically language impaired children. *Journal of Speech and Hearing Disorders* 55, 101–117.

Van der Lely, H.K.J. and Stollwerck, L. (1993). Language modularity, binding theory and specifically language impaired children. Paper presented at Generative Approaches to Language Acquisition Conference, University of Durham, September.

Wheldall, K., Mittler, P. and Hobsbaum, A. (1987). *Sentence Comprehension Test – Revised Version*. Windsor: NFER-Nelson .

Wiig, E.H. and Secord, W. (1985). *Test of Language Competence*. New York: Psychological Corporation .

Wilcox, S. and Palermo, D.S. (1975). 'In', 'on' and 'under' revisited. *Cognition* 3, 245–254.

Chapter 8
Assessment of Semantics

JENNY LANDELLS

Introduction

Semantics has been defined as the study of meaning in language (see Chapter 2). Meaning may be seen as central to the communication process; without meaning the purpose of communication is lost. Yet the assessment of meaning in the clinical setting has traditionally been poorly executed. Clinicians are aware of semantic problems in the language-impaired population but have lacked a systematic approach to their analysis and remediation. The major reason for this is the complexity of semantic organisation in comparison with the more readily defined levels of phonology and grammar.

There are many different aspects of semantics with roots in philosophy and psychology as well as linguistics. For introductions to linguistic semantics see Crystal (1981, Ch. 5), Leech (1974), Hurford and Heasley (1983). Structural semantics, a branch of structural linguistics, considers language as a set of interrelated elements which are not valid, i.e. are meaningless, except in relation to each other (see Chapters 1 and 2, this volume). Meaning in language has thus been found to be hierarchically organised and rule-governed in a similar way to syntax and phonology. This chapter will concentrate on the application of the principles of structural semantics to the clinical assessment of semantics. Throughout the chapter the reader will note frequent references to the overlap of semantics with other areas of linguistic organisation. Indeed, in the clinical analysis of utterances, semantics is sometimes included in syntactic assessment (see Chapters 6 and 7, this volume). However, in this chapter an attempt will be made to isolate and clarify specific semantic areas requiring assessment in the language-impaired individual. The first step is to clarify the division between lexical and relational semantics.

Lexical Semantics

Lexical semantics refers to the meaning of individual words, or, more

185

specifically, lexemes. A lexeme is defined as a minimal unit of vocabulary (see further Chapter 2). The clinical application of the study of lexical semantics involves looking at the vocabulary or 'personal dictionary' of an individual. As has been stated in Chapter 2, whereas a dictionary is organised according to alphabetical order, vocabulary is considered to be organised in terms of semantic fields. Semantic fields are further divided into subfields:

> ...each lexeme will cover a certain conceptual area, which may in turn be struc-
> tured as a field by another set of lexemes (as the area covered by 'red' in English
> is structured by 'scarlet', 'crimson', 'vermillion' etc). (Lyons, 1977, p 254)

Semantic field theory is not the only possible analysis of word meanings. Componential analysis sees word meaning as the sum of a number of features. For example, woman could be analysed as + human - male + adult (see Lesser, 1978, Ch. 5; Crystal, 1981). The method of considering the relationship between lexemes, of which semantic field theory is a part, is known as sense relations.

The clinical application of lexical semantics also needs to consider issues such as how we learn, store and access words and how these skills differ between adults and children. A good introduction to these topics is provided by Aitchison (1987) in a very readable book, with an extensive reference list for follow-up study.

Relational Semantics

Relational semantics refers to the relation between semantic categories in an utterance. There is an overlap of linguistic levels of organisation here. Utterances may be analysed in terms of grammatical or semantic categories. For example, the utterance 'The boy kicked the ball' would be analysed grammatically as a sequence of three clause elements: Subject, Verb and Object. It can also be analysed semantically as a sequence of three semantic elements: Actor, Dynamic and Goal. A change of grammatical category will not always result in a change of semantic category. For example, the above sentence could be altered to a passive, i.e. 'The ball was kicked by the boy'. Here 'the ball' becomes the grammatical subject of the sentence but 'the boy' remains the actor in semantic terms. Relational semantics thus studies the meaning of vocabulary in different contexts. 'Context' here relates to linguistic context, i.e. the syntagmatic relationship between semantic elements. This needs to be seen as quite distinct from the situational context (see Chapter 2), which refers to the situation in which the utterance occurred and its function. A number of other terms may be found in the literature which are synonymous with relational semantics. For example, *sentence meaning, grammatical meaning, semantic functions* and *participant roles*.

The assessment of semantics needs to consider both the lexical and relational aspects and we will return to this later in the chapter. In the following section, aspects of semantic disorders will be discussed with reference to assessment in key areas.

Semantic Disorders

The paucity of research in the area of semantics and our lack of knowledge of semantic development is reflected in our limited understanding of semantic disorders. A discussion of some of the features of semantic disorders follows. These features may well be found in the presence of other language problems.

Word Retrieval versus Word Learning

Word-finding problems may be observed in language-impaired children (and adults). A distinction needs to be made between word retrieval and word learning. The question is, 'Does the child know the word but have difficulty accessing it in his or her mental dictionary, or is the word not sufficiently familiar to the child to have been learned and is therefore not stored in the lexicon?' It is clearly important to attempt a distinction here in order to plan remediation. If the language-impaired child has restricted lexical knowledge, cueing to help find a word will be of no use because the child will search for a word which is not available. The use of overt *search behaviours* may indicate that the child is attempting to find a word which *is* known. There are a number of such behaviours, summarised by McCartney, Flower and Meteyard (1986):

1. the use of initial speech sounds or silent articulatory gestures preceding the target word;
2. giving semantic information, e.g. 'I see one of them, Mrs Walker got';
3. using a 'filler' or empty word, e.g. 'Serve thingies and cook';
4. self-correcting, starting, stopping and restarting, e.g. 'A woman is going in... a woman is going in... in the station';
5. gesturing, signing, miming or using symbolic noise;
6. extra verbalisations and starters;
7. frustration gestures.

It may be helpful to consider whether a particular search behaviour predominates and assists the child in accessing the word. If so, the child could be encouraged to use the effective search behaviour when difficulty occurs. Alternatively, it may be that the child does not attempt a search and may need to be taught to do so. It is interesting to note that one of the most effective cues in the study by McCartney *et al.* was for the adult to indicate that the child's response was incorrect or had not been understood. It is possible that the child was prompted to undertake a lexical search at this point.

One assessment which can assist in the identification of word-finding problems is the *Test of Word Finding* (TWF) (German, 1986). This is a standardised assessment which aims to assess accuracy and speed of naming in children. Naming ability is tested in five different ways: picture naming of both nouns and verbs, sentence completion, naming of an object from a given description and naming the category a group of objects belong to (e.g. *pliers, axe* and *screwdriver*: **tools**). In addition to a standard score result, analysis of the naming behaviour and obser-vation of gestures and extra verbalisations is undertaken. Analysis of the naming behaviour involves looking at the *substitutions* the individual produced and dividing these into categories. For example, substitution of the word *game* in place of *domino* would be recorded as a *Superordinate* response, *seasons* instead of *weather* would be in the category of *Associations*. These categories could be useful for monitoring the child's naming behaviour in informal testing and spontaneous language. German emphasises that the test is not a complete analysis but that it will allow hypotheses to be made which can be further tested informally. The test also incorporates a comprehension section, to be administered following the test of word finding, to check whether errors are a result of the child not knowing the word. The TWF is a useful assessment to aid the analysis of word finding and it includes a comprehensive bibli-ography of the subject. The main disadvantage for clinicians in the UK is that a number of American terms are included, which would cause diffi-culty for normally developing children in this country. For example, from the sentence completion section: 'It's fun to watch the band march in the fourth of July —?' (**parade**). Alteration of these would, of course, affect the validity of the test. For the diagnostic model, literature review and discussion of the test itself, see German (1989).

Current studies into word finding and word learning are concentrat-ing on the relationship between lexical and phonological knowledge (see also Chapter 13, this volume). For children to acquire a new item of vocabulary, they have to understand its conceptual attributes (which semantic field it belongs to, which contexts it can be used in, etc.). They also must be able to perceive and produce its phonological form and then store this in memory in order to access it later. Children with normally developing language do this readily. Carey (1978) found they are often able to gain the basic conceptual knowledge necessary to fit the new item into their developing lexicon after only one hearing. She terms this 'fast mapping'. Additionally, their abilities to segment and repeat new words are superior to language-impaired children. Dollaghan (1987) found there was no difference between language-impaired children and normally developing children in their acquisition of the *conceptual* knowledge. However, the normally developing children were much better at producing the phonological form of the word. Gathercole (1993) discusses the significance of this work and the role of short- and long-term memory in the learning of new words. She concludes that language-impaired children have exceptional difficulty in the short-term retention of new words. This information should make us think again about our intervention procedures with this group of children. Gathercole makes some practical suggestions for working on memory skills and indicates that research should further investigate the short-term retention of new words and effective remediation for this problem. For more information of the relationship between working memory and vocabulary see Gathercole and Baddeley (1993).

Much remains unknown about how children learn words and processes of word retrieval procedures but research is now being directed to these areas, thereby giving us new directions. (See further: Haynes, 1992; Chiat and Hunt, 1993; Hyde Wright *et al.*, 1993.)

Overextensions

Overextensions, where a lexical item is used to refer to a larger category of objects than in adult usage (see further Chapter 2), are often present in the speech of children with developmental language delay and are generally recognised as characterising an immature semantic system. They are well documented in linguistic literature, for example (Bloom, 1973; Clark, 1973; Rescorla, 1981). A review of competing theories of overextension can be found in Dromi (1987).

Developmental studies record overextensions occurring in the vocabulary of the normally developing child, between the ages of 1;1 and 2;6 years, which have usually disappeared by the age of 3 years. Clark's (1973) hypothesis of semantic feature acquisition suggests that the child has identified an object by one particular perceptual feature, e.g. 'apple' by the fact that it is round. The term 'apple' becomes overextended when the child names another round object (e.g. *a plate*) as 'apple'. It thus becomes necessary for the child to perceive another feature which distinguishes *apple* from *plate*. This could be, for example, the fact that apples are edible whereas plates are not. According to Clark, shape is the first perceptual attribute to control word meaning, followed by size, sound, movement, texture and finally, to a lesser extent, taste.

There are other explanations for overextensions. These include the use of a known word, or even a preferred word in place of an unknown, or less well-liked word (Hoek, Ingram and Gibson, 1986). This study also showed the use of a phonologically simpler word for one that was more difficult. Similar results are provided by Schwartz and Leonard (1982), who found that young children are selective in the words they attempt to say. Words which were consistent with the limited phonological development of the children studied were more likely to be acquired than words with phonological characteristics considered to be outside their systems. It is therefore likely that a child with a restricted phonological system will have a limited vocabulary which may not necessarily imply a problem in the semantic system. This needs to be considered during assessment and treatment planning (see further Chapter 13, this volume).

Confusion of Polar Opposites

A second, common feature of delayed language development is confusion of polar terms, e.g. *more* and *less, high* and *low, before* and *after*. For example, the immature child will choose a tree containing more apples in response to a request for 'more' *and* will choose a tree containing more apples in response to 'less',(Donaldson and Balfour, 1968). Clark (1973) considers this to be another form of overextension. Her explanation is that both items of the pair have a large number of semantic features in common and differ in respect of one feature only. At the stage of confusion, the child has realised that 'more' and 'less' are both measurements of quantity but not that 'more' refers to positive quantity and 'less' to negative quantity.

More and *less*, of course, do not refer to constants. For example, three may be 'more', if compared with two but 'less' if compared with five. The terms are therefore completely arbitrary; the meaning of 'more' can only be understood in the context of the opposing term 'less'. (Cf. the arbitrary nature of the sign, Saussure, Chapter 1, this volume.)

Semantic-Pragmatic Disorder/Difficulties

Rapin and Allen (1983) coined the term *semantic-pragmatic disorder* in their classification of developmental language disorders. 'semantic-pragmatic disorder without autism' is used to describe a group of children who present with very fluent expressive language, yet are not effective communicators. They are described as generally able to produce utterances which are syntactically and phonologically well formed. However, what superficially appears to be 'good language' is revealed on closer examination to be not really communicative. In fact, the children demonstrate severe difficulties with language processing and language use. Problems of discourse comprehension, irrelevant responses to questions, echolalia, disruption of syntax and prosody were all noted.

Semantic-pragmatic disorder has been the subject of much debate since the term was coined and much remains to be resolved. It is not clear that a homogeneous group can be identified and therefore the term *semantic-pragmatic difficulties* is now preferred. Some authors, for example, Smith and Leinonen (1992) object to the close linking of the terms semantic and pragmatic. Their objections are twofold. First, the linking can suggest that the two concepts are inseparable. Second, there is an implication that a pragmatic disability has its roots in language rather than in a deeper failure to make sense of the world. Other authors consider semantic-pragmatic difficulties as part of the autistic continuum. For a critique of this view see McTear and Conti-Ramsden (1992). Although a large amount of data have been collected from this group, we have still not determined how far the semantic difficulties extend, or whether the pragmatic element is the key. The picture may well differ across children. Work such as that of Adams and Bishop (1989) and Bishop and Adams (1989), in attempting to pinpoint the features that typify children with semantic-pragmatic difficulties, is extremely helpful (see further Chapter 9, this volume). What is clear is that the clinician needs to consider the semantic component when confronted with a child who has pragmatic difficulties. It is important to look at the child's world knowledge through semantics to see if his or her semantic system is lacking in some respect.

Examination of the child's lexical system may reveal one or more of the following features.

1. Slow development and difficulty in acquiring semantic field boundaries

In the following example, a child aged 13 has been asked to list lexemes from the semantic field of *fruit*.

Child:	apple;
	banana;
	pineapple;
	cabbage.
Therapist:	Is cabbage a fruit?
Child:	No – carrots.
Therapist:	Are carrots fruit?
Child:	Yes.
Therapist:	No. Cabbage and carrots are ___?
Child:	Vegetables.

Here, although the child appears to know both the superordinate terms 'fruit' and 'vegetable', she is unsure which lexemes belong in each of these semantic fields.

2. Rigid concept boundaries

One example is of a child who, when told a butcher sold meat, listed beef pork and chicken as types of meat but would not accept the suggestion of sausages as he considered these to be food and not meat. Smedley (1989) discusses rigid concept boundaries in some detail. He has observed many instances of preposition or particle error in children with semantic-pragmatic difficulties. For example, the child who said 'the clock is *by* the wall' had a rigid boundary for 'on'. He interpreted 'on' as a concept for a *horizontal* plain and therefore would not use 'on' to refer to a clock in a *vertical* plain.

3. Incorrect semantic ordering in part–whole relationships

For example: 'What's got a roof on?'
                   'Chimney'.

This may be caused by poor knowledge of the associations between words, in this example, the knowledge that a chimney is a part of a roof which is, in turn, a part of a house. Alternatively, the error may be a failure to comprehend the syntax of the question, so that the child interprets 'roof on' as 'on roof' and selects a logical response to this.

4. Overuse of deictic terms

Deixis is the term used for lexemes whose meaning is dependent on shifting referents. For example, the meaning of the personal pronouns 'I' and 'you' changes according to who has said them; the meaning of 'here' and 'there' varies over distance. Crystal (1982) suggests four categories of deictic terms:

Animate: 'him', 'she' 'I' etc.
Inanimate: 'it' ,'that' etc.
Scope: 'then','there', 'now', 'down' etc.
Other: includes where deixis has an unclear reference,
                   for example 'one' may be animate or inanimate.

Overuse of deictic terms can result in ambiguities. Analysis of this overuse may suggest a semantically based problem, i.e. poor lexical knowledge, or it could be that the speaker has failed to appreciate the listener's state of knowledge (listener perspective). This would therefore seem to be a good example of the interface between the semantic and pragmatic elements of semantic-pragmatic difficulties.

5. Lexical access difficulty

As well as word-search behaviours (discussed above), Smedley (1989) notes that problems with lexical access can result in: *literal paraphasias* (words which contain at least 50% of the same sounds as the target

items); *semantic paraphasias* (words which belong to the same semantic category as the target item); *neologisms* (made up words) (see
further Chapter 11, this volume.

In addition to specific lexical assessment, it is recommended that the
child's reasoning ability be investigated. It is can be difficult to determine the boundaries between semantic, pragmatic, syntactic, and world
knowledge. Our understanding of a particular word meaning in a given
utterance is doubtless affected by our individual experiences, by our
expectations of its possible contexts both in terms of syntax and situation, as well as the particular context given. It is suggested that the child
with 'semantic-pragmatic difficulties' fails to integrate this information
successfully and therefore his or her reasoning through language is
affected. The following features may be observed:

(a) *failure to make inferences*:
    The child finds it difficult to interpret information which may be
    given in visual or verbal form. For example, the child is shown a
    picture of an accident victim being put in ambulance but is unable to
    answer the question, 'Where will the ambulance go next?'. This
    implies that the child is in some way unable to use the information
    provided in the picture to assess the situation, integrate this with
    knowledge of the world, i.e. where ambulances normally take acci-
    dent victims and reach a conclusion of *hospital*;
(b) *literal interpretations*:
    Clinicians frequently note literal interpretations of idiomatic
    phrases, e.g. 'pull your socks up', as a feature of the language behav-
    iour of children with semantic-pragmatic difficulties. However, a
    recent study (Vance and Wells, 1994) found no evidence that chil-
    dren judged to have semantic-pragmatic difficulties had a greater
    problem with the interpretation of non-literal language in a struc-
    tured situation than other children with specific language impair-
    ment. Literal interpretation cannot therefore be cited as an
    identifying feature of semantic-pragmatic difficulties. Further
    research needs to determine whether there is a distinction between
    the two groups in their understanding of non-literal language during
    conversational interaction;
(c) *Reasoning may be logical but idiosyncratic*:
    McTear (1985) reports on a conversation with a child where the child
    seemingly repeatedly fails to understand the interviewer's questions.
    However, when the child's half of the conversation is analysed, it is
    shown to progress logically but not in the way the adult expects. (For
    further discussion see Chapters 9 and 13, this volume.)

Careful assessment and data collection are essential, and should not be
restricted solely to the areas of semantics and pragmatics. Because the

problem involves the breakdown of conversational interaction, it is important that conversational analysis is undertaken. The reader is directed here to Chapters 9 and 13. Further suggestions for semantic assessment, including the assessment of non-literal meaning, can be found in Lund and Duchan (1983, Ch.7).

Semantic Disorders in Adults

One linguistic description of aphasic impairment (Jakobsen, 1956) has divided disorders into two broad categories; those of *selection* and *combination* (see also Lesser, 1978; Code and Müller, 1983). Semantic problems may be observed in both of these categories. Word-finding/access difficulties may be seen as a problem of selection, along the *paradigmatic axis* (see Chapter 1, this volume). At the *syntagmatic level*, problems in linking linguistic elements to form larger units, e.g. sentences, are classed as combination difficulties. Of course, the division is a very simplistic one. The complexity of aphasic disturbances is reflected in the diversity of typological classification of aphasic impairment. Some of these classifications are taken from linguistics, others from anatomy, physiology and psychology (see Whurr, 1982 for a review).

When working with an adult who has acquired a semantic deficit following brain injury, the assumption is made that, pre-trauma, the individual was functioning with a mature semantic system. The workings of the system, including theories on organisation and access, plus the development of the individual's unique system, are well outlined by Aitchison (1987). Additionally, the 'hiccups' that can occur in a mature and functioning system are explained, e.g. *tip-of-tonguedness, mala-propisms* etc. Brain injury can cause disruption to the semantic system at any of the levels which had reached maturity during development.

It has become accepted that a *linguistic* description of the communicative ability of the person with aphasia is required before therapy is planned. However, developments through *cognitive neuropsychology* and *processing theory* have highlighted the necessity for *psycho-linguistic* assessment.The influence of cognitive neuropsychology is affecting our thinking about semantics, current research and clinical practice. Cognitive neuropsychology studies patterns of behaviour in brain-injured individuals, i.e. which aspects of behaviour have become abnormal and which remain intact. For example, a brain-injured person may have no reading skill but still understand the spoken word. It attempts to explain the patterns in terms of damage to one or more parts of a model of normal cognitive functioning. The cognitive neuropsychology model is based on the assumption of an internal processing system and that this system is modular. Separate cognitive activities are carried out by separate modules. Each module works independently of other modules, unless in direct communication. For a good introduction to cognitive neuropsychology and language impairment see Ellis and Young (1988). The modular system is disputed by the connectionist theorists, for example Stemberger (1985), who argue that processes can be carried out in parallel.

Cognitive neuropsychology was used initially to investigate lexic disturbances, was later applied to brain-injured adults with aphasia, and is now also being applied to developmental disorders of speech and language.

The *Psycholinguistic Assessments of Language Processing in Aphasia* (PALPA) (Kay, Lesser and Coltheart, 1992), as its title explains, is a battery of tests to assess language processing in aphasia. It is based on a model of processing which considers the semantic system as central, with access to the system via the auditory and visual pathways of spoken word, written word and pictures. The assessments within the section entitled 'Picture and Word Semantics' can help to determine whether or not the semantic system is impaired but also how, and to what extent, it may be impaired. One assessment requires the subject to match a picture to a word spoken by the tester. In addition to the target picture on the page, there are four distractor pictures: a close semantic distractor, a distant semantic distractor, a visual distractor and an unrelated distractor. Frequent selection of the visual distractors may suggest visuo-perceptual difficulties, whereas selection of close semantic distractors implies relatively high-level semantic impairment. Other assessments in the battery look at factors that may affect lexical storage and retrieval, for example, the effect *word frequency* has on the ability to name objects. Another example is the effect of a word's *imageability* on the skill of judging whether two words have the same meaning or not. The PALPA battery is an extremely useful tool for the clinician, well laid out with clear instructions for administration, implications of results and suggestions for further assessment.

Another assessment that can provide insight into the semantic system of the aphasic person is *Pyramids and Palm Trees* (Howard and Patterson, 1992). The subject is required to judge which picture goes with another, from a choice of two, e.g. 'does saddle go with goat or horse?' If it is administered as a pure picture assessment (and the subject is asked not to name the pictures), it bypasses the spoken or written word, where breakdown may occur, to directly access the individual's semantic knowledge. Additional tasks to access this route are categorisation of pictures and simple picture sequencing. For further discussion of assessment for intervention in aphasia consult Chapter 11, this volume.

Assessment of lexical semantics

A test of receptive vocabulary often administered in the clinic is the

British Picture Vocabulary Scale (BPVS) (Dunn, Dunn, Whetton and Pintillie 1982). Although useful as a screening device for identifying children with poor vocabularies, this test is not based on linguistic principles. A random selection of vocabulary items is used, which provides little information about the subject's semantic *system* and offers no approach for remediation. It is essential to take a detailed look at vocabulary if patterns of use and problem areas are to be determined.

Crystal's *Profile in Semantics* (PRISM) (1982) provides the opportunity to examine both the lexical and relational aspects of an individual's lexicon. It is divided into two sections: *Prism-Lexicon* (PRISM-L) and *Prism-Grammar* (PRISM-G). PRISM-L is an attempt to provide a structured way of looking at vocabulary. It forms a basis for vocabulary counting but, much more importantly, it looks at the organisation of vocabulary in terms of semantic fields and sense relations. The linguistic theories on which the profile is based are explained in detail in Crystal (1981). His work is a logical but intuitive extension of the work of Lyons (1977) and Palmer (1981).

The ideal profile needs to be able to record any vocabulary item which may be used by the subject. In attempting to meet this criterion, PRISM-L is 16 pages long. It therefore appears as an unwieldy and somewhat daunting document to the clinician. However, although Crystal states that PRISM-L can be used as an assessment tool, it is in no respect something which should be administered and then put to one side. Rather it provides an ongoing assessment and record of the subject's progress.

The PRISM-L profile is organised in semantic fields which move from concrete to abstract. This layout was based on child studies of lexical development (e.g. Clark, 1979; Rescorla, 1981), which found that early vocabulary was likely to be drawn from the semantic fields of *food* and *drink, body parts, clothing, animals, vehicles, living routines, bodily functions, household items* and *people*. However, development is to a large extent idiosyncratic, particularly in the early stages when it is totally dependent on the child's concrete experiences. For example, the vocabulary of a child who lives on a farm is likely to include a greater number of terms from the subfield of *farm animals* at an earlier age than a child from an urban environment. There are therefore no norms on the expected acquisition or development of particular fields. However, PRISM-L enables careful recording of data which can detect 'gaps' in the system, e.g. a sample from a language-impaired child included the body part items 'arm', 'wrist' and 'fingers' but not 'hand'. These items may then be selected to be taught to the child.

Built into the PRISM-L procedure is the use of a type–token ratio. *Type* refers to the number of different vocabulary items used by a subject and *token* to the number of examples of that particular item. This can be a useful measure over a period of time, to see if the child begins to use a greater number of types either across all fields or within particular fields. As there are no norms for expected number of tokens per type, the type–token ratio cannot be used to compare the language-impaired population with the normally developing one. It may therefore be more helpful to look at individual vocabulary items which have a high number of tokens: for example, there may be frequent use of relatively 'empty' verbs such as 'go' and 'got' rather than more specific verbs. Therapy goals may thus be indicated.

As well as looking at the distribution of vocabulary in terms of semantic fields, PRISM-L enables the clinician to record the relationship between the items used. The final page of PRISM-L looks at the lexicon as a system of contrasts (sense relations). This is the section which is likely to be the most helpful in identifying disordered lexicon – where it is possible to record 'expected' developmental errors and also errors which do not fall into usual patterns. It is divided into three sections:

1. *Paradigmatic relations*:
   Under the paradigmatic section it is possible to record examples of synonymy, opposition, hyponymy and incompatibility (see also Chapter 2).
2. *Syntagmatic relations*:
   Syntagmatic errors are defined as instances where the vocabulary does not collocate correctly, e.g. 'the teeth is open', instead of 'the mouth is open'. In normally developing children this is relatively rare although in neurologically impaired adults it is quite common.
3. *Developmental error*:
   Developmental errors are very common in children with delayed language. For example, see the preceding discussion on *overextensions*.

Profiles can be used over time to record data and monitor progress. However, standardised assessments can sometimes provide information more quickly, as well as giving an objective measurement of progress. The *Test of Word Knowledge* (TOWK), (Wiig and Secord, 1992), aims to explore semantic knowledge, covering both receptive and expressive skills. It is an American test, with norms for 5–17 years and testing can commence at either Level 1 (5–8 years) or Level 2 (8–17 years). Subtests cover three aspects of word knowledge. First, *Referential Meaning*: the ability to match a spoken word to a picture (referent) and to name pictures. Second, *Relational Aspects*, tested by the ability to provide word definitions and to recognise opposites and synonyms. A further subtest (Level 2) can probe understanding of conjunctions and transition words. (Note that Wiig and Secord's use of the term 'relational' here is not as defined by me under Relational Semantics.) Third, *Meta-linguistic Knowledge*, (Level 2 only) tests multiple contexts; the ability to provide more than one meaning for a word, e.g.:

cold – the opposite of hot;
– sickness causing sneezing and coughing.

The final subtest of metalinguistic knowledge checks understanding of figurative language:

e.g.:   Which one tells about someone who is not being noisy?
(a) busy as a bee;
(b) **quiet as a mouse**;
(c) sly as a fox;
(d) eats like a bird.

The TOWK can be a difficult assessment for non-readers as many of the subtests are presented through the written word. Although the tester also reads the material out loud, the auditory memory loading required for the non-reader is very high, as in the above example. An additional difficulty for the British market is the number of Americanisms. For example, a *'litterbug'* is defined as 'a person who leaves *garbage* on the streets'. These criticisms aside, the TOWK can be a useful clinical tool. The subtests provide a range of information about the individual's semantic system and a comparison of receptive and expressive skills. The record sheet is clear to use and good guidelines for scoring are found in the manual.

Vocabulary Collection

The collection of a good sample of vocabulary by the clinician is bound to be limited by both time and situation. Half-hour recordings are likely to produce a mere fraction of the child's actual vocabulary. There is now evidence to suggest that children's vocabulary may be grossly underestimated. Developmental checklists often refer to vocabulary counting. For example, a child at age two years 'uses 50 or more recognisable words and understands many more' (Sheridan, 1960). However, recent advances in recording techniques have made it possible to record children's utterances throughout their waking day (e.g. Wagner, 1985). Wagner's study, discussed by Crystal (1987), showed that Andreas, aged 2;1 years, used a total of 20 200 tokens of 2210 types of different words in one day's utterances. Crystal (*op. cit.*) feels it is likely that the vocabulary of language-impaired children is similarly underestimated. Bearing such evidence in mind, it would seem essential to obtain a number of recordings in a variety of circumstances. Crystal further suggests that parental diaries of vocabulary can be particularly helpful. Parents are simply asked to list the vocabulary they hear the child use, noting down context, to avoid ambiguities e.g. 'top' (referring to a *toy* or to *the opposite of bottom*).

Assesment of Relational Semantics

Detailed analysis of the lexicon, using PRISM,-L can be complemented by the PRISM-G procedure (Crystal, 1982), which provides a profile of relational semantics. It is divided into five stages which correlate with the five stages of LARSP (Crystal, Fletcher and Garman, 1989) but there are no age norms given. Clause constituents are analysed as *semantic elements*, e.g. 'My sister is going to the circus today' would be analysed as follows:

'My sister'	– *Actor*
'is going'	– *Dynamic*
'to the circus'	– *Locative*
'today'	– *Temporal*

Phrase constituents are given the label *specifications*. The above sentence has the following specifications:

'sister' specified by 'my'	(*Possessive*)
'going' specified by 'is'	(*Other*)
'circus' specified by 'to'	(*Scope*)
and 'the'	(*Definiteness*)

The number of elements is deliberately restricted by Crystal to those which he feels are of most significance. Additional semantic functions are recorded under 'Other'. He points out that roles are often difficult to determine in the early stages of development and that theorists are not in agreement as to the kinds and number of semantic roles to use in later stages. (Cf. *Content/Form Analysis*, Bloom and Lahey, 1978; the *Derbyshire Language Scheme*, Knowles and Masidlover, 1982; and the *Bristol Language Development Scales*, Gutfreund, Harrison and Wells, 1989 – discussed below.) Stage I of PRISM-G thus has a different range of categories compared with the later stages.

Stage V involves the analysis of sequences of clauses. Eight types of semantic relationship are identified, e.g.:

Contrast: 'I was going to go out but it rained'
Temporal: 'I want to see you before you leave'

PRISM-G will show which clausal elements are being used by the subject and in what combinations, the amount and type of phrasal specification; and details, such as the number of deictic items.

The two PRISM profiles can be used separately, or as complementary procedures. Over time, they can indicate whether a lexical item is used in every semantic role or has restricted usage, e.g. 'man' may only be used as an *Actor*, never as *Experiencer* or *Goal*. (The interrelationship with grammar must always be considered, as this could be due to lack of ability to express the appropriate syntactic construction.) It is also possible to see if semantic elements have a good lexical range. The PRISM procedures are the only structured linguistic profiles available which tackle the area of semantics. They can be used with both adults and children for assessment and as a basis for remediation programmes. As such, although extremely time-consuming to administer, their selective clinical use can help us to tackle the complexity of semantic problems. As a research tool, they should also be of valuable assistance in the objective analysis of data.

The *Bristol Language Development Scales* (BLADES) (Gutfreund *et al.*, 1989) enable a comparison of the development of sentence meaning against other linguistic levels. BLADES provide what is believed to be the only integrated picture of the development of three aspects of language: *functions, sentence meaning* and *syntax.* The child's individual utterances are thus analysed on three levels: *pragmatics* – what the utterance is for; *semantics* – what the utterance is about; and *syntax* – the grammatical form of the utterance. There are two scales: the *Main Scale* and the *Therapy Planning Form.* The Main Scale consists of selected items from across the three areas and is used for initial assessment and progress checks. The Therapy Planning Form is used when more detailed analysis is necessary and as a model on which to base therapy. Under semantics, coding is divided into three sections:

1. *Sentence meaning* – the topic of the utterance or what the person is talking about.
2. *Time* – past or future and *Aspect* – the organisation of time within the event (e.g. 'going' – continuous).
3. *Modality* – which is divided into the degree of certainty (e.g. 'certain', 'probable') and constraints placed on sentence meaning ('can', 'ought').

To be able to compare the child's expressive language across linguistic levels is most helpful. It is possible to see strengths and weaknesses, e.g. the child may be able to convey a range of sentence meanings despite limited syntax. It is also easy to see 'gaps' in the child's developing system. Because the assessment compares three linguistic levels the coding is complex and time-consuming. The manual, however, contains detailed *Keys* to help with coding and a comprehensive sentence-meaning glossary. Additionally, The *Diagrams* show the order of emergence of linguistic items and are an aid to planning intervention. For further discussion of BLADES, see Chapters 6 and 9, this volume.

Semantic-based Language Programmes

As discussed above, it is most important to take into account the different levels of linguistic organisation when assessing language. Bloom and

Lahey (1978) attempted to bring together grammatical and semantic development in their Content/Form analysis. They point out the underlying semantic meanings possible in a single syntactic form, for example, in the development of negation. Negatives analysed grammatically as being at LARSP Stage II, are interpreted as having four different meanings:

Non-existence:	'no pocket' (there is no pocket)
Disappearance:	'soup all gone'
Rejection:	'no drink' (I don't want a drink)
Denial:	'no dirty' (that's not dirty)

These meanings may not appear simultaneously. Bloom's (1970) study of three children showed that the syntactic expression of nonexistence was learned before the syntactic expression of denial.

The Content/Form analysis codes utterances according to semantic categories but also notes grammatical details. Bloom and Lahey emphasise that it is intended as a 'clinical tool' to aid the planning of remediation for language-impaired children and not as a means of comparing such children with the normally developing child.

Similar types of semantic categories to those found in the Bloom and Lahey analysis are used in the *Derbyshire Language Scheme* (Knowles and Masidlover, 1982). For example, the four categories used for negatives are:

Rejection:	'don't want it'
Prohibition:	'don't touch'
Inability:	'won't go on'
Denial:	'not my coat'

The scheme includes assessments of both comprehension and expression, analyses being taken from a semantic viewpoint, but at the same time taking into account the appearance of grammatical structures. They are not strictly linguistic assessments but are based on developmental research such as that of the Bloom (1970) study cited above. Following assessment, the scheme provides a well-structured, detailed programme for the user to follow. The development of comprehension and expression is cross-referenced and teaching suggestions are provided for each step in the programme. The theoretical background is presented alongside teaching ideas. The Derbyshire Language Scheme was developed in a school for children with severe learning difficulties and is recommended for use with this group of children. It may also be appropriate for the child with a fairly straightforward delay but should not be seen as the answer to all problems. The scheme is a very practical clinical tool but it is not a detailed linguistic assessment and therefore additional assessments will be necessary for the analysis of complex problems.

In contrast with these structured schemes which tackle the area of relational semantics, very little attention has been given to the teaching of the lexicon. Early stages of the Derbyshire Language Scheme provide a suggested teaching vocabulary but after this the introduction of vocabulary is left to the discretion of the user. The authors make it quite clear that this is the case. In fact many language schemes rely on lexical development to appear naturally, as sentence meaning and grammar increase in complexity. Clinicians recognise that this frequently does not occur and the necessity for structured vocabulary teaching is evident.

We have much to learn about the acquisition of word meaning in the child. Rice (1980) gives a comprehensive review of the appropriate literature. She concludes that we cannot standardise an early vocabulary to be taught to all children. Each child builds a set of words based on their own unique environment and communicative needs. The choice of vocabulary to be taught must therefore be dependent on the individual. Crystal (1987) argues that although the clinician must engage in guesswork when planning remediation, this guesswork can be 'informed' by careful study of the child's environment, interests and needs.

The assumption is often made that vocabulary can readily be taught in simple activities by indicating the association between a word and its referent. Carey's (1978) observation of 'fast mapping' by the young child (see above) showed that the initial stage of lexical acquisition is rapid. However, the process of learning the complete meaning was completed only slowly, over months, and required protracted experience. Crystal (1987) discusses the complexity of individual word meanings and how these meanings are gradually acquired. In addition, he outlines an approach to vocabulary teaching which may prove valuable in remediation programmes.

Making the Link between Linguistic and Cognitive Knowledge

There is without doubt an intricately bound relationship between the child's developing linguistic knowledge and conceptual knowledge. Bloom (1973) argued that the child's first word reflects their already established perceptual awareness. It would therefore seem inappropriate to look at the child's linguistic knowledge without also taking into consideration cognitive development. As already stressed, semantic development must be seen in relation to other linguistic levels but it must also be seen against a background of cognitive knowledge. Bloom (1970) described her approach as an analysis of what the child said in relation to what they were talking about and the behaviour that co-occurred with what was said.

We can look at the child's behaviour in various situations but in particular through play. The major consideration should be: Is the language appropriate for the situation or is there a mismatch? For example, a 5-year-old engaged in symbolic play with cars hitched one car up to a breakdown lorry and was then heard to say: 'Car's got a broken leg. Going to hospital.'

It is possible that there are gaps in this child's 'knowledge of the world'; that cars do not have legs, they have wheels and are taken to garages when they break down. Further, language sometimes appears appropriate when studied out of context but when the situation is known it can become meaningless. For example, the child who was saying, 'Car's going round the roundabout', was actually pushing a car in a straight line down the road. Clinicians are therefore advised to make detailed notes whilst recording data or to videotape sessions.

Conclusion

The clinical application of the study of structural semantics is still in its infancy. Much further research is needed to improve our understanding of semantic problems. However, it is pleasing to record that since the first edition of this book was published there has been increased interest and research directed towards semantics. Clinical studies are looking at learning the lexicon, as yet with few conclusive results, but in numerous further directions. In spite of the absence of an agreed theory, structural semantics has now provided a framework within which an individual's semantic system may be investigated. The use of this linguistic framework in assessment, supplemented by information from psycholinguistic and cognitive studies, is helping us to achieve a more accurate description of disordered language and a more disciplined approach to remediation.

Acknowledgements

Thanks are due to Jean Racktoo for her helpful comments and especially to Ian for his continued patience.

References

Adams, C. and Bishop, D.V.M. (1989). Conversational characteristics of children with semantic-pragmatic disorder, 1: Exchange structure, turntaking, repairs and cohesion. *British Journal of Disorders of Communication* 24, 211–239.

Aitchison, J. (1987). *Words in the Mind: an Introduction to the Mental Lexicon*. Oxford: Blackwell.

Bishop, D.V.M. and Adams, C. (1989). Conversational characteristics of children with semantic-pragmatic disorder, II: What features lead to judgement of inappropriacy? *British Journal of Disorders of Communication* 24, 241–263.

Bloom, L. (1970). *Language Development: Form and Function in Emerging Grammars*. Cambridge, MA: MIT Press.

Bloom, L. (1973). *One Word at a Time: the Use of Single-word Utterances before Syntax*. The Hague: Mouton.

Bloom, L and Lahey, M. (1978). *Language Development and Language Disorders*. Chichester: Wiley.

Carey, S. (1978). The child as word learner. In: M. Halle, J. Bresnan and G. Miller (Eds.), *Linguistic Theory and Psychological Reality*. Cambridge, MA: MIT Press.

Chiat, S. and Hunt, J. (1993). Connections between phonology and semantics: An exploration of lexical processing in a language-impaired child. *Child Language Teaching and Therapy* 9, 200–213.

Clark, E.V. (1973). What's in a word? On the child's acquisition of semantics in his first language. In: T. Moore (Ed.), *Cognitive Development and the Acquisition of Language*, pp. 65–110. New York: Academic Press.

Clark, E.V. (1979). Building a vocabulary: words for objects, actions and relations. In: P. Fletcher and M. Garman (Eds.), *Language Acquisition*, 1st edn. Cambridge: Cambridge University Press.

Code, C. and Müller, D.J. (1983). *Aphasia Therapy*. London: Edward Arnold.

Crystal, D. (1981). *Clinical Linguistics*. Vienna: Springer-Verlag.

Crystal, D. (1982). *Profiling Linguistic Disability*. London: Edward Arnold.

Crystal, D. (1987). Teaching vocabulary: the case for a semantic curriculum. *Child Language Teaching and Therapy* 3, 40–56.

Crystal, D., Fletcher, P. and Garman, M. (1989). *The Grammatical Analysis of Language Disability*, 2nd edn. London: Whurr Publishers.

Dollaghan, C.A. (1987). Fast mapping in normal and language impaired children. *Journal of Speech and Hearing Disorders* 52, 218–222.

Donaldson, M. and Balfour, G. (1968). Less is more: A study of language comprehension in children. *British Journal of Psychology* 59, 461–472.

Dromi, E. (1987). *Early Lexical Development*. Cambridge: Cambridge University Press.

Dunn, L. M., Dunn, L.M., Whetton, C. and Pintillie, O. (1982). *The British Picture Vocabulary Scale*. Windsor: NFER-Nelson.

Ellis, A.W. and Young, A.W., (1988). *Human Cognitive Neuropsychology*. London: Lawrence Erlbaum.

Gathercole, S.E. (1993). Word learning in language-impaired children. *Child Language Teaching and Therapy* 9, 187–199.

Gathercole, S.E and Baddeley, A.D. (1993). *Working Memory and Language*. Hove: Lawrence Erlbaum.

German, D.J. (1986). *Test of Word Finding*. Allen, TX: DLM Teaching Resources.

German, D.J. (1989). A diagnostic model and a test to assess word-finding skills in children. *British Journal of Disorders of Communication*, 24, 21–39.

Gutfreund, M., Harrison, M. and Wells, G. (1989). *Bristol Language Development Scales*. Windsor: NFER-Nelson.

Haynes, C. (1992). Vocabulary deficit – one problem or many? *Child Language Teaching and Therapy* 8, 1–17.

Hoek, D., Ingram, D. and Gibson, D. (1986). Some possible causes of children's early word overextensions. *Journal of Child Language* 13, 477–494.

Howard, D. and Patterson, K. (1992). *The Pyramids and Palm Trees Test*. Bury St. Edmunds, Suffolk: Thames Valley Test Company

Hurford, J.R and Heasley, B. (1983). *Semantics: a Coursebook*. Cambridge: Cambridge University Press.

Hyde Wright, S., Gorrie, B. Haynes C. and Shipman, A. (1993). What's in a name? Comparative therapy for word-finding difficulties using semantic and phonological approaches. *Child Language Teaching and Therapy* 9, 214–229.

Jakobsen, R. (1956). Two aspects of language and two types of aphasic disturbances. In R. Jakobsen and M. Halle (Eds.), *Fundamentals of Language*. The Hague: Mouton.

Kay, J., Lesser, R. and Coltheart, M. (1992). *PALPA: Psycholinguistic Assessments of Language Processing in Aphasia*. Hillsdale, NJ: Lawrence Erlbaum.

Knowles, W. and Masidlover, M. (1982). *Derbyshire Language Scheme*. Ripley, Derby: Educational Psychology Service.

Leech, G. (1974). *Semantics*. Harmondsworth: Penguin.

Lesser, R. (1978). *Linguistic Investigations of Aphasia*. London: Edward Arnold.

Lund, N.J. and Duchan, J.F. (1983). *Assessing Children's Language in Naturalistic Contexts*. Englewood Cliffs, NJ: Prentice-Hall.

Lyons, J. (1977). *Semantics*. Cambridge: Cambridge University Press.

McCartney, E., Flower, P. and Meteyard, J. (1986). A study of word retrieval difficulties in language disordered children. Paper presented at ICAA Conference, Advances In Working With Language Disordered Children.

McTear, M. (1985). Pragmatic disorders: a case study of conversational disability. *British Journal of Disorders of Communication* 20, 129–142.

McTear, M. and Conti-Ramsden, G. (1992). *Pragmatic Disability in Children*. London: Whurr Publishers.

Palmer, F.R. (1981). *Semantics*. Cambridge: Cambridge University Press.

Rapin, I. and Allen, D. (1983). Developmental language disorders. In U. Kirk (Ed.), *Neuropsychology of Language, Reading and Spelling*. New York: Academic Press.

Rescorla, L.A. (1981). Category development in early language. *Journal of Child Language* 8, 225–238.

Rice, M. (1980). *Cognition to Language...Categories, Word Meanings and Training*. Baltimore, MD: University Park Press.

Schwartz, R.G. and Leonard, L.B. (1982). Do children pick and choose? An examination of phonological selection and avoidance in early lexical acquisition. *Journal of Child Language* 9, 319–336.

Sheridan, M.D. (1960). *The Developmental Progress of Infants and Young Children*. London: HMSO.

Smedley, M. (1989). Semantic-pragmatic language disorder: a description with some practical suggestions for teachers. *Child Language Teaching and Therapy* 5, 174–190.

Smith, B.R. and Leinonen, E. (1992). *Clinical Pragmatics*. London: Chapman & Hall.

Stemberger, J. P. (1985). An interactive activation model of language production. In: A.W. Ellis (Ed.), *Progress in the Psychology of Language*, Vol. 1. London: Erlbaum.

Vance, M. and Wells, B. (1994). The wrong end of the stick: language-impaired children's understanding of non-literal language. *Child Language Teaching and Therapy* 10, 23–46.

Wagner, K.R. (1985). How much do children say in a day? *Journal of Child Language* 12, 475–487.

Whurr, R. (1982). Towards a linguistic typology of aphasic impairment. In: D.Crystal (Ed.), *Linguistic Controversies: Essays in Linguistic Theories and Practice in Honour of F.R. Palmer*. London: Edward Arnold.

Wiig, E.H. and Secord, W. (1992). *Test of Word Finding (TOWK)*. Psychological Corporation/Harcourt Brace.

Chapter 9
Assessment of Pragmatics

GINA CONTI-RAMSDEN AND MICHAEL F. McTEAR

The order of authors is alphabetical as the work represents the equal contribution of both co-authors.

Introduction

Pragmatic assessment is such a new concept in speech and language therapy that a few preliminaries need to be covered before we examine some of the tools which have recently become available for the assessment of pragmatics. It is probably the case that many clinicians are unsure what, exactly, the term 'pragmatics' means and how an approach to language assessment and intervention might profit from work in pragmatics. For this reason we devote the first two sections of this chapter to a brief outline of those phenomena normally covered in pragmatics followed by a discussion of the relevance of this work for speech and language therapists. This will then provide a basis for the main concern of this chapter, which is to evaluate some currently available procedures for pragmatic assessment. In the final section we will discuss some of the ways in which these tools might be improved, as well as some of the directions which future research in pragmatic disability might take.

What is Pragmatics?

Pragmatics has been described as *the study of the rules governing the use of language in a social context* (Bates, 1976). Yet, simple as this definition might appear, it conceals a wide range of linguistic and non-linguistic phenomena which have been traditionally assigned to this area. In his textbook on pragmatics, Levinson (1983) concludes a lengthy discussion of definitions of pragmatics by listing the major phenomena which a pragmatic theory should account for: deixis, implicature, presupposition, speech acts and some aspects of discourse structure. These are in turn complex concepts and a chapter is devoted to each in Levinson's book. The other main definitions which are considered include the following:

1. the study of relations between language and context which are encoded in the structure of a language;
2. the study of aspects of meaning which are not captured in a semantic-theory;
3. the study of relations between language and context which support a theory of language understanding;
4. the study of the appropriate use of language.

Whilst none of these definitions is sufficient on its own, it can be argued that all of these aspects of pragmatics contribute to a theory of language use. We will return to this point in the final section.

One useful distinction, which cuts across these definitions, is that of the difference between narrow and broad views of pragmatics (Craig, 1983). In the narrow view, pragmatics is seen as an additional level of language above phonology, syntax and semantics, and attention is directed in developmental and clinical studies towards those skills which can be described as discourse or conversational – for example, turn-taking, producing and understanding speech acts, making reference, telling stories and repairing conversational breakdowns.

The development of conversational skills in young children has been documented by McTear (1985), and there is a fast emerging literature on several aspects of language usage by language-impaired children (see Fey and Leonard, 1983; and McTear, 1985; for reviews). There has, however, been little attempt to integrate work in pragmatic disability with results from other studies of development and impairment in traditional areas of linguistic analysis such as phonology, syntax and semantics. For this reason it can be concluded that the narrow view of pragmatics is concerned with an additional set of rules for using language which are quite separate from rules of linguistic structure.

The broad view of pragmatics, on the other hand, is concerned with the integration of linguistic structure and conversational rules. Here questions arise such as whether particular conversational problems are the result of structural deficits or whether structural deficits are a *reflection of problems* at the pragmatic level. For example: does a child have difficulty in making reference to non-present persons or objects because of an inability to construct relative clauses, or does the need to develop the ability to construct relative clauses only emerge when the child becomes aware of his/her communicative functions? Much of the literature on communicative and functional explanations of language development is concerned with questions such as these (Bates and MacWhinney, 1982). This aspect of the broad view of pragmatics overlaps with Levinson's first definition outlined earlier. Another aspect of this broader view, which has particular relevance for speech and language therapy, is concerned with the study of situational effects of language usage. This involves examining all those features of context that might have a bearing on the child's linguistic performance, such as the nature of the task and the setting, and the role played by the child's conversational partner(s). A concern with these aspects of context has lead to greater awareness of how a child's performance can be adversely affected in traditional clinical interviews, so that the tendency now is to create a relaxed and non-threatening context in order to maximise the child's linguistic output. This more general insight informs the methodology employed in the assessment tools to be discussed later. In addition to this, it has also been recognised that the production of particular linguistic structures can be influenced by context. For example, in an asymmetrical situation, such as a traditional clinician–child interview, it is usually the case that the clinician falls into the role of asking questions to which the child often gives the most minimal of answers. In such a case it would not be possible to observe the child's usage of interrogative forms or of the particular speech acts which they realise. Similarly, as it is quite normal in such an interaction to use elliptical sentences, this would militate against the assessment of the child's ability to construct full sentences. As with the other aspects of context described earlier, clinicians and researchers are becoming increasingly conscious of the need to recognise how the use of particular language forms is context-dependent.

A final aspect of this broader view of pragmatics is concerned with methodological issues such as data collection and transcription. We have already alluded to the need to consider different contexts in which language is used. What is also important is the methods used to collect language samples. Many researchers use video-recordings in order to capture significant non-linguistic features; however, it is important to be aware of the constraining effects of obtrusive recording methods in terms of their effects on the participants and on the range of activities which can be easily recorded. As far as transcription is concerned, findings from pragmatic studies, particularly those within the more narrow view, have established the importance of a detailed transcription which includes previously disregarded features of performance such as self-repetitions, pauses and overlapped turns, not to mention non-verbal behaviours (Ochs, 1979).

Bringing these points together, we can see that pragmatics may involve the following aspects of language use:

1. the study of discourse and conversational skills;
2. the study of relationships between pragmatic and other levels of language;
3. the study of situational determinants of the use of language.

The pragmatic assessment tools which we will discuss later address the first of these aspects primarily and are thus concerned with the more narrow view of pragmatics, although in their methodology and underlying philosophy they have taken account of the third aspect, especially in relation to methods for the successful elicitations of naturally-occurring samples for children. The second aspect has not been addressed to any great extent in this work, and we will discuss this failing in greater detail in the final section. But before looking at some procedures for the assessment of pragmatics, we will outline in more detail some of the pragmatic implications of assessment.

Three major implications can be drawn from a pragmatic approach to the assessment of communication disorders in children. First, the realisation that language is fundamentally an integration of structural and pragmatic knowledge and that communication also involves the integration of linguistic, social and cognitive knowledge (Prutting, 1982; Prutting and Kirchner, 1983) has brought home to all of us the importance of natural language use. Children use language mainly when they feel the need to communicate and it is in this context that they need to be assessed. Clinicians have long been aware of the generalisability problems brought about by decontextualised intervention where structures are taught without regard to their context and use (Leonard, 1981). This same idea is now being applied to assessment. It is necessary that we collect valid, representative and relevant data about the child's communicative strengths and weaknesses and the pragmatic perspective suggests that this cannot be done successfully without paying attention to the child's ecology. Naturalistic assessment is now the most central element of the whole assessment procedure. Clinicians may well want to use standardised tools, interviews, tasks, etc., but the information gathered in this way, which usually comprises a categorisation of what the child can and cannot do, needs to be integrated within a pragmatic framework which emphasises an interactive approach in order to understand how the child's communicative behaviours are related to one another (Muma, 1983). Thus, we need to develop and refine the tools available to clinicians to enable them to gather, systematically describe, and understand natural communicative interaction. Indeed, speech–language pathologists have always believed in the value of 'an informal chat' with the child and parents. This informal chat, which usually took place at the beginning or end of the session, is now assuming the central core of our assessment protocols.

Second, assessment cannot involve one member of the dyad only, be it the child or the adult (usually a parent). Communication is an interactional, interpersonal process and as such it involves as a minimum two people: the dyad. Thus, we can no longer view communication disorders in children from an intrapersonal perspective, trying to find out what is wrong with the child's communication so that we can help that child overcome it alone. We need to consider the important role significant others play in facilitating or constraining communication, as the effects are always bidirectional, from child to significant other and from significant other to the child. In Chapter 13 the authors provide a framework for the development of the possible interactive alignments experienced by the child under 'Significant Social Contexts in the Child's Development'. This framework provides us with guidelines as to appropriate contexts in which assessment should take place. Thus, for example, assessment of a very young child should include *caregiver–child* interaction and the assessment of a young adolescent should include *adult–child* and *child–child* peer contexts.

Third, assessment of any particular aspect of language needs to amalgamate the contribution of pragmatic knowledge with the contribution of structural-semantic knowledge. Thus, at an initial assessment visit, a failure on the part of the child to produce a particular syntactic structure in the clinic, with the clinician as the conversational partner, signifies that the child is not able to produce that particular syntactic structure, in a strange environment (the clinic) and with a non-familiar conversational partner (clinician). It does not necessarily mean that the child does not have that structure in his or her linguistic system, or that, given a different context, for example with a parent at home, this structure will not be used. The opposite situation can also occur. In a home visit, a clinician may note comprehension on the part of the child to parental use of commands involving 'before' such as 'before you go to bed, brush your teeth', or 'before you sit for dinner, wash your hands'. This observation tells us that in parent–child interaction at home and with reference to everyday, repetitive routine activities, the child understands structures referring to the order of events in time. This does not necessarily mean that the child's linguistic system is such that it can cope with this type of information or that, given different structural-semantic information, for example the sentence 'before you touch the red block, touch the blue block', the child will be able to understand. Assessment thus has to be more comprehensive in that it always needs to integrate the pragmatic factors in the situation with the structural-linguistic knowledge necessary to participate in it.

Assessing Pragmatics

A narrow view of pragmatics has brought forward an additional set of skills that are the concern of speech–language pathologists. Clinicians are actively seeking information about how children acquire the rules necessary to use language appropriately in a variety of contexts and how these skills are learned and used by language-impaired and other atypical populations. This additional set of language skills that the child acquires during development also needs to be assessed and understood within the interactional framework discussed in the previous section. Narrow pragmatics needs to be understood within broad pragmatics.

Prutting and Kirchner (1987) suggest that the paradigm necessary for conceptualising pragmatic aspects of language is only just evolving and currently much of what is available involves the beginning stages of fact-gathering and description.This, none the less, should not hinder us as clinician-researchers from actively trying to apply what we know in order to assess pragmatics in language-disordered populations. As will be seen in this chapter, procedures, materials and tests are being developed to help the clinician provide a profile of the pragmatic abilities and deficits of different groups of language-learning children.

We can distinguish between three main approaches to the assessment of pragmatics: the ethnographic method, the checklist approach and the standardised test. We will examine each of these approaches in the following sections.

The Ethnographic Method

Ethnography refers to a method of study of events and persons in which one of the main aims is to discern underlying rules and patterns which operate for the participants (Ripich and Spinelli, 1985). The ethnographic method can be seen as an alternative to more traditional approaches to assessment in which the main focus is on the results of assessment: for example, the number of times a child performs a task correctly. In the ethnographic approach, on the other hand, the emphasis is on the processes of assessmen: for example, how the child seems to arrive at a particular task performance, especially in cases where the child's answers are incorrect.

The ethnographic approach can be characterised in the following ways. First, it is *inductive*. What this means is that the analyst makes observations of a subject in selected contexts, collects data – for example, in the form of transcripts of interactions – and draws conclusions from a careful examination of the data. Thus the method requires keen observational skills and the ability to generalise from particular examples. A second characteristic is that the method involves *qualitative* as opposed to quantitative analysis. Rather than being concerned with the number of times a subject performs a particular action, the analysis involves a detailed examination of how the action gets performed. Third, the approach is *naturalistic*, which means that it is considered important to observe events in their natural settings. Thus, if a child is reported as having difficulty with communication in everyday settings, it would not be considered sufficient to observe the child's behaviour while interacting with a speech and language therapist in a clinic; instead, it would be necessary to observe the child in a variety of contexts which reflected the child's everyday communicative situations. A fourth aspect is that the analyst needs to be able to *adopt the perspective of the subject under analysis*. In the case of a child with pragmatic disability, this would involve a child-centred perspective in which an attempt would be made to view the communicative context from the viewpoint of the child. This perspective contrasts with the more normative view typical of an adult-centred approach in which the child's performance is measured against norms of expected or desired behaviour. Thus, instead of judging a child inadequate because the child fails to use a particular communicative skill in the way a child of the same age or an adult would do, the analyst examines the way in which the child actually uses the skill in question, and attempts to assess its effectiveness (or lack of effectiveness) in terms of the child's perspective. The identification of avoidance strategies in children who have linguistic and communicative difficulties owes much to this more child-centred approach to analysis. Finally, the ethnographic approach is *constructionist*. What this means is that the analyst examines the processes of an event rather than its outcome. In the case of an interaction involving an adult and a child, the emphasis would be on how both adult and child actively contribute to the interaction that evolves, rather than treating the interaction as directed by one of the participants – usually the adult.

Ripich and Spinelli (1985) outline an ethnographic approach to classroom assessment and intervention which could be generalised to the study of interactions in the clinic as well as everyday situations outside the clinic in which the child is involved. Their approach consists of the following stages:

1. identify the child to be studied, on the basis of reports, questionnaires, checklists, or referrals from people involved with the child, such as parents, teachers, or clinicians;
2. make a preliminary description of the communicative problem based on these sources of information, which may be supplemented by interviews with the people concerned, including the child;
3. develop a summary of the problem;
4. observe the child in the relevant communicative contexts;
5. summarise the observations and identify patterns of communication breakdown;
6. validate these observations in consultation with the teacher, parent or clinician and the child.

It might be useful to summarise a case-study which Ripich and Spinelli (1985) present as an illustration of the ethnographic method. The child they examined was unable to follow classroom instructions and had a low level of participation and attention in the classroom. The initial step of identification of the child and his problem was taken by the child's teacher. Next, the clinician set about describing the communication problem, asking the teacher to elaborate on the nature of the problem as well as interviewing the child. The interview with the teacher was structured around a Classroom Communication Checklist (Ripich and Spinelli, 1985, p. 209), in which the teacher was asked to rate the child's effectiveness across a number of parameters, such as participation, manner and frequency of interruptions, ability to maintain attention and follow instructions, questioning and descriptive ability. This information was supplemented by more specific information concerning different contexts in which the child's particular difficulties were observed. In this case, for example, it was found that the child never responded in whole-class contexts, seldom participated in reading group discussions, and was more interactive in one-to-one situations.

In the interview with the child, each area of communicative breakdown was discussed and an attempt was made to elicit from the child the possible motivations for his behaviour. The following example illustrates how some useful information was gained on the child's perspective on classroom participation (Ripich and Spinelli, 1985, p. 209):

Clinician: Why do children not always answer in class?
Child: They don't know the answer or they don't think fast
             enough. My mum says it's better to listen.
Clinician: So do you try to listen?
Child: Yeah, that's the best way.

On the basis of these initial observations, the clinician concluded that the child's low level of classroom participation was due to the fact that he had overgeneralised the rule that it is important to listen, whereas his difficulty with following classroom instructions was possibly related to processing difficulties. These conclusions were then tested and supported in classroom observations, following which it was concluded that the child only communicated when highly motivated – for example, when he needed information to complete his work – and that his difficulties in following instructions were due partly to the way the teacher presented the instructions and partly to his processing difficulties. These problems were intensified in larger groups. The observations were validated in further interviews with the teacher and the child, and options for a plan of intervention were discussed, which involved the teacher attempting to be more systematic in giving instructions and the child practising 'doing his work right and talking more in class'. Indeed, the intervention strategy which was implemented involved developing the child's ability to make clarification requests appropriately, thus facilitating both classroom participation and attention.

We have exemplified the ethnographic approach in some detail as it illustrates the strengths as well as the weaknesses of this method of assessment. One general point is that it is difficult to assess communicative skills outside natural communicative contexts. The ethnographic method provides a way of overcoming this problem. It is important to emphasise that what is involved is not just a set of good observation skills, but rather the ability to generalise from these observations and to avoid being biased by prior assumptions. In this way it is possible to focus on the particular problems of an individual child, without having to interpret these problems within a predetermined theoretical framework.

However, the other side of the coin is that the approach lacks generality as it cannot benefit from knowing what typical problems are that children encounter. It is for this reason that several investigators have developed checklists of pragmatic skills which observers can try to identify as they watch the child interact.

Checklists of Pragmatic Skills

Checklists serve to heighten the clinician's awareness of pragmatic issues which arise in everyday conversational interaction. Typically, a checklist requires the observer to note the number of times a set of behaviours occurs in an interaction or sometimes simply whether it occurs or not. This can be done while the interaction is taking place, but more usually audio- or video-recordings are used so that a more accurate and a more easily verifiable analysis can be made.

There are now several checklists available for the analysis of pragmatic behaviours. We will examine a selection of these checklists, summarising their strengths and weaknesses (for a description of a wide range of pragmatic assessment procedures, see also Smith and Leinonen, 1992). Following this, we will assess the usefulness of checklists in general as a method for assessing pragmatic ability and disability and will outline some problems with the use of checklists. We will begin with two procedures that are used to elicit information from parents and others interacting with a child about the child's communicative behaviours – in other words, reports about the child's communication. We will then examine checklists which are used to analyse recordings and samples of actual communicative situations involving children. As we will see, both types of checklist are potentially useful as sources of information about a child's communicative abilities.

Pre-assessment Questionnaire

The Pre-assessment Questionnaire (Gallagher, 1983) is an attempt to address the problem of obtaining a representative sample of a child's language, given that a child's language performance varies across different contexts. These contexts may include the child's communicative partner or physical context variables such as the activities or materials used to elicit language samples. The Questionnaire is to be used as a means of obtaining information from parents and other significant persons in the child's life about the child's use of language in these different contexts.

The first part of the procedure is concerned with basic information, such as children and adults who live in the child's home. The next part includes questions about the nature of the child's communicative difficulties, based on reports of different persons. There follow questions concerning how the child's behaviour changes when interacting with different partners – friend, younger and older sibling, teacher, mother, father, familiar adult, unfamiliar adult, small group – as well as in different contexts such as talking about things he has done, things he will do, things he is doing, things someone else is doing, and familiar and unfamiliar toys or activities. Finally, there are questions about the child's best and most frequent communicative situations.

The Pre-assessment Questionnaire is intended as a supplement to standard assessment procedures. It provides basic information about contextual factors influencing the child's communicative behaviours and is to be used prior to language sampling, so that more representative samples of the child's language may be obtained. Gallagher cites some examples of how useful this information can be in obtaining representative samples of children's language. One child had an MLU value of 1.6 in the clinician–child sample but an MLU of 3.96 when talking with her brother. One boy produced his most structurally complex utterances while playing with water toys in a plastic bucket filled with water, whereas for another it was when playing with a younger friend, and for yet another it was talking about pictures in a family album. An awareness of the influence of these contextual factors on performance also helps to clarify therapy goals by indicating the contexts in which the child appears to have greater difficulty.

The Pragmatics Profile of Early Communication Skills

This profile (Dewart and Summers, 1988) is also concerned with obtaining information about children's use of language in a variety of contexts, based on a questionnaire which is administered in an informal interview with parents or other caregivers.

The Pragmatics Profile is concerned with four aspects of the child's communication skills: communicative intentions, responses to communication, interaction and conversation, and contextual variation. Communicative intentions covers the range of speech acts a child uses, such as requesting, rejecting, protesting, greeting, naming, commenting and giving information. Response to communication addresses questions such as how the parent gets the child's attention, how the child responds in interaction, whether the child understands gestures, acknowledges previous utterances, understands a speaker's intentions, and responds to 'no' and occasions when the parent says things like 'in a minute'. Interaction and conversation includes questions about interactive aspects of the child's communication, such as how exchanges are initiated and maintained, how the child initiates and responds to conversational repair, how the child terminates and joins conversations. The final aspect, contextual variation, examines the persons, places, times and topics which produce the child's best communication, how the child uses language intrapersonally in play as well as interpersonally with peers, and the child's awareness of social conventions. Each category is illustrated with examples to help prompt the parent in providing information.

This profile is concerned with qualitative information about a child's communication skills. It is intended for use with infants and pre-school children as a means of helping the therapist identify those aspects of the child's communication which need to be developed or modified, or where further, more detailed investigation is warranted. There is a possible objection that parental reports may be unreliable, as parents often do not know which aspects of the child's communication are important to report and which are not important. Moreover, parents may also either over-estimate or under-estimate their child's abilities as they are unaware of developmental norms. Against this the authors argue that parents know their children well and have wide experience of trying to communicate with them, so that information from the parents provides a useful guide to how the child communicates in everyday interactions outside the clinical situation.

Assessing the Pragmatic Ability of Children

Roth and Spekman (1984) provide an organisational framework for the assessment of the pragmatic abilities of children. They divide communication skills into three levels of analysis: communicative intentions, presupposition and the social organisation of discourse. Communicative intention refers to the intended illocutionary acts which a child produces, such as requesting, naming, greeting and responding. Two aspects of communicative intention are investigated: the range of different illocutionary acts used and understood by the child, and the child's ability to use and understand indirect as well as direct speech acts.

The term *presupposition* is used in a confusing way by Roth and Spekman. The usual definition within pragmatics involves inferences or assumptions which are built into linguistic expressions (for example, that if someone *managed* to do something, this presupposes that they *tried* to do it). Roth and Spekman use the term presupposition to refer to the ability of children to make inferences about their conversational partner's knowledge. More usually this ability is referred to as *role-taking*. The child's ability to make these inferences is reflected in the *content* and *form* of his or her messages – for example, the use of different styles for different communicative partners or for different physical contexts, such as face-to-face interaction as compared with telephone conversations. The third level of assessment – social organisation of discourse – deals with the ability to maintain a dialogue over several turns and includes conversational turn-taking, topic initiation, maintenance, termination and shift as well as conversational repairs.

The main value of this framework is that it draws the attention of clinicians new to pragmatics to the major findings of the past fifteen years or so. The main criticism of the framework is that it is not organised as a protocol with discrete, non-overlapping and well-motivated categories. Rather, a series of categories is presented based on comprehensive reviews of studies of pragmatic behaviour in normally developing children. Terminological distinctions arising from differences in theoretical orientation are disregarded and there are no guidelines as to how the results of the analysis should be interpreted and translated into proposals for intervention.

An Approach to Developing Conversational Competence

Bedrosian (1985) presents a two-level approach to data analysis. His molecular level involves a fine-grained analysis of the child's behaviour and focuses primarily on topic. Each topic initiation is coded according to its subject-matter, participant orientation (whether self-orientated or other-orientated), its communicative intent (as in Roth and Spekman), and whether eye contact is used for attention-getting. Subsequent turns are coded according to whether they are continuous or discontinuous for the discourse. Finally the interaction is coded according to the dimension of control, which is expressed by items such as interruptions and interrogatives. The second level of analysis, the molar analysis, is more global and is recommended for those observers operating under stricter time constraints. The molar level consists of a discourse skills checklist with sections for topic initiations, topic maintenance, use of eye contact, turn-taking, politeness and some non-verbal behaviours. The categories in this checklist are simpler than those of Roth and Spekman and consist mainly of observational points such as: initiates new topics on a daily basis, talks mostly about self, responds to questions, interrupts others, uses commands, or uses non-verbal head nods to acknowledge. These are categorised by the observer.

Like the other checklists discussed earlier, Bedrosian's scheme covers a wide range of conversational behaviours and consists of categories which are largely self-explanatory. Furthermore, Bedrosian presents some useful ideas for improving deficient conversational skills. These consist of discourse goals and a series of teaching procedures which are clearly illustrated. So, for example, one goal might be to increase the child's frequency of topic initiations and the teaching procedures for this goal include practice in greetings, departures, ways of getting the listener's attention, expressing needs, making requests for information and for repair. Whilst most of the discourse goals have the aim of increasing frequencies of behaviours, there is also a goal for decreasing the frequency of inappropriate topic initiations involving practice in items such as turn-taking, listening and decreasing interruptions. Thus the results of the checklist have to be interpreted by the observer according to their perceived appropriateness in order to determine what the discourse goal should be. This is perhaps the main weakness of this scheme, in that it leaves the most important part – the interpretation – to the observer's intuitions, although, to be fair, this weakness is shared by most other schemes and in any case it might be argued that most of the required interpretations can indeed be made by an insightful observer with sound common sense. How this problem might be overcome will be discussed presently.

Towards a Profile of Conversational Ability

The checklist presented in McTear (1985) is similar to that of Roth and Spekman, in that it is based on behaviours observed in normally developing children, although in McTear's checklist there is some attempt to motivate the categories in terms of a developmental sequence. The most basic category is turn-taking, which is a defining characteristic of conversation. Turn-taking precedes other pragmatic behaviours developmentally as it is possible for children to take turns in conversations before they have learned to fill out their turns with any meaningful linguistic content. Next comes the ability to produce contingently related turns. This involves at the minimum either the ability to initiate a conversational exchange, which includes getting the listener's attention and directing it to the objects and persons being referred to, or the ability to produce an appropriate response. At a more advanced level there are devices for introducing and reintroducing discourse topics and for drawing on background and shared knowledge (what Roth and Spekman describe as presupposition). Each of these skills can be seen in terms of their appropriateness, and in the case of this checklist requests for action are identified as a speech act whose appropriate usage requires a complex assessment of social considerations such as the role of the addressee and the nature of the requested task. Finally there is a section dealing with the main ways in which conversational breakdown can be repaired.

The main strength of McTear's scheme is that it presents a detailed summary of many of the key points of interest in developmental pragmatics, which is potentially useful in the analysis of disordered conversation. What is lacking, however, is a set of guidelines for the interpretation of results. Observers may quantify the frequencies of the many behaviours listed in the checklist but there is no suggestion as to how these frequencies are to be interpreted. Indeed, as we will see later, it is not clear whether frequency is a useful index for conversational analysis in any case.

The Pragmatic Protocol

The Pragmatic Protocol (Prutting and Kirchner, 1987) is a descriptive taxonomy covering 30 pragmatic aspects of language. This protocol is designed mainly for use with children aged 5 years or older, though it has also proved useful as a means of providing an overall communicative index for adults. In this protocol each of the pragmatic skills falls under one of the following categories: verbal, paralinguistic and non-verbal. Verbal aspects include speech-act pair analysis (taking speaker and listener roles appropriately), variety of speech-acts, topic management (selection, introduction, maintenance and change), and turn-taking, whilst paralinguistic aspects include intelligibility and fluency, and non-verbal aspects include physical proximity, body posture and facial expressions. All of these items are coded according to whether they are used appropriately or inappropriately in the discourse.

The main strength of the Pragmatic Protocol is its comprehensiveness and its attempt to integrate verbal with paralinguistic and non-verbal behaviours. Each of the items is clearly defined and references are provided to indicate how the categories are motivated by the research literature. However, as with several other such taxonomies, there is no mention of how the different levels in the taxonomy relate to one another. Are some levels more general and others more specific? For example, is turn-taking initiation more specific than cohesion? Related to this, do some problems at one level predict problems at another level? For example, does a problem in topic maintenance affect turn-taking contingency?

Analysis of Language-Impaired Children's Conversation (ALICC)

This procedure (Adams and Bishop, 1989; Bishop and Adams, 1989) is based on the empirical studies involving group comparisons consisting of specific language-impaired children. The procedure consists of two parts: a quantitative analysis of aspects of children's conversational abilities and a detailed analysis of inappropriate language use.

The analysis of children's conversational abilities is based on the framework developed by McTear (1985) and involves applying procedures developed for the analysis of normal conversational behaviour to children with language impairment. The aspects which are examined are exchange structure, turn-taking, repairs and cohesion. Exchange structure is concerned with different ways of initiating and responding in conversational sequences. Initiations are subdivided into questions, requests for action and statements, whilst responses are coded as minimal or extended. The analysis of turn-taking is concerned with the identification of gaps and turn-taking violations. A distinction is made between inadvertent overlap, where the child has attempted to predict a turn completion point, and interruptions, in which turn-taking rules are violated. Repairs include responses to requests for clarification, whether appropriate or inappropriate, the production of clarification requests, corrections of the other person's utterances, and self-repairs. Finally, cohesion focuses on the use of pronouns and demonstrative terms, distinguishing between cases where the pronoun is recoverable from the linguistic context, the situation, or is ambiguous or unrecoverable.

Although these conversational features, when examined in the speech of language-impaired children, and especially those with pragmatic disability, can help to indicate the nature of the child's problems by indicating how the child's conversational behaviours differ from those of normal children, the authors argue that it is necessary also to examine the ways in which a child's language is inappropriate. The analysis of inappropriateness constitutes the second part of the procedure.

As a basis for the analysis of inappropriateness, transcripts of language-impaired and control children were examined and instances were identified of utterances where the normal flow of conversation appeared to be disrupted because the child's utterance was inappropriate in some way. These inappropriate utterances were then subcategorised as follows:

1. *Expressive problems in syntax/semantics*: This category occurs where the child's utterance is inappropriate because of a linguistic problem, such as the wrong use of a lexical item.
2. *Failure to comprehend literal meaning*: This category includes cases where the child gives an inappropriate response to a question, which may have been because of misinterpretation or because the child only had a vague notion about what was being asked.
3. *Pragmatic problems I: violation of exchange structure*: This category concerns failure to obey conversational sequencing rules, either by not responding at all or by ignoring the other person's initiation and continuing with an unrelated utterance.
4. *Pragmatic problems II: failure to use context in comprehension*: The most typical example of this category is where a child responds to the literal meaning of a partner's utterance but misses its intended meaning: a meaning which can only be understood if the linguistic or situational context is taken into account, as in an indirect speech-act.
5. *Pragmatic problems III: too little information provided to partner*: In this case the child fails to provide information which the partner requires in order to make sense of an utterance. This could be as a

result of leaving out some important words on the wrong assumption that the listener has knowledge of them; the use of an unestablished referent, for example, by wrongly using a pronoun; or by omitting a logical step or crucial piece of information when telling a story or giving instructions.

6. *Pragmatic problems IV: too much information provided to partner*: In this case the child over-elaborates on a topic saying more than is necessary to answer the question, repeats unnecessarily, or fails to use ellipsis appropriately.

7. *Unusually or socially inappropriate content or style*: This category covers cases where the child goes off at a tangent and changes the topic inappropriately, fails to mark changes in topic, uses stereotyped language, asks questions to which the conversational partner could not possibly know the answer, or makes socially inappropriate remarks: for example, remarks which are over-friendly or over-personal. This notion is particularly difficult to pin down, and research (Bishop and Adams, 1989) shows that it is not easy to obtain inter-rater agreement on precisely what inappropriacy is.

8. *Other problems*: This category covers examples where the child lacks knowledge or experience that is required for an adequate response.

All of these categories reflect aspects of pragmatic disability which have been reported in the literature. Bishop and Adams (1989) found that these categories could be used reliably to distinguish children with pragmatic disability from normally developing as well as language-impaired children. They point out that many of the categories involve problems which are not specifically linguistic. For example: providing too much or too little information would appear to be a consequence of an inability to assess what the listener needs to know, whereas inappropriate questioning results from an inability to assess the listener's knowledge state. In both cases the problem is socio-cognitive. On the other hand, when the child is unable to answer adequately because of a lack of knowledge or experience, this reflects a cognitive disability.

Taken together, these two sets of measures can provide a profile of a child's conversational abilities and difficulties. The measure of conversational abilities is useful for providing a quantitative index when comparing subgroups of children or investigating how conversational competence varies in different settings. The analysis of inappropriateness provides a basis for a detailed investigation of specific areas of pragmatic difficulty and how these difficulties relate to the child's levels of linguistic, cognitive and sociocognitive development. In this way this procedure addresses the issue of different types of pragmatic disability to a much greater extent than other checklists.

BLADES

BLADES (Bristol Language Development Scales) (Gutfreund, Harrison and Wells, 1989) provides a comprehensive approach to the assessment of language production in children, involving the following areas: the purposes for which language is used in conversation (pragmatics), the meanings that are expressed (semantics), and the form and structure of the language used (syntax). We will focus on the first of these aspects here; the semantic aspect is addressed in Chapter 8, and the syntactic aspect in Chapter 6, this volume.

The assessment of pragmatics in BLADES involves the analysis of the functions of utterances. Functions are defined as the purposes which utterances serve in conversation: to control the speech or actions of others (control function), exchange information (representative function), express feelings and attitudes or ask about the feelings and attitudes of others (expressive function), and to facilitate the channel of communication (procedural, social and tutorial function). Each of these main functions is broken down into sub-functions. For example, control functions include requests for action, requests for permission, suggestions, statements of intention, offers. Each of these functions is assigned a level, based on the order of emergence of that function in a longitudinal study of a large group of children. Thus it is possible to compare the use of functions by a child and to determine whether the child's use of language is at average level for age. It is also possible to identify gaps in a child's functional use of language and to use the Therapy Planning Form, which sets out the functions according to type and level, to plan for the items which the child should learn next. The manual also includes detailed guidance as to the elicitation, transcription and coding of utterances.

The potential value of BLADES becomes apparent when utterances are analysed at all three levels – pragmatics, semantics, and syntax – as it is then possible to determine links between a child's difficulties at these different levels. However this cross-analysis of levels is not part of the procedure, although it would be possible to examine coded utterances to see which particular syntactic structures are used by a child to express a particular function, and, by comparing with samples from other children, to judge whether the child's range of structures for that function is restricted. As with similar schemes for coding the functions of utterances there is the problem of identifying what function a particular utterance might have. The scheme allows for multiple coding of utterances. As an example: the utterance *I am going out now because it is raining* can be coded as both INTEND and GIVE EXPLANATION. This is a realistic approach, as clearly utterances may serve several functions simultaneously. However, there is the practical problem of knowing when to draw the line with multiple coding, as the coding scheme would permit utterances to be coded in many different ways and there is no way of deciding when the process is complete or whether some functions should be considered primary and others secondary. Obviously such considerations are important when it comes to making comparisons across samples. Notwithstanding these problems, the BLADES scheme provides a useful tool for the assessment of children's language production as a basis for diagnosis and therapy planning.

Some Problems with Checklists for Pragmatics

As should be apparent from this brief review of checklists for pragmatics, all of these schemes cover roughly the same ground, with the main differences being in emphasis and grouping of items. This is hardly surprising, as the schemes have evolved out of extensive reviews of the developmental literature. The fact that there is this congruence and that the categories are well motivated is encouraging. However, there is still the problem that these categories may not be the most appropriate for pinpointing the types of problem which arise for language-impaired children. It may be the case that language-impaired children experience specific hurdles with certain aspects of language which are not specific hurdles for the normally-developing child. For example, language-impaired children show marked problems with initiating conversations which are above and beyond what would be expected from normal controls of the same MLU (mean length of utterance). For this reason case studies and ethnographic approaches will still be valuable. Furthermore, few of these checklists have been tested extensively with language-impaired subjects. A notable exception is the Prutting and Kirchner (1987) study. One of the main findings from this study was that there appeared to be different clusterings of pragmatic disabilities as well as wide variations within diagnostic groups. Bishop and Adams (1989) make a similar point.

The other main problem associated with checklists arises in their implementation. The simplest approach would seem to be to count frequencies of behaviours. However, the frequency or even the presence or absence of a behaviour may not be the most important factor. Scores such as 80% do not make much sense and it is not even clear whether in some cases 80% is that much better than a score of 50%, as it may be the deficient 20% that has a devastating effect on communication. Indeed, in one case discussed by Prutting and Kirchner (1987), a single behaviour, where a client entered the room and proceeded to lie down on the couch, had a dramatic effect on the subsequent interaction even though it occurred only once.

Related to this is the question of the scoring method, in particular, how judgements on appropriateness are made. Viewed abstractly by an outside observer certain behaviours may appear inappropriate yet they may not have any adverse effect on the interaction. For this reason Prutting and Kirchner (1987) recommend the more conservative approach which only scores items as inappropriate if they have a perceived detrimental effect on the interaction. This allows for those cases where an individual produces unusual compensatory strategies to further the interaction. What still cannot be accounted for, however, is the use of compensatory strategies by the person's conversational partner. It is possible to make someone's behaviours appear better than they might have been – the converse is also possible, of course. The paradigm case of this is where mothers of very young infants make their babies appear to be more competent conversationalists than they really are by building conversations around whatever gestures or sounds they happen to produce. This is a paradox inherent in the study of interaction, which is, after all, *interpersonal* rather than intrapersonal and for this reason any checklist which focuses on only one side of the interaction is bound to run into difficulty.

Standardised tests

From what has been said so far it might seem premature to think of standardised tests in the area of pragmatic disability, as the field is so young and little is known about the range of disabilities which might fall under this general umbrella. However, it is also possible that the use of pragmatic tests in research might contribute to our understanding of pragmatic disability. Standardised tests have a further, more practical, value in that clinicians often require the support of such tests in demonstrating the need for a course of treatment for language disability and until recently this was only possible in the more traditional areas of phonology, syntax and semantics. In this section we will look at two tests: one for pragmatics which is in fairly wide use: the Test of Pragmatic Skills (Shulman, 1985) and The Pragmatic Screening Test (Prinz and Weiner, 1987).

The Test of Pragmatic Skills

Shulman's Test of Pragmatic Skills is intended for children suspected of having impairment in the appropriate use of conversational intentions or with a limited range of such intentions. Thus the focus is on the child's usage of illocutionary acts such as requesting information, requesting action, refusing and denying; and on their ability to choose an appropriate act in different communicative contexts. The main task for the tester is to elicit appropriate communicative intentions from the child in four standardised assessment tasks: playing with puppets, playing with a pencil and sheet of paper, playing with telephones, and playing with blocks. Some examples should make clear what is involved.

The puppet task involves two puppets, one of which the child is allowed to choose. Following this the clinician presents a series of probes which are intended to elicit a variety of illocutionary acts from the child including greeting, answering, informing and naming. For example, the following are the probes for this task (for details of the other tasks, see Shulman, 1985):

1. Let's talk! Hi!
2. How are you today?
3. I like to watch TV.
4. Tell me what your favourite TV show is.
5. I've never watched that show. Tell me about it.
6. Do you know what my favourite show is?
7. I like _____ .(clinician names a television show)
8. Who are the good guys on your favourite TV show?
9. Why are they good guys?
10. Thank you for talking with me. Bye-bye.

It should be fairly obvious what sorts of responses the child is required to make and in the test instructions sample responses and the illocutionary acts to be observed are set out for each probe. The child's response is scored on a six-point scale, as follows:

0 no response
1 contextually inappropriate
2 contextually appropriate non-verbal/gestural response only
3 contextually appropriate one-word response without elaboration
4 contextually appropriate response with minimal elaboration (two or three words)
5 contextually appropriate response with extensive elaboration (more than three words)

The child's total raw score on all four tasks is calculated and then divided by four to obtain the Mean Composite Score (MCS) which is then used to determine the child's Percentile Rank. This is based on information obtained from a standardisation sample of 650 children (see Shulman, 1985, for further details), which provides normative data across individual assessment tasks and mean composite scores.

The first point to note in the evaluation of this test is that it deals only with communicative intentions, which the author claims are an important foundation for functional communication. Communicative intentions are probably easier to elicit in standardised tests than other conversational behaviours but, even so, a wide range of responses could be predicted from even the fairly tightly-constraining probes presented earlier, as the imaginative reader will no doubt have ascertained. This raises the question of scoring. Given that it is difficult to predict the full range of responses, rather too much has to be left to the tester in determining what score to assign. To take an example: one sample response to the probe 'I've never watched that show. Tell me about it' is 'I don't want to'. This is described as rejection/denial but what score should be given? If the response is judged to be appropriate, (and it is difficult to see why not), then should it receive maximum points on the grounds that it contains more than three words? How does this compare with a response which gives a long description of the show, which can only receive five points at a maximum? Indeed the child could go through most of the probes giving this type of response and score as well as a child who was more cooperative. In the same vein it can be argued that complexity is not necessarily a function of the length of an utterance and that a distinction between utterances of one word, two to three, and more than three words in length is too simplistic.

A further problem relates to what scores from this test really tell us about a child's pragmatic abilities. Shulman puts forward the hypothesis that the scores might be used to predict young children's use of early discourse rules such as turn-taking, speaker dominance, topic mainten-ance and topic change, on the assumption that the child has demon-strated in the test the ability to express conversational intent. However, this hypothesis begs the question of the nature of the relationships between communicative intentions and these quite diverse discourse rules. It is possible to imagine children who might score well on this test but who still perform poorly in everyday conversations. In other words, the Test of Pragmatic Skills covers a restricted set of conversational behav-iours, although it does provide a standardised and norm-referenced assessment instrument for measuring these behaviours. There is also a Language Sampling Supplement, covering turn-taking, speaker domi-nance, topic maintenance and topic change, which operates more or less along the lines of the checklists discussed earlier and which can be used to glean further information about the child's conversational abilities.

The Pragmatics Screening Test

Like the Test of Pragmatic Skills, the Pragmatics Screening Test (Prinz and Weiner, 1987) involves eliciting illocutionary acts from the child but, in addi-tion to this, it is concerned with the ability to take the listener's perspective and to process and initiate conversational discourse and narratives. The test is intended as an initial screening instrument in pragmatic abilities for children aged between 3;6 and 8;6 and the elicitation procedures are presented as game-like activities. The test consists of the following items:

Pretest Training
Absurd Requests
Ghost Trick
Referential Communication Task

Before beginning the test the child's teacher is asked to complete the Pragmatics Teacher Rating Scale, in which the child is rated on dimensions such as verbally interactive, cooperative, attentive, follows direction, confident. This is to ensure that children who are quiet or shy will not be disadvantaged in the test, which requires an ability to indicate discourse at appropriate points. The Pretest gives the tester a further chance to ascertain the child's suitability and to prepare the child for the humorous and informal nature of the subsequent tasks. The child is presented with some incongruities so as to elicit uninhibited responses. For example, the tester points to a picture of a dog and says 'I'm going to tell you a story about this picture. *There was once a little cat.*' Any response, non-verbal or verbal, is acceptable, but if the child fails to respond to this and subsequent prompts, then the test is discontinued.

The point of this Pretest becomes apparent when we look at the first test item – Absurd Requests. The materials for this part of the test include a teddy bear without arms and a pair of scissors taped together and the child is asked to do things which are impossible in this situation, such as 'Show me his hand' and 'Cut the paper'. Several pragmatic categories are listed as possible response types to these requests: statement of fact; attitude of belief; denial; request for action or object; request for information or clarification; interpretive response; no response. Each is illustrated with sample responses. Each response type is coded and the tester enters the response codes on a standardised record form which is then sent off for analysis by the publishers. As the criteria for this analysis are not available in the published version of the test, it can only be assumed that the responses are ranked in some scale of complexity and that the total scores are computed over all the test items. It would also be possible to isolate from the record form those areas in which the child appeared weakest as a basis for subsequent intervention work.

The remainder of the tasks can be described briefly. The Ghost Trick involves a small conjuring trick with a handkerchief and is meant to elicit a series of responses from the child, some of which seem to be a little unrealistic. Indeed at some points an attentive child might not feel the need to make any verbal comment while the trick is being performed, yet such a child would presumably score lower than a child who says something like 'My uncle does tricks'. When the trick is finished, the tester promises the child a sticker but keeps it out of reach, thus attempting to elicit a response. If the child does ask for the sticker, he or she is prompted to ask even more nicely, so as to elicit politeness markers. Then the tester tells a short ghost story and asks the child to retell the story. The child's story is scored according to whether it contains the basic elements of the narrative: beginning, goal, outcome and ending.

The Referential Communication Task is similar to the many tasks of this type familiar from the literature. In this case the child has to construct a face from a set of pieces and to instruct the tester, who is separated by a screen, how to construct the same face from an identical set of pieces. However, in order to elicit various pragmatic categories from the child, the tester constructs the wrong face and also rephrases the child's subsequent instructions inappropriately: for example, if the child says, 'Put the nose in the middle' the examiner might say, 'Put the mouth in the middle'. Possible child responses to this are listed as request for action, 'Do you want me to do it for you'; denial, 'No'; and revision or clarification of the original instruction, 'No, put the nose in the middle'. The test concludes with a final inappropriate request, 'Take that mouth and put it next to the cat'. This is inappropriate because there is no cat and appropriate responses include related statements, information or clarification requests, or denials that one of the objects mentioned is present.

From this brief description it is possible to see that the Pragmatics Screening Test aims to elicit a range of illocutionary act types, politeness devices and a narrative structure. The illocutionary act categories are represented more than once across the tasks (unlike the Test for Pragmatic Skills), so that the child is given several opportunities to produce the desired response. This also makes the test procedure rather more naturalistic. A further interesting feature is the attempt to elicit some of those illocutionary act types, such as denials or clarification requests, which occur regularly in spontaneous discourse (see many examples in McTear, 1985) but which are difficult to elicit in a test situation. The success of this attempt depends to some extent on the virtuosity of the tester as well as on the degree to which the child feels at ease in the test situation.

In comparing these two tests it can be seen that both focus primarily on the elicitation of illocutionary acts, although the Pragmatics Screening Test deals with a wider range of illocutionary act types and also includes other aspects of pragmatic disability such as perspective-taking and narrating. There is also an attempt in both cases to stimulate a natural context in keeping with one of the aims of the broad view of pragmatics. However, we can see how restricted the range of pragmatic categories is when we compare them with the categories covered in pragmatic checklists. Naturally a test has to be constrained in order to be standardised and practical to administer, but there is the danger, as with any test of language ability, that only those behaviours which can be standardly elicited will be examined. In the case of pragmatic abilities this leaves a lot of ground uncovered. Nevertheless, the designers of these tests should take credit for their ingenuity and originality and it is to be hoped that tests such as these will provide an impetus for further innovations in this area. Table 9.1 presents a summary of the checklists/standardised tests available at present.

Table 9.1: Checklists and standardised tests of pragmatic skills

Type	Description
Checklists:	
Pre-assessment questionnaire (Gallagher, 1983)	Obtains sample representative of child's language across different contexts, by use of questionnaire which indicates his or her communicative behaviours
The Pragmatics Profile of Early Communication Skills (Dewart and Summers, 1988)	Obtains information about children's language across different contexts by use of questionnaire concerning four aspects of communication skills: communicative intentions; responses to communication; interaction and conversation; contextual variation. Helps identify aspects of communication needing development/modification/investigation
Assessing the Pragmatic Ability of Children (Roth and Spekman, 1984)	Framework for assessment. Based on normal behaviours. Three levels of analysis: intentions; presupposition; social organisation of discourse
An Approach to Developing Conversational Competence (Bedrosian, 1985)	Two-level data analysis: first of child's behaviour focusing on topic; second of more global nature, for observers under time constraints. Covers wide range of behaviours; presents useful ideas for improving conversational skills
Towards a profile of Conversational Ability (McTear, 1985)	Based on normal behaviours. Three levels of analysis: turn-taking in conversation; producing related turns; introducing/re-introducing discourse topics. It is comprehensive and integrates verbal/non-verbal behaviours
The Pragmatic Protocol (Prutting and Kirchner,1987)	Descriptive taxonomy covering 30 aspects of language. Mainly for children over 5 years. Categorises each pragmatic skill as: verbal, paralinguistic or non-verbal, then codes them as to their appropriate use in discourse. Is comprehensive and attempts to integrate the three categories of behaviour
Analysis of Language-Impaired Children's Conversation – ALICC (Adams and Bishop 1989; Bishop and Adams, 1989)	Procedure based on empirical studies of SLI children. Two parts – quantitative analysis of abilities; detailed analysis of inappropriate language use. Addresses issue of different types of pragmatic disability
BLADES (Bristol Language Development Scales) (Gutfreund, Harrison and Wells, 1989)	Comprehensive approach to assessment of language production. Involves pragmatics, semantics, syntax. Possible to see links between difficulties at these three levels
Standardised tests:	
Test of Pragmatic Skills (Shulman, 1985)	For children suspected of impairment/limited range of conversational intentions. Focuses on eliciting illocutionary acts in different contexts. Based on four standard assessment tasks, playing with: puppets; pencil and paper; telephones; blocks. Problem is in interpreting the scores. Includes Language Sampling Supplement (like the checklists above)
The Pragmatics Screening Test (Prinz and Weiner, 1987)	Involves eliciting illocutionary acts, as Shulman test, but also concerns listener's perspective; process and initiate discourse/narratives. Intended as initial screening instrument. Based on game-like activities: pre-test training, absurd requests, ghost trick, referential communication task. Categories repeated more than once – enables several opportunities to produce desired response

Pragmatic Assessment: Future Prospects

The tools for pragmatic assessment which have been evaluated in this chapter have served the useful function of drawing the attention of clinicians to an important aspect of language which has until fairly recently been neglected in linguistics. However, this work must be seen as only the first stage in the development of realistic assessment instruments incorporating both the narrow and the broad views of pragmatics. Tests have the advantage that they can be administered quickly and can be standardised across a large sample to provide norm references, but they have the disadvantage that they focus on restricted aspects of language which are amenable to such testing. Checklists are more comprehensive, but they leave a lot to the clinician's intuitions in terms of making judgements about appropriateness as well as in interpreting the results. Ethnographic methods provide the most detailed analyses which permit individual and idiosyncratic profiles to emerge, but this method is too time-consuming for practising clinicians and, for researchers, there is the problem of comparability across studies.

Three problems have emerged from our discussion of pragmatic assessment. The first of these relates to the dimension of complexity. Many pragmatic functions can be accomplished in a variety of ways, all of which might be appropriate on a given occasion. Yet some of these devices will be more complex than others, either in terms of their linguistic or their conceptual complexity. Labelling items in terms of their illocutionary act function, such as request or denial, does not provide any information as to their complexity. At the moment judgements about complexity are made at a fairly intuitive level. There needs to be a more principled way of evaluating complexity in pragmatic categories (for one scheme which proposes a scale of conceptual complexity, see Blank and Franklin, 1980).

The second issue concerns the tendency to generalise from studies of normally developing children to a language-impaired population. As a first stage this strategy has been useful as a means of enumerating the factors that might be relevant. What is required now, however, is more research on language-impaired children in order to pinpoint those areas where problems tend to arise. If results were to emerge with any clarity this would result in less redundancy in assessment procedures, as clinicians could focus on the most relevant categories within a more tightly constrained range.

Finally, there is a need to adopt, to a greater extent, the broad view of pragmatics and to integrate other aspects of language – phonological, syntactic and semantic – with information on pragmatics. Most researchers pay lip-service to this principle, advocating that scores from tests at other levels should be considered, but there needs to be more research on exactly how these different levels are to be integrated. For example, is a particular pragmatic deficit a consequence of a deficiency at some other level? Related to this is the question of how problems in pragmatics can be recast as deficits in conceptual and socio-cognitive domains. For example, is the failure to take the listener's perspective a problem of language or of social cognition? The answers to questions such as these will determine the direction that therapy should take.

In this respect it might be useful to outline briefly the approach being used in an ongoing project at the Wolfson Centre in London (Allen, Jolleff and McConachie, 1990). This research is concerned with the assessment of children who seem to have problems with the semantic and pragmatic areas of language. More specifically, it had been noticed that several of the children in the study had similar behaviour characteristics, such as obsessions and uncooperativeness, so that a major concern of the research was to investigate links between language and behaviour in these children. Some examples are:

1. using obsessions to make the world predictable when reasons for change or new events are hard to understand;
2. becoming upset when told off, and not understanding why;
3. becoming upset when unable to explain what they want, or why something is important.

To investigate these relationships between language and behaviour, the investigators used a three-part assessment strategy:

1. history-taking, e.g. social interaction in the first year, reason for first referral, previous language assessments, previous cognitive assessments, current behaviour such as attention span, nature of imaginative play, obsessions, home/school differences in behaviour;
2. standardised assessment, e.g. performance skills, reading, drawing, language tests;
3. observation in unstructured and structured play situations.

This research is still in progress and the assessment strategy is still being developed. However, it illustrates the main points which we have been making in this chapter and more generally throughout the book:

1. it is important to gain a complete picture of the child's pragmatic abilities in different contexts;
2. it is important to collect information which will enable us to consider relationships between the child's use of language and other potentially determining factors, such as (in this case) behavioural problems;
3. in order to explain a child's pragmatic difficulties, it will be necessary

to have information about earlier development and assessments, as the child's current difficulties may well be a consequence of earlier problems which themselves are no longer apparent.

In summary, there is a need for further work which takes into account both the narrow and the broad views of pragmatics, using a variety of methods, including longitudinal case-studies and comparative samples, and integrating information from linguistic, social and cognitive domains. This is an area where speech and language therapists will be able to make a valuable contribution, both in the evaluation and improvement of currently available procedures and in the conduct of pragmatically orientated studies of language-impaired children. The present overview of assessment procedures should provide a guideline as to the tools which are currently available as well as indicating the sorts of assessment strategies which will prove most useful in future work.

References

Adams, C. and Bishop, D.V.M. (1989). Conversational characteristics of children with semantic-pragmatic disorder, I: Exchange structure, turn taking, repairs and cohesion. *British Journal of Disorders of Communication* 24, 211–239.

Allen, J., Jolleff, N. and McConachie, H. (1990), Semantic-pragmatic disorder: behaviour language links. Paper presented at First Workshop on Semantic-Pragmatic disorders, Wolfson College, London, January.

Bates, E. (1976). *Language in Context: the Acquisition of Pragmatics*. New York: Academic Press.

Bates, E. and MacWhinney, B. (1982). Functionalist approaches in grammar. In: Wanner, E. and Gleitman, L.R. (Eds.), *Language Acquisition: the State of the Art*. Cambridge: Cambridge University Press.

Bedrosian, J.L. (1985). An approach to developing conversational competence. In: Ripich, D.N. and Spinelli, F.M. (Eds.), *School Discourse Problems*. London: Taylor & Francis.

Bishop, D.V.M. and Adams, C. (1989). Conversational characteristics of children with semantic-pragmatic disorder, II: What features lead to a judgement of inappropriacy? *British Journal of Disorders of Communication* 24, 241–263.

Blank, M. and Franklin, E. (1980). Dialogue with preschoolers: A cognitively based system of assessment. *Applied Psycholinguistics* 1, 127–150.

Craig, H.K. (1983). Applications of pragmatic language models for intervention. In: Gallaher, T.M. and Prutting, C.A. (Eds.), *Pragmatic Assessment and Intervention Issues in Language*. San Diego: College Hill Press.

Dewart, H. and Summers, S. (1988). *The Pragmatics Profile of Early Communication Skills*. Windsor: NFER-Nelson.

Fey, M.E. and Leonard, L.B. (1983). Pragmatic skills of children with specific language impairment. In: Gallagher, T.M. and Prutting, C.A. (Eds.), *Pragmatic Assessment and Intervention Issues in Language*. San Diego: College Hill Press.

Gallagher, T.M. (1983). Pre-assessment: a procedure for accommodating language use variability. In: Gallagher, T.M. and Prutting, C.A. (Eds.), *Pragmatic Assessment and Intervention Issues in Language*. San Diego: College Hill Press.

Gutfreund, M., Harrison, M. and Wells, G. (1989). *Bristol Language Development Scales*. Windsor: NFER-Nelson.

Leonard, L.B. (1981). Facilitating linguistic skills in children with specific language impairment. *Applied Psycholinguistics* 2, 89–118.

Levinson, S. (1983). *Pragmatics*. Cambridge: Cambridge University Press.

McTear, M. (1985). *Children's Conversation*. Oxford: Basil Blackwell.

Muma, J.R. (1983). Speech–language pathology: emerging clinical expertise in language. In: Gallagher, T.M. and Prutting, C.A. (Eds.), *Pragmatic Assessment and Intervention Issues in Language*. San Diego: College Hill Press.

Ochs, E. (1979). Transcription as theory. In: Ochs, E. and Schieffelin, B. (Eds.), *Developmental Pragmatics*. New York: Academic Press.

Prinz, P. and Weiner, F. (1987). *The Pragmatics Screening Test*. Ohio: Psychological Corporation.

Prutting, C.A. (1982). Pragmatics or social competence? *Journal of Speech and Hearing Disorders* 47, 123–134.

Prutting, C.A. and Kirchner, D.M. (1983). Applied pragmatics. In: Gallagher, T.M. and Prutting, C.A. (Eds.), *Pragmatic Assessment and Intervention Issues in Language*. San Diego: College Hill Press.

Prutting, C.A. and Kirchner, D.M. (1987). A clinical appraisal of the pragmatic aspects of language. *Journal of Speech and Hearing Disorders*, 52, 105–119.

Ripich, D.N. and Spinelli, F.M. (1985). An ethnographic approach to assessment and intervention'. In: Ripich, D.N. and Spinelli, F.M. (Eds.), *School Discourse Problems*. London: Taylor & Francis.

Roth, A. and Bliss, L.S. (1981). A comparison of verbal communicative skills of language impaired and normal speaking children. *Journal of Communication Disorders* 14, 133–140.

Roth, F.P. and Spekman, N.J. (1984). Assessing the pragmatic ability of children, Part 1: Organisational framework and assessment parameters. *Journal of Speech and Hearing Disorders* 49, 2–11.

Smith, B.R. and Leinonen, E. (1992). *Clinical Pragmatics*. London: Chapman & Hall.

Shulman, B. (1985). *Test of Pragmatic Skills*. Arizona: Communication Skill Builders.

Chapter 10
Linguistic Assessment of Prosody

BILL WELLS, SUE PEPPÉ AND MAGGIE VANCE

Introduction

The focus of this chapter is on the functional value of prosody for effective communication. Prosody is central to communication, not something 'stuck on top' of the words and sentences, as is sometimes implied by linguists whose orientation is to the written form of language. The centrality of prosody is evident if we consider that it can be used to convey different emotions or attitudes, to signal the difference between illocutionary acts such as questions and statements, to make grammatical distinctions, and to handle subtle aspects of interaction. Prosodic breakdown or problems with prosodic development can affect all these aspects of communication, with major consequences for the individual. Prosodic difficulties, receptive and expressive, have been found in a wide range of developmental and acquired clinical conditions, including dysarthria (Vance, 1994), aphasia and right hemisphere damage (Bryan, 1994), hearing impairment (Parker and Rose, 1990), learning difficulties (Heselwood, Bray and Crookston, 1995), autism, (Baltaxe and Simmons, 1985, Local and Wootton, 1995), developmental speech and language disorders (Hargrove and Sheran, 1989; Wells and Local, 1993). The chapter begins with an outline of the functions of prosody in communication, followed by an account of the phonetic parameters involved. The second part is devoted to a more detailed discussion of assessment of one important prosodic system in English: that of accentuation, as it relates to the function of information focus and emphasis.

The scope of the term 'prosody' varies from linguist to linguist, but is usually held to refer to those phonetic and phonological features that are not 'segmental', i.e. not attributable to consonant and vowel places in the phonological structure. Many contemporary linguists thus refer to the syllable as a prosodic unit. The broadest conception of prosody was Firth's: he introduced the terms 'prosody' and 'prosodic' to refer to features that might extend over anything from a single segment to a whole utterance, such as nasality, aspiration, palatality or retroflexion, as

234

well as accent, intonation etc. (Firth, 1948; Waterson, 1987). The focus of the present chapter is principally on what is commonly referred to as *intonation*, i.e. on prosodic features which have implications for units above the word, such as phrases, clauses, sentences and interactional sequences. Intonation forms part of what is often referred to as suprasegmental phonology, which, as the name implies, is concerned with the sounds of language at levels hierarchically above segments. The basic unit is generally considered to be the syllable and the prime concern is the relation between syllables. This can be illustrated by looking at accentuation, which is part of suprasegmental phonology: a syllable is said to be accented when contrasted with a (normally adjacent) syllable that is unaccented. Accent is thus relational, and as such has no absolute value. At the phonetic level, prosodic features do have an absolute value: pitch, for example, is present on every syllable and corresponds to an absolute value expressed in terms of fundamental frequency, which can be measured in hertz (Hz). Considerations of absolute value may be of clinical interest, for example in the case of voice patients with habitually high or low pitch. However, the emphasis of the present chapter, which has the *linguistic* assessment of prosody as its topic, will be on phonology, and thus on relational value. The phonetic parameters considered here include pitch, loudness, length, and silence, but not voice quality, which does not impinge so directly upon linguistic meaning (Laver, 1980). The assessment of voice quality is reviewed by Wirz and Mackenzie Beck (1995).

Functions of Prosody

What prosody contributes to successful communication is dependent to some extent on how it interacts with other factors. Assessing whether a person's prosody is functioning adequately therefore requires some familiarity with the interplay of linguistic levels. For example, it is often assumed that there is a relationship between prosody and the linguistic activity of questioning: that questions, as well as being (often) distinguishable from statements by their grammatical form (presence of 'wh-words' or inversion of subject and auxiliary verb), also have a characteristic intonation that differs from the intonation of statements. Because of this, a questioner can dispense with the question form and use questioning intonation instead, and still accomplish the business of questioning (Weber, 1993). The fact that questioning can be achieved by intonation and/or by the presence of certain lexical items and/or syntactic forms suggests that all these factors interact, and that the contribution of one may be more or less important for the functions of language according to the amount or type of contribution from the others.

Bearing this in mind, we can look at the approaches which linguists have adopted towards looking at the role of prosody in communication, in relation to the various levels of organisation of language: phonology, grammar and lexis (for more detailed reviews of functions that involve prosody see Couper-Kuhlen, 1986; Cruttenden, 1986). Prosody can perform *indexical* functions such as sex-grouping: in some English-speaking communities, for example, particular types of pitch movement are associated with women rather than men (McConnell-Ginet, 1980). Prosody can also be indicative of age-grouping: for example, Local (1982) found that the pitch patterns of Tyneside children take on more specifically regional characteristics as the children get older. More grossly, the pitch characteristics of speakers change with advancing age (Baken, 1987). The most pervasive indexical function is probably the socio-regional one: different regional varieties of English have strikingly different prosodic characteristics (Cruttenden, 1986). The need to take this into account in prosodic assessment is illustrated later in the chapter.

In addition to conveying relatively permanent indexical information about a speaker, intonation is thought to communicate temporary emotional, attitudinal or *affective* states. Crystal (1969) deplored the fact that concentration on the grammatical context of intonational patterns had deflected focus away from their role in affective language. However, his own attempt to explore the links bears witness to the problems involved in defining and labelling emotions: he points out that the total number of affective labels used in two key studies total over 300. Couper-Kuhlen (1986) reviews what is known about the relationship between intonation and attitude, stressing that it is not really possible to separate out the contribution of intonation from that of lexis and the context. Given such methodological problems in researching the relationship between prosody and attitude or emotion in normal speech, it is difficult for the clinician to assess how the ability to use prosody to convey emotions or attitudes is affected in clients with speech and language disorders. Nevertheless, some studies have been carried out. For example, Courtright and Courtright (1983) found that a group of specifically language-impaired (SLI) children between 3 and 7 years old were less accurate than aged-matched normal children, at interpreting emotional meaning from vocal cues in utterances recorded by actors to illustrate different emotions. (It is interesting to note that this difference disappeared when language age was controlled for, indicating that the poorer performance of the SLI children was a function of their immature language, rather than of a specific deficit in interpreting prosody.)

Grammatical functions of prosody have received much attention, and many disambiguating roles performed by prosody have been identified. Some of these are usefully grouped together as *information structure*. This includes the delimitation of where one piece of information ends and another begins. On a large scale, this can involve the grouping of several utterances into topics, as explicated within discourse analysis research (Brazil, Coulthard and Johns, 1980; Brown, Currie and Kenworthy, 1980).

In particular, topic demarcation and turn delimitation can be closely linked. Work within conversation analysis has also shown how prosodic features are used within speakers' turns to mark continuity and discontinuity (Local, 1992). It can also be considered to operate on a smaller scale, in the grouping of words into larger prosodic units, known as tone-units (Crystal, 1969), or tone-groups (Halliday, 1967), which normally coincide with grammatical units such as the clause or sentence. Within information structure, much attention has been paid to *focus* (or information focus) – the use of accentuation to indicate the most important points of an utterance. This function is discussed in detail later.

Prosody has a role in several areas of language that are normally grouped under the heading of *pragmatics*, which includes aspects of interaction, deixis, presupposition and speech acts (Levinson, 1983). The role of prosody in the realisation of *illocutionary acts* has already been touched upon: questioning was the case in point. Other illocutionary acts are statements, offers, promises, requests, orders, exclamations etc., some of which, like questions, have associations with specific grammatical structures, and possibly also specific intonation patterns. The pragmatic functions of prosody are closely related to grammatical functions: thus questions constitute a type of speech act characterised by particular grammatical structures, and also by particular intonation patterns (Halliday, 1967).

One of the most important *interactional* functions in which prosody plays a part is the management of the system for the exchange of speaker turns (Sacks, Schegloff and Jefferson, 1974). Prosodic features have been shown to contribute to turn-yielding and turn-holding (Beattie, Cutler and Pearson, 1982; Cutler and, Pearson 1986; Local, Kelly and Wells, 1986; Wells and Peppé, in press), and also to turn-competition: interruptions, the fending off of interruptions, and the relinquishing of turns are routinely accompanied by specific sets of prosodic features (French and Local, 1983). In theory, a prosodic difficulty could therefore cause a client considerable difficulty in maintaining conversational interactions. The application of this research in the clinical domain is likely to reap benefits, but to date there has been little published work that attempts to do so. The interactional function of prosody will therefore not be considered in any detail in the present chapter.

Phonetic Framework

When discussing any aspect of phonology, including prosodic systems, it is important to distinguish between the communicative *functions* that are being realised and the phonetic *forms* that are used to realise them. Some of the functions of prosody have already been mentioned. From the formal point of view, at the phonetic level prosody consists of phonetic parameters such as pitch, loudness, rate of speech, silence. The link between the communicative functions of prosody and these phonetic parameters is provided by phonological systems, which phonologists set up in order to show how speakers of a language make systematic use of these phonetic parameters for communicative purposes. Such systems vary from description to description, depending on the functions that the analyst is particularly interested in. For example, Halliday (1967) concentrated on three systems (tonality, tonicity, tone) to capture the grammatical functions of intonation that were his concern; whilst Brazil, Coulthard and Johns (1980) introduce a further system of 'key', to handle aspects of discourse intonation.

The need for three levels of description – functional, phonological and phonetic – has sometimes given rise to confusion of terminology. For example, it is sometimes thought that 'stress' refers to a phonetic parameter, whereas it is most accurately used to refer to an inherent phonological property of a lexical item, as in 'the stress in *window* is on the first syllable'. Often, the stressed syllable will indeed be realised as prosodically more prominent than adjacent unstressed syllables, through features such as pitch obtrusion, length, loudness etc. However, there are many occasions when the stressed syllable is no more prominent than the following unstressed syllable, as in the word *window* in 'Someone's broken the window', where *window* occurs in post-tonic position. Because of the confusion of terminology, it is helpful to provide a framework that sets out the terms used for different levels of analysis. The framework presented in Table 10.1 is derived from Barry (1981) and Brewster (1989).

Phonetic Parameters: Definition and Notation

In this section, brief notes on the phonetic parameters in Table 10.1 are

Table 10.1: Prosodic terminology

Physiological Activity	*Acoustic Properties*	*Auditory Parameters*
Respiratory drive	Amplitude	Loudness
Absence of activity	Silence	Silence
Time taken for articulation	Duration	Length
Rate of vibration of vocal folds	Fundamental frequency	Pitch height
Variation in rate of vocal fold vibration	Fundamental frequency change	Pitch movement
Articulatory setting	Spectral structure	Timbre

followed by a summary of the notational conventions provided in the most recent revisions of the International Phonetic Alphabet, together with the extensions to the IPA for atypical speech (Duckworth, Allen, Hardcastle and Ball, 1990), referred to henceforth as ExtIPA (see Chapter 2, this volume). A useful discussion of transcriptional issues relating specifically to non-segmental aspects of disordered speech can be found in Ball, Code, Rahilly and Hazlett (1994). Exemplification of some of the notational devices is provided in the extracts presented in the second part of this chapter.

Loudness

The loudness of speech can be measured on a perceptual scale, in sones (Moore, 1989) whilst amplitude is measured in decibels, but for linguistic prosodic assessment judgements of *relative* loudness of syllables are the most useful, and the notation system reflects this.

Notation: braces {} labelled *f* (loud), *ff* (very loud), *p* (quiet) at the start and end of the stretch of speech thus described. To indicate the relative loudness of individual syllables, IPA stress marks {ˌ '"} could be used, as they have no other phonetic interpretation in the IPA system (cf. Wells, 1994).

Loudness, with length and silence, contributes to the impression of rhythm (Couper-Kuhlen, 1993). It also contributes to the impression of accent, although Fry (1958) found it was less important for this than length and pitch height.

Silence

Silence manifests in speech as breaks in phonation, some of which are heard as pauses. How long a break needs to be before it is perceived as a pause depends upon the context in which it occurs: within a tone group, as little as 80 msec, but at a tone group boundary, as much as 220 msec (Butcher, 1981, cited in Garman, 1990). Pauses do not always consist solely of silence: they may include pause fillers such as those orthographically notated as 'er', 'um' etc.

Notation: ExtIPA : (.) short pause; (..) medium-length pause; (...) long pause. An alternative is Crystal's 'beat' system: one dash (–) accounts for one beat of a speaker's normal speech rhythm (Crystal, 1969); though Garman (1990, p.131) gives Crystal's notation an explicit durational interpretation, in terms of msec. Particular attention is given to pause in conversation analytic (CA) research, using notation conventions devised by Gail Jefferson (Atkinson and Heritage, 1984). Here, pause is measured in tenths of a second, (e.g. 1.2). In all three systems, a dot (.) indicates a minimal pause.

Pauses can coincide with inhalation, and with cognitive planning. In terms of communicative effect, the breaks for inhalation are more likely to coincide with pauses at major syntactic and prosodic boundaries, thus having a delimitative function; whereas breaks for cognitive planning (such as word-finding), which tend to occur within major grammatical units such as clauses but before major lexical class items such as nouns (Garman, 1990), are more likely to be heard as hesitations .

Silence can have other phonological functions: for example, the 'hold' phase of plosive consonants manifests acoustically as silence. Some of these phonological functions are prosodic. For instance, silence can have a rhythmic function, as in the notion of 'silent stress' or 'silent beat' (Abercrombie, 1971). It can also combine with loudness, length, pitch range, pitch height and glide to enhance the effect of accentuation in conveying information focus (Wells, 1986).

Length

When vowels, consonants and syllables are lengthened relative to adjacent units (beyond what is required for purposes of segmental contrast, e.g. *bit vs. beat*) they acquire contrastive (functional) potential at the prosodic level.

IPA notation: lengthening [:] shortening [ˇ]. Length marks can be incorporated into a transcription of speech rhythm that indicates the relative length of syllables using conventions drawn from the description of poetic metre: − and ∪ for relatively long and short syllables respectively.

Length makes a (relatively minor) contribution to accentuation for focus purposes (Wells, 1986). Together with other prosodic features, it contributes to the delimitation of larger linguistic units (Kreiman, 1982).

Length also contributes to *tempo*: changes in tempo (slow and fast speech) are signalled when groups of syllables are all speeded up or slowed down by comparison with adjacent groups of syllables.

ExtIPA notation: braces { } labelled *lento* (slow) or *allegro* (fast).

Pitch height

Pitch is the perceptual correlate of fundamental frequency (Fo), which is measured in hertz (Hz). The aspect of most linguistic interest is the pitch-height relation, between one syllable and another or between one stretch of speech and another. The amount by which pitch height can vary is known as the pitch range. One speaker's pitch range includes the highest and lowest pitch heights habitually used by that speaker.

Notation: lines showing relative pitch height iconically, between staves representing the normal extremes of the speaker's pitch range.

The pitch height a speaker selects can have functional consequences for topic structure: a high point in the range is generally used at the start of a topic (Cruttenden, 1986). Crystal (1969) suggests that wide pitch range tends to denote a high degree of emotional involvement. Width of pitch range over a constituent is the prosodic feature that correlates best with degree of perceived information focus (Wells, 1986).

Pitch movement

Henceforth referred to as *glide*, pitch movement is effected by change in fundamental frequency in the course of a syllable. The pitch can simply move up or down (rise or fall), or it may change direction in the course of a syllable (fall–rise, rise–fall). Sometimes the glide is initiated on one syllable and continued in subsequent syllables, which can thus be seen as part of the same glide (as in the system of tones proposed by Halliday, 1967).

Notation: lines showing direction of pitch movement, iconically, between staves.

From a functional point of view, glide is probably the aspect of prosody for which most claims have been made. Glide is a common exponent of accentuation, as used to convey information focus: words which display a perceptible pitch movement, particularly when combined with a wide pitch range, or when taking the form of a complex glide such as fall–rise, are normally heard as conveying a high degree of information focus (Wells, 1988). However, in some English accents, such as that of the Black Country (West Midlands), the accented syllable of the informationally most important word in the utterance usually has level pitch (Wells, 1989).

Strong claims have been made for the communicative strength of particular pitch directions. Thus it has been proposed that rising pitch is associated with questioning and also with non-finality, whereas falling pitch is associated with statements, and with finality. Whilst there is undoubtedly some truth in such claims for some varieties of English, these need to be hedged about with many provisos regarding context (both grammatical and sequential/conversational), and modified radically for different regional accents, such as Ulster (Jarman and Cruttenden, 1976; Wells and Peppé, in press) and Tyneside (Local, 1986; Local, Kelly and Wells, 1986), where the ends of speakers' turns are characterised by rising or non-low pitch terminations, rather than falling or low pitch.

One of the aims of prosodic assessment is to identify which phonetic parameters the client is able to manipulate for communicative purposes. Assessment can be done informally, by observation of habitual speech, or by reading standardised passages, and instrumental analysis can be particularly useful in quantifying the phonetic strengths and limitations of the client at the prosodic level (Baken, 1987; Ball, 1991). Because, as has been shown, there is often more than one prosodic parameter involved in the exponency of communicative functions, some prosodic cues are potentially redundant. Thus, if a client's ability to perceive and produce one parameter is weak, they can therefore be encouraged to use another parameter to compensate for the weak one.

With this in mind, Peppé (in preparation) has devised a test battery for the different phonetic parameters involved in prosodic systems. This gives the clinician a profile of the client's strengths and weaknesses, as well as material for more qualitative analysis. The different prosodic parameters tested include Loudness, Pause, Length, Pitch, Range and Glide, as well as more complex phonological systems of Rhythm, Accent and Juncture. For each parameter, there is a receptive as well as an expressive section, and within each of these there are two subtests, one of which tests the client's ability to manipulate the phonetic parameter in question, and the other the ability to use the parameter in a communicative task. This enables the clinician to identify whether a client's communicative problem with prosody stems from an underlying inability to use the prosodic parameter in question, or from a difficulty at a higher linguistic level.

The Assessment of Accentuation

So far, we have been mainly concerned with the phonetic ingredients of prosodic systems. This is a prerequisite for considering the role of prosody in communication, and particularly for considering ways in which difficulties with prosody can impair communication. It is beyond the scope of a single chapter to cover all the possible communicative functions of prosody, or even to cover the various (prosodic) phonological systems involved in the realisation of a single function. We have therefore selected one system which is generally recognised as central to our understanding of the role of prosody in English: *accentuation*, as it relates to utterances (rather than to single words as in word stress or accent). This system is variously referred to in the literature as tonicity (following Halliday, 1967), sentence stress, sentence accent or nuclear stress. Accentuation will be discussed primarily in relation to its role in conveying *information focus*, and this system will therefore be referred to as the *focus accent* system. The main advantages of concentrating on the focus accent system are that it is relatively well understood in phonological and semantic terms (compared, for example, with the system of glides), it is relatively robust with regard to dialect variation (though see below), and it is a favourite of researchers and clinicians when carrying out prosodic assessment. It therefore provides an opportunity for considering wider issues surrounding the assessment of prosody.

Accentuation and Utterance Completion

As has been indicated, the assessment of prosodic accentuation will be discussed in relation to the way in which accentuation is used to high-light important information in the utterance. In English, however, as in many other languages, accentuation simultaneously fulfils another function – that of delimiting stretches of talk: when the point of major prominence is reached, the listener knows that potentially the stretch of talk is, or is nearly, completed. Indeed, it could be argued that this is the primary function of accentuation, more important than the focusing function, on the grounds that the speaker has to accent something in the utterance to mark it as complete, even if the utterance actually contains no new information. This phenomenon is referred to as 'default accent' (Ladd, 1980). Thus, in the following extract (1), *read* is 'given', but is nevertheless accented, as this is the least unacceptable place for the accent to fall – all other positions would give rise to unwanted contrastive implications:

Extract (1)

> Cue: Has John read *Slaughterhouse Five*?
> Response: He doesn't **read** books.

In the following discussion of accentuation in relation to information focus, it should therefore be borne in mind that for speakers of most varieties of English, accentuation has a dual function: delimitative and focusing. For some speakers with communication difficulties, the two functions may become dissociated; in particular, accentuation may be reserved for its delimitative function, and not used at all to convey information focus. Examples of this will be presented later, but it is important to stress at the outset that a client who fails to use accentuation appropriately to highlight the important elements of the utterance may still be using it for other communicative purposes.

Information Focus

The Focus Accent System in Southern British English

Focus refers to the highlighting of a part or parts of the utterance as particularly important, the concomitant being that the remainder of the utterance is assumed to be less important. In many cases, the focused portion corresponds to 'new' information, and the non-focused portion to information that is 'given' by the linguistic or non-linguistic context (Halliday, 1967). Focus can be achieved by various linguistic devices, which vary from language to language, and which can combine within a single language: these include word order, choice of syntactic structure, particles and prosodic accentuation. Accentuation is a particularly important focusing device in English, as can be illustrated from the following elicited data, from Wells (1988). The subject, an adult female speaker of the standard southern British English variety, was asked to read the target sentence 'The sun was shining' in response to a series of

selected to illustrate different locations and degrees of semantic focus.
(In the original study, there were nine target sentences, and order of
presentation was randomised to avoid ordering effects.). The subject's
responses are given below in Extract (2):

Extract (2)

(a) Cue: What was it like?

          ‾   \   –   \ –

Response: The 'sun was "shining
             ⏑ – ⏑ – ⏑

(b) Cue: Describe the sun that morning

          – \ – \ –

Response: The ' sun was 'shining
         ⏑ – ⏑ – ⏑

(c) Cue: Of course, if the sun had been shining I'd have felt a lot
happier.

          –   ‾
                \ –

Response: The 'sun "was 'shining
        ⏑ – – – ⏑

(d) Cue: As Mary stepped out into the garden, the moon was shining up above her ....

           \
       –   – \ –

Response: The "sun was 'shining
        ⏑ –: ⏑ – ⏑

(e) Cue: I'm pretty sure the sun was hidden by a cloud

        – ‾ \ –

Response: The 'sun was 'shining
        ⏑ – ⏑ – ⏑
          { allegro }

The responses display different prosodic patterns, for example with
regard to the locus of greatest prosodic prominence: compare (d) with
(e). These differences can be related fairly straightforwardly to the
'newness' of the semantic items in the response sentence, as determined
by the particular cue that the subject heard: thus *was shining* is 'given' in
(d), whereas it represents the new information in (e). However, it is
noteworthy that the responses share certain phonetic features: for
example, the pitch contour always ends low, at the base of the speaker's

normal range; and prominence is achieved either by an upward obtrusion of pitch on the focused word, e.g. *was* in (c), or by a relatively wide falling pitch movement, e.g. *shining* in (e), or by both, e.g. *sun* in (d).

Assessing the Focus Accent System

Difficulties in using accentuation to convey appropriate information focus are evident in clients presenting with a range of different communication disorders, acquired and developmental. One such client is John, who is 23 years old, with an acquired aphasia and accompanying dysarthria. In Extract (3), he and the therapist have been talking about John's dislikes with regard to TV programmes:

Extract (3)

1T: what sort of things 'do you watch

2J: it's er (1.0) 'first of all it's (.) er (0.5) 'not er good (0.5)

{*allegro*} {*lento*}

er (.) 'watching (.) the

3   box hh and er (.) like (1.5) 'mystery (.) er (1.5) or s er (0.5)

de'tective er hh

4   'but

lento}

5 T: you 'don't like 'Starsky and 'Hutch then

6 J: (laughs) yeah I 'watch it (.) yeah (.) hh (0.5) you watch it

```
\ - - - - \   - - . -  \ -
```

7 T: 'no actually I 'don't but I watch 'Kojak

```
-  ̄      -     -  \     - - \      \ -
```

8 J: I 'can't (.) und (.) ers 'can't (.) under'stand (.) 'Kojak

```
- -  -  -  -  -  -  ᴗ  ᴗ  -  - -  - -
```

In John's first turn, he repeatedly gives considerable accentual prominence to the lexically stressed syllable of the first word of a breath group: *first, not, watching, mystery, detective, but*. This is sometimes semantically appropriate, e.g. on *mystery, detective*, which represent new information, and also *not*, as the negative polarity is important informationally. The accent on *watching* seems inappropriate, as this clearly represents a well-established topic: the therapist presented it as 'given' in her prior turn by accenting *do* rather than *watch*. It would not have been any more appropriate to accent *box*, as the given topic is *watching the box*, not just *watching*: in such cases, the whole phrase is generally spoken without any prominence, for example on a level low pitch, and as such it would not constitute a separate tone group. Even more anomalous is the prominent falling pitch on *but*, a word almost never accented in this way in normal speech. It appears that in this (quite extended) first turn, accentuation is determined by a phonetic constraint – the need to speak in short breath groups, which are preceded by a pause and start with a major initiatory effort. Where John is able to locate breath group boundaries before a semantically new word as in *detective* and *mystery*, this does not cause problems, but when this is not possible, the resulting accentual pattern appears anomalous in terms of information focus. John is similar in some respects to the dysarthric speaker D., described by Vance (1994), who routinely paused for inhalation in the middle of a clause, then produced a falling pitch movement; though it appears that D. was more successful than John in ensuring that the falling pitch occurred on the word that needed to be focused.

A similar pattern of short breath groups, each containing a major accent, is found in John's final turn. The result is that *can't, understand* and *Kojak* all appear to be presented as individually important, as if contradicting three separate assertions, e.g. that *I can (vs. can't) tolerate (vs. understand) Starsky and Hutch (vs. Kojak)*. This is again anomalous, as *Kojak* is clearly 'given' in the therapist's prior turn; furthermore, it is the proposition *can't understand* as a whole that is 'new', so a single accent on *understand* would be adequate.

John manages his prosodic resources to greater effect in his second turn (6 J). In the first phrase, the accent is on *watch*, which is the preferred default location given that all three items are in some sense 'given'. The location of the accent on *watch* also suggests a contrast with *like* in the therapist's question: John doesn't go so far as saying that he likes it, only that he watches it! In the second phrase, he accents *you*, which helps to point up the function of this phrase as a question: the focus on *you* indicates that the therapist is the point of interest, and that *you* does not merely have an impersonal reference (i.e. *one*). The questioning function is further reinforced by the rising pitch contour. In the absence of syntactic inversion ('do you watch it'), John is dependent on prosodic means to convey the function of the utterance, and in this he is successful: the therapist's next turn is clearly designed as a response to a question.

John's pattern of accentuation has some features in common with the speech of Phillip (C.A. 8;07), who has a specific developmental language disorder and attends a residential school for language-impaired children. He is generally able to use accent appropriately to mark focus, but occasionally also accents a word that clearly represents 'given' information. In Extract (4) this occurs on the word *questions* in line 10, which is accented even though *questions* has clearly been established as the topic by Phillip in line 8, and confirmed as such by the therapist in line 9:

Extract (4)

1 T: you did some reading
2 P: (only) reading and number
3 T: only reading and number
4 P: yeah
5 T: oh

6 P: and I did er (.) do (1.0) er (.) er one or two 'big (.) uns (1.5)
    {lento   {f}   lento}

7 P: one or two 'big uns (.) one or two big 'questions

8 T: did you some 'long questions

9 P: yeah * * I did and I did do 'eight 'questions

10 T: eight questions

12 P: one- one or two ques- 'big questions

13 T: mhm

14 P: {dɔd} all the little

Note that Phillip's accenting of the same word questions is appropriate in line 8, as he is introducing 'questions' as a new topic, as is his failure to accent it in line 12, by which time 'questions' is established as a topic; and Phillip uses accent appropriately to contrast *big* with *little* (line 14).

Phillip and John have quite different diagnoses in speech and language pathology terms: John has an acquired aphasia and dysarthria, whilst Phillip has a specific developmental language disorder. Nevertheless, their speech has some features in common, including the occasional anomalous accent placement, which gives rise to anomalous information focus structure. Their speech also shares the feature of being slow, and chunked into more tone groups than is usual. In John's case, this appears to be related to phonetic problems, i.e. with breath support and control, whereas in Phillip's case, it seems likely that the rate of utterance is determined more by his difficulties in finding the words he wants and in formulating the correct grammatical structure. Comparison of the two cases illustrates the point that prosodic similarity at a linguistic or phonetic level of description should not be taken to imply identity, or even similarity, of underlying causation.

Len, who is at the same school as Phillip, demonstrates a different kind of problem with accentuation. In some respects he is quite similar to Phillip, displaying considerable difficulties with word-finding and sentence formulation. However, his utterances are generally more rapid, though often with pauses preceding and following. In the following extract (5), he is talking with a therapist about the things he buys when he goes to town:

Extract (5)

1. T: who are the other things for then (1.0)

2. L: other pe- other people in my family

3. T: oh I see d'you mean presents

4. L: no not presents (0.5)
       {ff   ff}

5. T: no (1.5)

6. L: things
       { ff }

7. T: things:

8. L: yeah that's - and food that 's what I (mean)- that's what I said

In lines 4 and 6, Len is engaged in correcting the incorrect inference the therapist made in line 3. This is done with an appropriate contrastive accentual pattern: a fall–rise on the item being contradicted (*presents*), and a rise–fall on the correct item in line 6, which is thus presented prosodically as the new item of information contrasting with *presents*. Unfortunately, the effect is spoilt by his choice of word for the correct item in line 6: *things*, being a superordinate of *presents* is not a seman-tically appropriate lexeme to contrast with it. Had he used the word *food* – subsequently produced in line 8 – the accentual pattern would have been quite appropriate. Thus whilst Phillip chose the appropriate lexis but used the wrong accentual pattern, Len used the right accentual pattern but chose the wrong word to go with it. The case of Len illustrates that, when assessing accentuation, and prosody in general, it is necessary simultaneously to take account of other levels of linguistic organisation, such as grammar and lexis.

Dialectal Considerations

When assessing a client's use of prosodic means to indicate focus, it is important not only to be aware of the prosodic variation that is attributable to focus, as has just been illustrated, but also to take account of prosodic differences that may be attributable to other sources, in particular the dialect or accent background of the speaker. This can be illustrated by comparing responses to just one of the cues presented in (2) above, when uttered by speakers of different accents of British English. The speakers in Extract (6), all female and in their early twenties, each heard the cue spoken on audiotape by a speaker from their own regional accent group.

Extract (6) Cue: If the sun had been shining I'd have felt a lot happier.

(a) South East (Surrey)

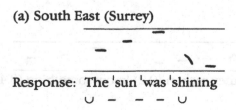

Response: The 'sun 'was 'shining

(b) West Midlands (Brownhills)

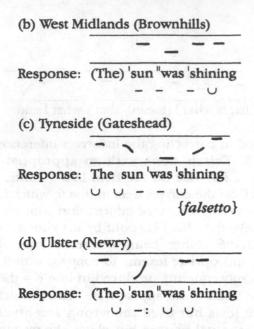

Response: (The) 'sun "was 'shining

(c) Tyneside (Gateshead)

Response: The sun 'was 'shining

{*falsetto*}

(d) Ulster (Newry)

Response: (The) 'sun "was 'shining

Each speaker marks the same item as prosodically prominent, and thus can be said to be operating with the same focus accentual system; but the way in which that prosodic prominence is achieved differs markedly, according to the dialect background of the speaker. Differences are particularly evident in pitch direction; and the use of level as opposed to gliding pitch on the focused word.

Dialectal differences in relation to the focus accent system are even more striking in the case of British speakers of dialects that are Afro-Caribbean in origin, such as London Jamaican. Although the lexis and syntax of this variety share many features with other indigenous varieties of British English, prosodically it is very different. With regard to accentuation, it appears that, unlike almost all other varieties of British English, accent is *not* associated with information focus: the main accent normally falls on the final syllable of the speaker's turn, irrespective of focus considerations, which means that a word representing 'given' information can, and will, be accented if it occurs in turn final position (Local, Wells and Sebba, 1985). This is evident in Extract (7), in which two adolescent males are talking. The fourth occurrence of the word *law* is accented, even though it clearly represents a well-established topic:

Extract (7)

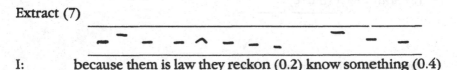

I: because them is law they reckon (0.2) know something (0.4)

> —   —   —   —   —   — —   — \
> ?all them p'licemen break the law you know (1.2)
>
> —   —   _   _   \   — — — — \
> hm   /   you call them law but they break the law (0.4)
>
>   \
> F: hhh   mm

It appears that in London Jamaican, accentuation is not related to the system of information focus, but is used exclusively to mark a speaker's turn as complete – hence the location of the main accent at the very end of the turn. In order to mark a word as informationally important, London Jamaican speakers therefore need to have recourse to other devices, such as lengthening of consonants, and subtle modifications of the pitch contour (Wells, 1992). It is therefore necessary to take dialect into account in prosodic assessment, in order to avoid the pitfall of labelling as 'deviant' a pattern that is merely non-standard: for example, the pattern of accentuation in an Afro-Caribbean person with dysarthria or aphasia would need to be assessed in the light of facts such as these.

Vance (1994) takes account of dialect factors in her case study of a dysarthric adult from Belfast, using the description of Belfast intonation in Jarman and Cruttenden (1976) as the basis for prosodic assessment. In the same vein, Wells and Local (1993) present a case study of a prosodically impaired child, David, from Sandwell (West Midlands), based on a description of the local prosodic systems in Wells (1989). This case study is of particular interest here, as David's prosodic difficulties affect his ability to mark information focus appropriately. The following extract (8) is taken from a recording made when David was aged 5;4. At the time he was having therapy on account of his severe speech and language difficulties. David is looking at some pictures with a student speech and language therapist.

Extract (8)

1 E: who's that there coming up the path

2 D: {pp (2 syll.) pp} (1.5)

>   —   /
3 D: postman (1.2)
>   {f}

4 E: what's he going to do

             _ _ _ _/

5 D: get out a letter: (1.0)
                 {f}

6 E: get out a letter

             /

7 D: yes

8 E: and what's he going to do with the letter (1.0)

             _ _ _   _ _ _ _ _ _/

9 D: put it in (1.7) put it the letter box (0.8)
                               {f}

10 E: he's going to put it in the letter box =

             /

11 D: = yes (1.0)

12 E: and who's this d'you think (1.0)

             /

13 D: girl:: (1.0)

14 E: 's it a girl

             _ _ _ _   _   /

15 D: I already [gɛd] that (0.8)
                         {f}

16 E: she's already (0.5)

             _ _ _ _ ﹀   /   _﹈

17 D: I already [dɛd] that (0.3) I did (5.0)
                         {f}   {f}

18 E: see what's on the next page oh who's this again

The main pitch movement, accompanied by slowing of tempo and increased loudness, regularly occurs at the end of David's utterances, specifically on the final syllable (cf. the London Jamaican system). The fact that the pitch movement is invariably rising, rather than falling, can be attributed to the local accent, where statements generally end with non-low (i.e. rising or mid/high level) pitch, as in Extract (6b) above. However, other aspects of this recurrent pattern have negative consequences for David's ability to communicate effectively, and particularly for his system of information focus. For example, in 'I already [gɛd] that', (8.15) [gɛd], which presumably represents a lexical verb such as *said* or *read*, would normally be focused at the expense of the following 'that', which would be backgrounded because it is an anaphoric pronoun. In David's version, however, it is the pronoun that is phonetically most prominent, by virtue of its utterance final position. In 8.16, E displays that she has not understood David's [gɛd] from the previous turn, and seeks clarification. In David's attempt at clarification in 8.17, once again the word at issue is not made salient. The attempt at clarification appears to be unsuccessful, as E gives no acknowledgment, explicit or implicit, of having understood what David was saying. By failing to accent, and thus make more salient, the informationally important word in 8.15 and 8.17, David may have reduced his chances of being understood.

However, the analysis so far has focused exclusively on the point of maximum phonetic prominence in the utterance, paying no attention to the phonetic characteristics of the remaining part. This can lead to the overlooking of potentially significant prosodic features. It was noted that in 8.15, the verb would normally receive the main prominence, because *that* is anaphoric. The same is true of the repetition in 8.17. In both cases, the greatest prominence is on *that*. However, it will also be observed that on both tokens of the verb, the pitch drops (in 8.15 a step down, and in 8.17 a narrow fall), to be followed by the rise on the final word. In this West Midlands accent, focus is regularly marked by a noticeable step down to the focused word, followed by a step up to level (see Extract 6b). David has in fact used some of the phonetic features associated with focus in his accent, and located them on the contextually appropriate word, though this is overshadowed by his idiosyncratic pattern of prominence on the utterance-final syllable. In David's case, it seems that his ability clearly to mark information focus is impeded by an overriding need to mark the ends of his turns phonetically, thereby indicating to the interlocutor that she may proceed – which may not otherwise be evident, given David's general unintelligibility (see Wells and Local, 1993, for further discussion). The case of David illustrates two important points for the assessment of accentuation in particular and prosody in general. First, it is necessary to take account of regional accent or dialect features, to avoid labelling as deviant a pattern that is merely non-standard. Second, it may be that a client adopts a strategy that has a negative impact on one prosodic system (in David's case, information focus), but which results in what he might perceive as a greater benefit in terms of a different system (for David, turn-delimitation).

Preservation of the Focus Accent System in Prosodically Deviant Speech

David's failure to use accentuation clearly to mark the main point of information focus can be contrasted with other speakers who manage to signal focus fairly clearly, even though their speech has other deviant prosodic features. A case in point is Christopher, an 8-year-old boy from Edinburgh, who when younger had severe problems with segmental phonology. Prosodically, his speech is strikingly different from that of his peers. It is characterised by a slow rate, and a tendency to give each syllable equal durational value, leading to an impression of syllable-timed rhythm. He uses level on-syllable pitch almost to the exclusion of dynamic rises and falls. Pitch change is effected by a jump (up or down) to another level syllable, rather than by a dynamic fall or rise as would be very often the case in Edinburgh English (described in Brown, Currie and Kenworthy, 1980). These features are illustrated in Extract (9), where Christopher (C) is playing with his friend (F).

Extract (9)

1 F: 'I'm gonna make a - 'I'm 'na draw a 'puzzle (1.0) a 'jigsaw

d'you know

2 C: yes I think that I'll make a puzzle (.) a numbers countdown

puzzle (.)

3   thanks   now I've got one with my name on it

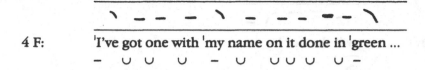

4 F: 'I've got one with 'my name on it done in 'green ...

F. uses dynamic pitch and rhythm to highlight focused words, such as *I*, *my* and *green* in line 4. Christopher, by contrast, uses level on-syllable pitch exclusively, and syllable-timed rhythm. In spite of this, he manages to mark focused words as prominent. In the second part of line 2, *puzzle* is by now 'given' information, and is realised by low-level pitch, both syllables on the same level at the bottom of the range. *Numbers countdown* constitutes the new information and, for both words, the first (i.e. the lexically stressed) syllable is on a slightly raised pitch level compared with the preceding and following syllables. As a result, *numbers* and *countdown* are heard as accented, whereas *puzzle* is not. In line 3, *I've* is made prominent, not only by being obtruded in pitch from the rest of the utterance, all of which is spoken on the same pitch level, but also by increased loudness. On this evidence, Christopher appears to have the ability to mark words as focused by accentual means which have some features in common with the local system, even though his prosody is atypical in many respects. However, it is not clear whether Christopher's ability to accent focused words is consistent. For example, in line 2, the context would suggest focus on *I'll*, but Christopher fails to make it prominent.

Elsewhere, there is even clearer evidence that Christopher is able to marshal the prosodic resources at his disposal to realise communicative functions normally associated with accentuation. One common situation in which accentuation is used for focusing purposes is where a speaker seeks to clarify a misunderstanding (illustrated in Extract 8 in relation to David). In Extract (10), F., for whatever reason, fails to comprehend Christopher's utterance in line 1. Christopher repeats it in line 3:

Extract (10)

1. C: she won't allow us to get one

2. F: what

3 C: ʃi wunt . ʔə.lau ʔʌs. təg:etʰwʌn
            she won't allow us to get one (2.0)
            {lento   lento}

$$\overline{-\ ^-\ ^-\ ^\searrow\ _-}$$

4. F: <u>will she not let us</u>

$$\searrow$$

5. C: <u>no</u>

In the repetition, Christopher focuses on every syllable of the utterance, by using very slow tempo, pause and glottal stop to segment the utterance into individual syllables, by segmental lengthening, by pitch ob-trusion (on *allow* and *to get*), and – most unusually for Christopher – even by using falling pitch, on the final word. Having thus combined a range of phonetic resources for focusing purposes, Christopher's attempt at clarification is successful: the friend displays his understanding in line 4.

Formal Assessment of the Focus Accent System

In the five cases illustrated in Extracts (3) to (5) and (8) to (10), problems with accentuation and their impact on the system of information focus have been discussed through the analysis of tape-recorded naturally occurring interactions, mainly between client and therapist. This approach to assessment has the advantage of naturalness, and permits fine-grained qualitative analysis. In many respects it follows Crystal's approach to prosodic assessment, formalised in his Prosody Profile, known as PROP (Crystal, 1982). PROP examines the grouping of information into *tone-units* (Juncture); the location of tone, or *tonicity*; and the type of *tone* (glide direction). The main concern is with intonation or pitch matters, because according to Crystal 'pitch causes most linguistic difficulties...the linguistic use of pitch is usually referred to as intonation, and indeed it is intonation with which we are most regularly concerned, in clinical settings' (1982, p.114). Length, Accent, Range and Juncture are considered in so far as they interact with Pitch. PROP does not address the functions of Loudness, Tempo, Rhythm, and Voice Quality ('paralinguistic features'), but provision is made for them to be noted if they strike the therapist as being inappropriately used. For all the prosodic systems included in PROP, there is provision for stating frequency of occurrence and whether this seems to be greater or less than one would expect to find in prosodically normal speakers. This is extremely useful, as it is not always the case that disordered prosody manifests as demonstrably odd prosodic patterns (as in the case of Christopher and David described above). Often, prosodic phenomena that do occur, but rarely, in prosodically normal speech seem to occur to excess; or else the proportion of (for example) one tone to the rest is unusual – as in the case of the dysarthric patient described in Vance (1994).

One limitation of PROP, discussed by Crystal (1982, p.123), arises from the use of spontaneous data: there is no way of checking what communicative task the client had in mind. There is also no way of deciding whether the disturbed or deviant prosody featured in the profile actually detracts from communication. For this reason, functional issues are relatively peripheral to PROP. The approach illustrated in the present chapter draws on the behaviour of other participants in the interaction as a resource for showing whether or not a particular communicative function has been conveyed. Examples are the therapist's response to David's repetition in Extract (8), which showed it was unsuccessful as a clarification; or the therapist's response to John's second turn in Extract (3), which indicated that she had indeed heard it as a question. This approach derives from Conversation Analysis (Drew, 1994), and has been applied recently to the study of prosody in normal conversational interactions (Couper-Kuhlen and Selting, in press), though there are as yet relatively few studies which use the approach to look at prosody in a clinical context (Wells and Local, 1993; Local and Wootton, 1995).

Like PROP, the approach to prosodic assessment illustrated here is time-consuming, and requires a relatively high degree of phonetic expertise; furthermore, it only addresses prosodic production, not perception or comprehension skills; and it provides no formal means of comparing the client's performance to that of other populations, normal or impaired. The PROP profile does include some tentative developmental norms although it is accepted that the empirical basis for these is as yet rather slight. An alternative would be to use more formal tests or assessments, but few are currently available. In the PETAL Speech Assessment Procedure for deaf people, (King, Parker and Wright, forthcoming), there is a structured procedure for eliciting contrastive focus accentuation, which can save the clinician time. For example, the child is shown a picture of a red car and asked if it is a blue car. A typical response might be 'No (it's a) red car'. A series of such responses is elicited, together with conversational material, and transcribed, with instrumental analysis if appropriate. On this basis the clinician can evaluate the client's ability to manipulate accentuation, at least for the purpose of correcting an incorrect proposition (Parker and Rose, 1990). Although this is not intended to constitute a formal test, and does not give a quantitative measure, similar procedures have been formalised as tests for experiments on normally developing children (Hornby and Hass, 1970; Hornby, 1971; MacWhinney and Bates, 1978).

Peppé (in preparation) has devised a formal test instrument for accentuation, as part of a comprehensive battery of prosody tests to be standardised on 90 adult English speakers. Once the standardisation is complete, it will be possible to compare clients quantitatively with normal and atypical populations. In one of the production subtests for accentuation, there are 15 'postcode' items. The subject reads the item aloud e.g. 'N7 1PB', and the tester displays that she is unsure about one element: 'E7?'. Subjects have to demonstrate that they have understood which element is being queried, then they have to correct it: 'No, N7'. Responses can be scored on a right/wrong basis.

Assessing Comprehension of the Focus Accent System

The assessments described so far are primarily concerned with the production of correct accentuation. There have also been some attempts to assess the comprehension of accentuation. For instance, Highnam and Morris (1987) devised a judgement task which they administered to 10 normally developing and 10 language-impaired children, the two groups being matched on chronological age. Subjects listened to dyads such as those in Extract (11).

Extract (11)   (a)   What did the man drink?
                                 The man drank **tea**.

                 (b)   What did Kathy throw?
                                 Kathy threw the ball.

Subjects had to decide whether the two sentences in the pair sound 'good together' (as in 11a) or not (as in 11b). The language-impaired children performed less well than the controls. More extensive control data, on a very similar task, was collected by Myers and Myers (1983), from 140 normally developing children from kindergarten to sixth grade. They found a developmental progression, whereby kindergarten children performed at chance level, but sixth-grade children scored 85% correct. Such tasks, and the data that have already been collected using them, are helpful for clinicians wishing to assess receptive prosodic skills and to compare their clients' performance with normal populations. By doing so, it may be possible to determine whether a client has a prosodic deficit, and also whether this deficit is specific, or part of a more general language disorder.

These issues, which are particularly important for the assessment of prosodic abilities in children, are addressed in a recent study of the comprehension of accentuation in an SLI population (Vance, 1993). Vance administered a test similar to those used in the studies by Myers and Myers (1983) and Highnam and Morris (1987), to a group of 17 SLI children, aged between 7;10 and 13;1. Their receptive language age was between 6 and 8 years, as measured on three subtests of the Clinical Evaluation of Language Fundamentals – Revised (CELF–R) (Semel, Wiig and Secord, 1987). For the control group, rather than selecting on the basis of chronological age, Vance used younger children, between 6 and 7 years old and attending a mainstream primary school, who were matched with the SLI children on receptive language score using the CELF–R. Potential subjects for both groups were screened further on a simple test of semantic anomaly, to ensure that any incorrect responses on the focus accent judgement task could be attributed to prosodic factors, rather than to a more general inability to recognise anomalous sentence pairs (see Vance and Wells, 1994 for further details of subject selection).

The difference in group mean between the two groups on the tonicity judgement task was not significant, which suggests that the comprehension of accentuation is associated with general receptive language development. It is not something which is particularly badly affected in SLI children; nor, on the other hand, is it an aspect of comprehension that develops at a normal rate in spite of other receptive language difficulties. This interpretation is supported by the fact that, for the SLI group, the tonicity judgement score was significantly correlated with receptive language score but not with chronological age.

The results of this study point up the interest, for the clinician assessing a client's prosodic abilities, not only in comparing the client's performance with that of his or her peers (in the case of a child, other children of the same age, and for an adult, other adults), but also in comparing the client's prosodic abilities to his or her other language abilities – in this case, receptive language skills. The latter type of comparison enables the clinician to identify whether the prosodic problem is specific, and thus perhaps requiring targeted therapy, or whether it might be expected to improve steadily in line with other aspects of language, perhaps as the result of therapy that is directed at aspects of language other than prosody.

One limitation of tasks of the kind used by Myers and Myers, Highnam and Morris, and Vance, is that they require the child to reflect on prosodic appropriacy. This may not be a direct reflection of a person's ability to comprehend accentuation 'on-line', in normal conversation. Such methodological issues underline the fact that assessing receptive prosodic skills in a formal way is intrinsically problematic, because prosodic meaning is elusive and therefore hard to represent. For example, one traditional technique for assessing comprehension is the picture-pointing task, and this has been used in some prosodic research, such as Cruttenden's study of 10-year-old children (Cruttenden, 1985). However, the differences between the pictures have to be quite subtle, and may pose insuperable difficulties for younger normally developing children, or for children and adults with impaired language. For example, in Cruttenden's study, the items testing comprehension of contrastive accentual patterns such as 'John's got **four** oranges' vs. 'John's got four **oranges**' required the child to differentiate between pictures of (a) a boy with four oranges and a girl with two oranges; (b) a boy with four oranges and a girl with four bananas; and (c) a boy with three oranges and a girl with four oranges. Such heavy demands on inferential processing can be avoided by using an on-line word monitoring task, measuring children's response rate to accented vs. unaccented words heard in sentential contexts (Cutler and Swinney, 1987). This type of task obviates the need for the child to reflect on the meaning of a prosodic stimulus before making a response, and so constitutes a more direct assessment of linguistic, rather than metalinguistic, knowledge. Although valuable as an experimental tool, such procedures are impractical for routine clinical use outside the laboratory. Thus it can be seen that all methods for the assessment of receptive prosody have considerable drawbacks.

Linguistic Classification of Prosodic Disorders

Prosodic difficulties are conceptually no different from 'segmental' speech difficulties, in that it is useful to distinguish initially between phonetic and phonological levels. A client may use lateral fricatives instead of alveolar fricatives, without any impact upon the ability to signal the phonological oppositions in the consonant system, i.e. target *seat* remains distinct from target *sheet, feet, teat* etc. Such a 'problem' is purely at the level of phonetic exponency, without phonological consequences, and can therefore be appropriately dubbed 'phonetic' (cf. Chapter 14, this volume). Similarly, a client may habitually use an idiosyncratically narrow pitch range when accenting a syllable, but this does not affect his/her ability to mark the syllable as accented. Christopher (extract (9)) exemplified this type, described by Brewster (1989) as 'prosodic deviation'. As far as the accentual system is concerned, this can be referred to as a phonetic problem.

On the other hand, a client may realise target alveolar fricatives as alveolar stops, and, because of their perceptual similarity to his or her realisation of target alveolar stops, he or she may thus fail to signal phonologically the contrast between *sea* and *tea*. It is therefore appropriate to refer to such a case as a 'phonological' problem (see further Chapters 3, 5 and 14, this volume). Similarly, a client may fail to accent adequately a word which carries the information focus, as David did in extract (8), and thus fail to mark the phonological opposition between focused and unfocused items. This is therefore an example of a phonological problem in the prosodic domain. Another example would be John's use of a succession of contrastive accents in 'I can't understand Kojak' (extract (3)), where the context does not require them. Phonological problems are, then, those which are likely to lead to misinterpretation of the message by the listener.

In the case of such phonological problems, it is quite possible that the client is in fact, from his or her own side, consistently differentiating between target alveolar fricatives and target alveolar stops: it is just that the difference in articulation that he or she makes is not sufficiently perceptible to listeners (cf. Gibbon, 1990; Chapter 14, this volume). Similarly, in the case of the focus accent system, the client may in fact be making a consistent distinction between focused and non-focused items, or between contrastive and non-contrastive focus, but this is not perceptible to listeners. It was suggested earlier that David might be a case in point. In such cases, from the speaker's side, the phonological problem is not so very different from a phonetic problem: the distinction is in the ear of the listener (cf. Chapters 14 and 15, this volume).

These instances need to be differentiated from the case of a client who is not aware that a phonological opposition exists and needs to be made – between target fricative and target stop, or between target-focused and non-focused items, for example. Such instances can be referred to as problems of (underlying) phonological organisation, representation or processing, and can arise from developmental or acquired causes. There is evidence that problems of prosodic processing or representation are found in patients with right hemisphere damage (Bryan, 1994) and with Parkinson's disease (Scott, Caird and Williams, 1984). Some deaf children also seem unable to set up appropriate phonological oppositions for prosodic systems. For example, one of the accentual systems illustrated in Parker and Rose (1990) involved invariably placing the main pitch prominence on the final word of the utterance, even when a contrastive focus context required it to be on an earlier word.

Whether or not other client groups have prosodic problems at this 'deep' level remains to be shown by future research. In order to demonstrate that the client's prosodic production errors can be attributed to representational or processing deficits, it is necessary to assess receptive prosodic skills as well – by no means a straightforward business, as has already been indicated. In any case, it always has to be borne in mind that the relationship between clinical diagnosis and type of prosodic disorder is unlikely to be a simple one. In relation to deafness, this is clear from the description of six accentual systems in Parker and Rose (1990). Two show no evidence of a focus accent system in their production, and so a phonological representation problem could be hypothesised: investigation of receptive skills would be needed to substantiate this. A third has the full range of pitch contrasts, but within a very narrow and relatively high pitch range. A fourth locates the focus accent correctly, but realises it with lengthening, high-level pitch and loudness, rather than dynamic pitch. Both thus illustrate phonetic problems. Another shows appropriate focus accent on non-final focused words, but also invariably has falling pitch on the final word, irrespective of focus considerations (cf. David): this might well cause problems for the listener, and if so would constitute a phonological problem. Thus, even within a narrowly defined client group, a linguistic assessment of prosody reveals different types of prosodic problem, which will require different therapeutic approaches.

Complementary Approaches to Prosodic Assessment

This chapter has offered a linguistic perspective on the clinical assessment of prosody. It is important to recognise at the outset that a linguistic assessment, whilst necessary for planning a principled programme of therapeutic intervention relating to prosodic difficulties, is by no means sufficient. It is important for the clinician to take account of medical factors, such as a neurological condition, hearing impairment, or a psychiatric condition, e.g. depression, all of which may influence the client's prosodic output and/or comprehension. Such factors are outside the domain of clinical linguistics. Closer to this domain, but omitted for reasons of space, is the phonetic assessment of prosody using instrumental techniques such as acoustic or laryngographic analysis. Such techniques, comprehensively reviewed elsewhere (Baken, 1987; Ball, 1991) have proved invaluable for the objective measurement of prosodic parameters, and also as a visual feedback device for clients receiving therapy.

In the future, it is likely that the psycholinguistic or cognitive neuropsychological approach to prosodic disorders will be developed further. This approach focuses on identifying the level of breakdown, or deficit, that gives rise to the client's prosodic difficulties, using a theoretical model of speech and language processing (cf. Stackhouse and Wells, 1993). It has been touched on in the discussion of disorders of prosodic representation and processing, but has as yet hardly been developed with reference to prosodic problems as described here. As has been the case with segmental difficulties, this approach is likely to be of help to the clinician who is assessing prosodic problems with a view to planning appropriate therapy.

References

Abercrombie, D. (1971). Some functions of silent stress. In: A.J. Aitken, A. McIntosh and H. Palsson (Eds) *Edinburgh Studies in English and Scots*, pp 147-156. London: Longman.

Atkinson, J.M. and Heritage, J. (1984). *Structures of Social Action: Studies in Conversation Analysis*. Cambridge: Cambridge University Press.

Baken, R.J. (1987). *Clinical Measurement of Speech and Voice*. London: Taylor & Francis.

Ball, V. (1991). Computer-based tools for assessment and remediation of speech. *British Journal of Disorders of Communication* 26(1), 95–113.

Ball, M.J., Code, C., Rahilly, J. and Hazlett, D. (1994). Non-segmental aspects of disordered speech: developments in transcription. *Clinical Linguistics and Phonetics* 8(1), 67–83.

Baltaxe, C. and Simmons, J. (1985). Prosodic development in normal and autistic children. In: E.Schopler and G.Mesibov (Eds), *Communication Problems in Autism*, pp 95–125. New York: Plenum.

Barry, W.G. (1981). Prosodic functions revised again! *Phonetica* 38, 320–340.

Beattie, G.W., Cutler, A. and Pearson, M. (1982). Why is Mrs. Thatcher interrupted so often? *Nature* 330, 744–747.

Brazil, D., Coulthard.M. and Johns, C. (1980). *Discourse Intonation and Language Teaching*. London: Longman.

Brewster, K. (1989). The assessment of prosody. In: K. Grundy (Ed.), *Linguistics in Clinical Practice*, 1st edn. London: Taylor & Francis.

Brown, G., Currie, K. and Kenworthy, J. (1980). *Questions of Intonation*. Beckenham: Croom Helm.

Bryan, K. (1994). *The Right-hemisphere Language Battery*, 2nd edn. London: Whurr Publishers.

Butcher, A. (1981). Aspects of the speech pause: phonetic correlates and communicative functions. Doctoral dissertation, University of Kiel.

Couper-Kuhlen, E. (1986). *An Introduction to English Prosody*. London: Edward Arnold.

Couper-Kuhlen, E. (1993). *English Speech Rhythm*. Amsterdam: John Benjamins.

Couper-Kuhlen, E. and Selting, M. (Eds) (in press). *Prosody in Conversation: Ethnomethodological Studies*. Cambridge: Cambridge University Press

Courtright, J.A. and Courtright, I.C. (1983). The perception of non-verbal vocal cues of emotional meaning by language-disordered children. *Journal of Speech and Hearing Research* 26, 412–417.

Cruttenden, A. (1985). Intonation comprehension in ten-year-olds. *Journal of Child Language* 12, 643–661.

Cruttenden, A. (1986). *Intonation*. Cambridge: Cambridge University Press

Crystal, D. (1969). *Prosodic Systems and Intonation in English*. Cambridge: Cambridge University Press

Crystal, D. (1982). *Profiling Linguistic Disability*. London: Edward Arnold

Cutler, A. and Pearson, M. (1986). On the analysis of prosodic turn-taking cues. In: C. Johns-Lewis (Ed.), *Intonation in Discourse*, pp. 139–155. London: Croom Helm.

Cutler, A. and Swinney, D. (1987). Prosody and the development of comprehension. *Journal of Child Language* 14, 145–167.

Drew, P. (1994). Conversation analysis. In R.E. Asher and J.M.Y. Simpson (Eds), *Encyclopedia of Language and Linguistics*. Oxford: Pergamon.

Duckworth, M., Allen, G., Hardcastle, W. and Ball, M. (1990). Extensions to the International Phonetic Alphabet for the transcription of atypical speech. *Clinical Linguistics and Phonetics* 4(4), 273–283.

Firth J.R. (1948). Sounds and prosodies. Reprinted in Palmer, F.R. (Ed.) (1970). *Prosodic Analysis*, pp. 1–26. London: Oxford University Press.

French, P. and Local, J. (1983). Turn-competitive incomings. *Journal of Pragmatics* 7, 701–715.

Fry, D.B. (1958). Experiments in the perception of stress. *Language & Speech* 1, 126–152.

Garman, M. (1990). *Psycholinguistics*. Cambridge: Cambridge University Press.

Gibbon, F. (1990). Lingual activity in two speech-disordered children's attempts to produce stop consonants: evidence from electropalatographic (EPG) data. *British Journal of Disorders of Communication* 25, 329–340.

Halliday, M.A.K. (1967). *Intonation and Grammar in British English*. The Hague: Mouton.

Hargrove, P. and Sheran, C. (1989). The use of stress by language-impaired children. *Journal of Communication Disorders* 22, 361–373.

Heselwood, B., Bray, M. and Crookston, I. (1995). Juncture, rhythm and planning in the speech of an adult with Down's syndrome. *Clinical Linguistics and Phonetics*. 9, 121–137.

Highnam, C. and Morris, V. (1987) Linguistic stress judgements of language learning disabled students. *Journal of Communication Disorders* 20, 93–103.

Hornby, P. (1971). Surface structure and the topic-comment distinction: a developmental study. *Child Development* 42, 1975–1988.

Hornby, P. and Hass, W. (1970). Use of contrastive stress by preschool children. *Journal of Speech and Hearing Research* 13, 395–399.

Jarman, E. and Cruttenden, A. (1976). Belfast intonation and the myth of the fall. *Journal of the International Phonetic Association* 6, 4–12.

King, A., Parker, A. and Wright, R. (forthcoming). *PETAL Speech Assessment Procedure*.

Kreiman, J. (1982). Perception of sentence and paragraph boundaries in natural conversation. *Journal of Phonetics* 10, 163–175.

Ladd, D.R. (1980). *The Structure of Intonational Meaning*. Bloomington: Indiana University Press.

Laver J. (1980). *The Phonetic description of Voice Quality*. Cambridge: Cambridge University Press.

Levinson, S. (1983). *Pragmatics*. Cambridge: Cambridge University Press

Local, J. (1982). Modelling intonational variability in children's speech. In S.Romaine (Ed.), *Sociolinguistic Variation in Speech Communities*. London: Edward Arnold.

Local, J. (1986). Patterns and problems in a study of Tyneside intonation. In: C. Johns-Lewis (Ed.), *Intonation and Discourse*, 181–198. London: Croom Helm.

Local, J. (1992). Continuing and restarting. In P. Auer and A. Di Luzio (Eds), *The Contextualisation of Language*. Amsterdam: John Benjamins.

Local, J., Kelly, J. and Wells, W. (1986). Towards a phonology of conversation: turn-taking in Tyneside. *English Journal of Linguistics* 22(2), 411–437 .

Local, J., Wells, W. and Sebba, M. (1985). Phonology for conversation: phonetic aspects of turn delimitation in London Jamaican. *Journal of Pragmatics* 9, 309–330.

Local, J. and Wootton, A. (1995). Interactional and phonetic aspects of immediate echolalia in autism; a case study. *Clinical Linguistics and Phonetics*.

MacWhinney, B. and Bates, E. (1978). Sentential devices for conveying givenness and newness: a cross-cultural developmental study. *Journal of Verbal Learning & Verbal Behaviour* 17, 539–558.

McConnell-Ginet, S. (1980). Intonation in a man's world . In: D.Thorne, C. Kramarae and N. Henley (Eds.), *Language, Gender and Society*. Rowley MA; Newbury House.

Moore, B.C.J. (1989). *An Introduction to the Psychology of Hearing*. London: Academic Press.

Myers, F. and Myers, R. (1983). Perception of stress contrasts in semantic and non-semantic contexts by children. *Journal of Psycholinguistic Research* 12, 327–338.

Parker, A. and Rose, H. (1990). Deaf children's phonological development. In: P. Grunwell (Ed.), *Developmental Speech Disorders*, pp 83–107. Edinburgh: Churchill Livingstone.

Peppé, S.J.E. (in preparation). *Profiling Elements of Prosodic Systems*.

Sacks, H., Schegloff, E.A. and Jefferson, G. (1974). A simplest systematics for the organisation of turn-taking for conversation. *Language* 50, 696–735.

Scott, S., Caird, F.I. and Williams, B.O. (1984). Evidence for an apparent sensory speech disorder in Parkinson's disease. *Journal of Neurology, Neurosurgery and Psychiatry* 47, 140–144.

Semel, E., Wiig, E.H. and Secord, W. (1987). *Clinical Evaluation of Language Fundamentals – Revised*. London: Psychological Corporation/Harcourt Brace Jovanovich.

Stackhouse, J. and Wells, B. (1993). Psycholinguistic assessment of developmental speech disorders. *European Journal of Disorders of Communication* **28**, 331–348.

Vance, M. (1993). An investigation of non-literal comprehension and recognition of intonation patterns in specific language impaired children, including semantic-pragmatic disorder, and in receptive language age matched normal children, aged 6 and 7 years. Unpublished MSc thesis, Institute of Neurology, University of London.

Vance, J. (1994). Prosodic deviation in dysarthria: a case study. *European Journal of Disorders of Communication* **29**, 61–76.

Vance, M. and Wells, B. (1994). The wrong end of the stick: language impaired children's comprehension of non-literal language. *Child Language Teaching and Therapy* **10**(1), 23–46.

Waterson, N. (1987). *Prosodic Phonology: the Theory and its Application to Language Acquisition and Speech Processing*. Newcastle-upon-Tyne: Grevatt & Grevatt.

Weber, E.G. (1993). *Varieties of Questions in English Conversation*. Amsterdam: John Benjamins.

Wells, B. (1986). An experimental approach to the interpretation of focus in spoken English. In: C.Johns-Lewis (Ed.), *Intonation in Discourse*, pp. 53–75 London: Croom Helm.

Wells, B. (1988). Focus in spoken English. Unpublished DPhil thesis, University of York.

Wells, B. (1989). Prefinal focus accents in English: a comparative study of two varieties. In: D. Bradley, E.J.A. Henderson and M. Mazaudon (Eds), *Prosodic Analysis and Asian Linguistics: to honour R.K. Sprigg* , pp. 17–32. Canberra Pacific Linguistics C-104.

Wells, B. (1992). Phonetic aspects of focus in London Jamaican. Paper presented at the British Colloquium of Academic Phoneticians, Cambridge.

Wells, B. (1994). Junction in developmental speech disorder: a case study. *Clinical Linguistics & Phonetics* **8**(1), 1–25.

Wells, B. and Local, J. (1993). The sense of an ending: a case of prosodic delay. *Clinical Linguistics and Phonetics* **7**(1), 59–73.

Wells, B. and Peppé, S. (in press). Ending up in Ulster: prosody and turn-taking in English dialects. In: E. Couper-Kuhlen and M. Selting (Eds), *Prosody in Conversation: Ethnomethodological Studies*. Cambridge: Cambridge University Press

Wirz, S. and Mackenzie Beck, J. (1995). Assessment of voice quality: the Vocal Profiles Analysis Scheme. In: S. Wirz (Ed.), *Perceptual Approaches to Communication Disorders*, pp. 39–55. London: Whurr Publishers.

Section III

The role of linguistics in the management of clients with speech and language impairments

Chapter 11
Applying Linguistics to Acquired Aphasia

ALISON ROSS

Introduction

Aphasia is a communication disorder which occurs when damage (lesion) to the adult brain impedes the use of language understanding and production. Except in the severest forms of aphasia, ideas and meanings (messages) seem quite well preserved, but phonetic, phonological, syntactic, semantic and pragmatic processing and performance are affected in a range of ways. It is very common to meet people with aphasia who, in spite of observed linguistic impairments, are able to convey relevant and organised messages. This is often achieved by their use of non-verbal behaviours, such as facial expression, gesture, pointing, and drawing. As the linguistic deficit need not be confined to the expression and comprehension of spoken language, but may extend to the use of written, gestural and other symbols, aphasia is often described as a multimodal disorder. However, the discussion of linguistics and aphasia in this chapter will be largely confined to spoken language.

The neurological impairment causing aphasia is likely simultaneously to affect non-linguistic brain functions such as attention, memory, perception, and other aspects of cognition, sensory reception, motor skills and emotional responses. Also, in reaction to the trauma and its effect on personal lifestyle, secondary emotional responses will be experienced. It is a complex of linguistic, and more strictly aphasic, as well as non-linguistic factors that together reduce the effectiveness of communication in a range of situations as diverse as taking part in everyday conversation, composing a letter, following a radio programme, or reading a newspaper. A person with aphasia is idiosyncratic in neurological impairment, linguistic and non-linguistic behaviours, psychological response, and in his or her needs and ability as a communicator. Clinical management similarly must be idiosyncratic and based on a holistic and comprehensive understanding of the individual. While the focus of this chapter is on the linguistic aspects of aphasia and aims to demonstrate ways in which linguistics is applied in the management of the person with aphasia, it is not intended to imply that other facets of the disorder are of lesser importance.

From observations of language performance, and a knowledge of descriptive linguistics and linguistic theory, the clinician can begin to decide what level, extent and complexity of phonetic, phonological, syntactic, semantic and pragmatic problems contribute to the disorder in a particular individual, and determine appropriate therapy. The clinician should also look beyond descriptive and surface-level interpretation and consider what underlying processing deficit(s) is/are bringing about the language behaviours that have been observed. The use of explanations derived from psycholinguistics and cognitive neuropsychology (Caplan, 1987; 1992; Lesser and Milroy, 1993) play an important part in understanding the nature of problems.

In this chapter many of the speech characteristics and language behaviours observed in aphasia are identified and explained with reference to linguistics, psycholinguistics and cognitive neuropsychology in order to provide a knowledge-base for later discussion of assessment and treatment. Prior to this a brief background about the associations of neurological lesion and language breakdown, and the classification of aphasia gives a wider context for the linguistic disorder.

Theoretical Background to Aphasia

Brain damage resulting in aphasia can be caused by various problems including vascular disorder (e.g. stroke), tumour, blood clot (haematoma), abscess, trauma (e.g. gunshot wound, road traffic accident, surgical intervention), and, less commonly, infections (e.g. meningitis, encephalitis). The location and extent of damage influences the severity and symptom complex that results. Nevertheless, even relatively small lesions, not always in areas primarily recognised as being responsible for language function, have been found to cause quite significant aphasic problems.

In most people, the 'language centres' seem to be found mainly in the left hemisphere (side) of the brain within the convoluted nerve tissue on the brain's surface, the cortex. The areas in the cortex associated with different language functions, e.g. serial organisation and motor programming (Broca's area), spoken language comprehension (Wernicke's area), written and spoken language association (angular gyrus), receptive and expressive association of spoken language (arcuate fasciculus), identified in Figure 11.1, are rather theoretical and ill-defined, and when damage occurs will respond in a somewhat individual way. In addition, the right hemisphere of the brain contributes to language, particularly in prosody and pragmatics (Code, 1987; Myers, 1986), and thalamic and extrathalamic structures in the subcortex of the left hemisphere also have a role (Crosson, 1985; Kirk and Kertesz, 1994).

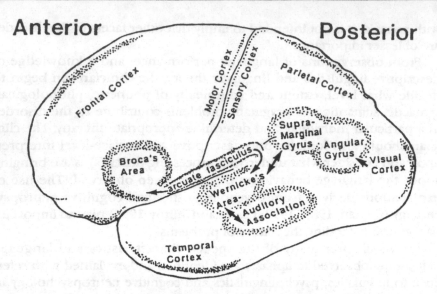

Figure 11.1: Diagram of the (left) cerebral hemisphere and cortical areas involved in language.

Many attempts have been made to classify a variety of types of aphasia on the basis of patterns of language behaviours or characteristics. The localisationalist model of Goodglass and Kaplan (1983) is currently the most widely used classification system. This model attributes certain patterns of aphasic characteristics to damage in a particular area of the brain making up the following classifications:

Broca's aphasia;
Wernicke's aphasia;
conduction aphasia ;
anomic aphasia;
global aphasia;
transcortical sensory aphasia;
transcortical motor aphasia;
mixed non-fluent aphasia;
subcortical aphasias;
aphemia;
pure word deafness;
pure alexia;
pure agraphia;
alexia with agraphia.

Another common system of classification is on a dichotomy of fluent and non-fluent. Aphasic speech is often described as either fluent or non-fluent according to the presenting features, such as speech rate, length of utterance, articulatory accuracy, presence or omission of function words, ease of word retrieval (Feyereisen, Pillon and de Partz, 1991). These speech patterns reflect the influence of different phonetic, phonological, semantic and syntactic dysfunction. In general the subtypes of aphasia resulting from lesions to the anterior part of the cortex are non-fluent, e.g. Broca's aphasia, and those from posterior damage are fluent, e.g. Wernicke's aphasia.

In reality it is difficult to define aphasic speech on this dichotomy, which fails to take account of a variety of linguistic phenonema. An individual speaker with aphasia can demonstrate a combination of fluent and non-fluent features within the same speech sample. In addition, in different contexts such as repetition, reading aloud, interview, referential communication or narrative, the same person is likely to demonstrate varying degrees of fluency. A label based on an overall impression of fluent and non-fluent tells us little about the nature of the problem or the management needs. Rather than look too closely for a category of fluency, an interpretation of the presenting characteristics and a comparison across contexts is a more effective approach. It is with this in mind that Feyereison *et al.* (1991) recommend that the clinician should analyse speech data using Garrett's (1980; 1982) model of speech production, which proposes a message level, a functional level, and a positional level to explain the psycholinguistic breakdown that relates to specific behaviours. This model has been modified by Schwartz (1987) who adds a phonetic level and a motor level, as described below.

1. A *message level*, which is conceptual rather than linguistic, is where decisions are made about ideas and meanings (messages) to be conveyed and depends on factors such as knowledge of situations, and speaking intentions, that is, the propositional aspects of language.
2. A *functional level* integrates three operations, the retrieval of the semantic representation of content words, the composition of the predicate argument structure, and the allocation of lexical items to role positions within the structure.
3. A *positional level* is concerned with the actual ordering of components prepared in the previous level into a syntactic planning frame. It is where all function words are accessed and a further lexical search retrieves the phonological forms of content words and places these into the planning frame.
4. A *phonetic representation level* is where the phonological information is recoded into its phonetic representations ready for articulation.
5. A *motor level* prepares the phonetic realisation into a neuromuscular code which can be articulated.

Use of this framework can guide treatment. Therapy might be to help the generation of ideas, or give strategies to improve word retrieval, or improve syntactic use, or slow speech to aid articulatory programming, depending on the level, and therefore the nature of difficulty identified.

Classification is potentially useful as a means of organising thinking about aphasia (Bartlett and Pashek, 1994) and in providing a convention to help communications between aphasiologists, e.g. 'This person has a predominantly Wernicke's aphasia but shows some signs of articulatory awkwardness more common in Broca's aphasia', or 'This person is generally fluent but elements of non-fluent speech occur when searching for specific content words', but has limitations. As Bartlett and Pashek (1994) explain, because the nature and severity of aphasia varies with each individual and it is rare for a syndrome to present in a pure form, alternative analyses are essential. Strong support is given for an analysis of linguistic behaviour and methods which specify the underlying psycholinguistic process which is affected.

Aphasic Characteristics and Behaviours: Linguistic and Psycholinguistic Explanations

The manifestations of linguistic impairment vary considerably between individuals with aphasia. When we meet a person with aphasia we can begin to specify their presenting features using terms that are used to describe the characteristics which occur in aphasic speech such as *articulatory awkwardness; phonemic paraphasia; neologism; circumlocution; semantic paraphasia; verbal paraphasia; anomia; automatism; recurrent utterance; stereotypy; agrammatism; paragrammatism*, which are explained below. At the same time, we can take account of behaviours that are associated with language use, e.g. turn-taking; appropriateness of response; perseveration; use of communication acts. The clinician also has to decide which of the verbal and non-verbal behaviours that the person exhibits are a direct result of impairments in linguistic performance and processing, and which are due to conscious or unconscious attempts to compensate for these deficits. From a thorough evaluation of the evidence deductions can be made leading to the provision of a therapy programme which will go some way to reduce the impact of the linguistic deficit. Linguistic and psycholinguistic explanations for the presenting features help our understanding of the nature of the aphasia and are discussed here under headings which relate to the surface-level description of the behaviours, i.e. *phonetics* and *phonology, semantics, syntax* and *pragmatics*.

Phonetics and Phonology

Problems in Language Expression

Articulatory awkwardness, as we have seen, is commonly used to describe the speech sound errors that contribute to non-fluent speech. The person is observed to search visibly and auditorily for articulatory positions, and to produce variable phonetic errors and also phonological errors which generally fail to comply with the phonotactics of the speaker's native language. These difficulties are not due to a neuromuscular disorder which would instead cause dysarthria, but due to a problem of phonetic planning. Several alternative terms and interpretations have been suggested for this problem, e.g. *apraxia of speech* (Wertz, La Pointe and Rosenbek, 1984; Square-Storer, 1989); *verbal apraxia* (Edwards, 1984); *aphasic articulatory defect* (Mackenzie, 1982); *speech apraxia* (Miller, 1992). (See also Chapter 15, this volume).

While the observed features demonstrate phonetic errors, argument persists about the underlying psycholiguistic breakdown, whether it is at a level of motor programming, the 'motor level', or an earlier stage of linguistic planning, the 'phonetic representation level'. A framework suggested by Caplan (1992) places the breakdown within a context of speech organisation. He identifies three operations needed to produce the sound pattern of a word: accessing the permanent lexical representation of the word; inserting the representation into a sentence; and preparing the representation for articulation. It is this latter aspect that would cause disturbances in programming the articulators and produce the phonetic errors seen in articulatory awkwardness.

People who present with this characteristic almost always have good monitoring abilities and are able to respond to feedforward and feedback information. The awkwardness observed is not only the outcome of linguistic breakdown but also is exacerbated by an anticipation of error and attempts to rectify errors as, or immediately after, they are made.

Phonemic paraphasia is demonstrated in speech by phoneme substitutions, rearrangements and additions, with consonants being affected rather than vowels, and segment production achieved with ease, or fluently. The phonemes and phoneme combinations that occur are always consistent with the phonotactic rules of the speaker's language, e.g. 'squottle' for 'bottle', or 'pusting' for 'putting'. There will also be sufficient phonologically accurate aspects of the target word remaining for it to be identifiable from the speech context: e.g. in a conversation about a person's interest in photography 'cagara' would be identified as a meaningful word.

Buckingham (1992) shows how phonemic paraphasias are qualitatively similar in features to the slips-of-the-tongue evident in non-aphasic speech and classified by Crystal (1987). The mechanism suggested to explain the phenonemon is a 'scan copier' (Shattuck-Hufnagel, 1979; Buckingham, 1992) which operates at the 'positional level' of speech production.

In phonological paraphasia, Garrett (1984) proposes that a word meaning is accessed but its phonological form, the phonological representation of the word, is impaired. As a result a 'word' of the same number of syllables, stress contour and even the same initial phoneme or syllable tends to be uttered, for example 'canderpillar' for 'caterpillar' or 'flowman' for 'snowman'.

There is a large degree of subjectivity attached to deciding whether a 'word' is the result of either phonological paraphasia, and an impairment in the ability to access the permanent lexical phonological representation of a target word (Caplan, 1992), or a breakdown at a semantic level. If the examples 'cagara' and 'flowman' were produced in a list of unrelated words or when the listener has not sufficient contextual knowledge to interpret the target it might be perceived as a neologism.

Neologism affects content words, making them appear bizarre and unlike any legitimate word in the speaker's language, unless by accident (Christman, 1992). The problem is generally believed to be the result of phonemic paraphasia of such severity that no real word can be recognised from the attempt. There can be a great structural resemblance to words in the language that could be used in the same position in the sentence (e.g. 'I'm wickling the pattle'), suggesting that the phonological form of a target word is known but phonemes are mis-selected and mis-ordered to such an extent that a meaningful word cannot be discerned. In other cases neologisms bear no relation to an appropriate type of word for the sentence structure (e.g. ' I'm swink that trid'), suggesting a failure even to access the phonological form of the word (Butterworth, 1979). An alternative interpretation is that neologisms may signal a semantic deficit; the meaning of the word is not accessed so a random selection of phonemes is made. The resulting neologism will contain acceptable phonological structures, indicating a certain degree of intactness at the phonological level, but problems in semantic access are evident because the attempt bears no relation to a meaningful word.

Problems in Language Reception

A disturbance in single word comprehension may be due to either a phonological- or semantic-level impairment. A phonological deficit affects the ability to activate the phonological structure reliably to recognise a spoken word. When a word is heard it will either fail to be recognised, or be misinterpreted as one with a similar phonological structure (Caplan, 1992). If word level comprehension is impaired, whether due to a phonological or semantic impairment, the person will have to rely on a range of other linguistic and non-linguistic information to gain meanings from longer units of speech (see further below).

A Central Problem of Phonological Processing

It is not uncommon to discover that the phonological deficit stems from a central phonological processing difficulty. In assessing a person it is important to establish whether the problem is confined to either the reception or production of language, or encompasses both.

Semantics

Problems in Language Expression

Word retrieval errors: Impairments in the ability to produce lexical items occur in every individual with aphasia whether in naming, spontaneous speech or reading. Different behaviours will present depending on the processing skills available to the person. The degree of awareness also contributes to the problem that we observe. Meaningful and non-meaningful word substitutions in unchecked fluent speech usually indicate a lack of awareness of errors, whereas different types of blocking and searching behaviours, such as pauses, hesitations and re-attempts at initial sounds and syllables or at whole words, are displays of awareness of difficulty. The following are some of the language features reflecting problems in lexical retrieval:

> *circumlocution*: In an attempt to retrieve a word, or at least convey its meaning, the subject talks around the target word. Intentional strategies are sometimes adopted, such as descriptions and definitions, as speech skirts round the specific word, and can seem like a delaying tactic. Where a person has extreme difficulty in accessing content words, empty runs of speech may be heard, such as 'It is over there, like the other one, the one he has';
> *semantic paraphasia*: A real word which has the same grammatical function as the target and also has semantic association with its substitute, for example 'walking' for 'running'; 'glass' for 'window'. As these examples show, the phonological structure of the substitute word will generally be dissimilar to the target;
> *verbal paraphasia*: A real word which has the same grammatical function but here there is no recognisable semantic association with the target. The error may show a degree of intactness of the structural features of the target word such as number of syllables,and some similarity in the phonemes, such as 'walking' for 'wishing'; 'chair' for 'chalk' or be unrelated in structure, for example 'quiet' for 'careful'; 'tree' for 'catapult';
> *perseverative paraphasia*: A word which has been expressed in a previous context is inappropriately repeated in a later utterance. As in other perseverative behaviours, both linguistic and non-linguistic,

this usually implies a failure in processing a new response which is more difficult than reproducing the former one;

anomia: This strictly refers to disorders of naming rather than word retrieval in running speech, and may be due to a failure to recall words from a variety of concept groupings, or may be restricted to specific word categories, notably body parts, colours and objects. As Caplan (1992) and study from cognitive neuropsychology (described below) explain, a naming impairment may be due to a range of possible processing deficits. The problem may be in:

(i)   visual perceptual analysis, causing visual agnosia;
(ii)   linking sensory and perceptual information with conceptual and semantic information;
(iii) accessing the semantic representation of an appropriate lexical item;
(iv)   eliciting the phonological structure of an appropriate lexical item.

Depending on the underlying difficulty, the anomic response may present as failure to evoke a word attempt, a semantic paraphasia, circumlocution, neologism, or feature phonemic paraphasia.

In a sample of aphasic connected speech, lexical retrieval problems will be realised by searching behaviour or any of the types of error described above. Additionally, there may be difficulties in placing the semantic representations, or themes that convey sentence meaning, into the sentence framework. In this case agrammatism, described below, is likely to be apparent. As will be explained in the discussion of syntax, there is a close interrelationship of semantics and syntax at sentence level which adds to the difficulty of determining the precise nature of deficit.

Problems in Receptive Language

If a spoken word heard by an individual with aphasia fails to evoke appropriate and sufficient sense relations, its meaning or referent cannot be accessed, or is only partially accessed from semantic memory. The word will be perceived as a meaningless nonsense word or may be interpreted as another concept from a related semantic field, for example 'turnip' for 'potato'; 'rake' for 'lawnmower'. A person with a lexical comprehension deficit generally has more difficulty correctly associating a heard word with one of two closely related pictures or items rather than with one of two unrelated pictures or items. For example, 'knife' is more likely to be recalled from pictures of a knife and a boat rather than from pictures of a knife and a fork. In the discussion of treatment at single word level below we will see that there are a variety of influences, including degree of imageability, abstractness and familiarity, that affect the ability to understand and use lexical items.

Often, difficulty arises in understanding single words because there is an absence of information to support any partial semantic processing. At a simple level, the word 'spade' is likely to be understood, or at least correctly guessed, if heard within a flow of speech containing associated words such as 'garden', 'dig', 'soil' from a person holding a tree that they intend to plant. As we have seen in the discussion of phonological impairment, linguistic and extralinguistic context is used to comprehend specific semantic and also syntactic information. As natural communication provides a great deal of contextual information this should be incorporated into therapy (Pierce, 1991).

Sentence meaning can also be affected by semantic comprehension problems. This occurs where there is an impairment in the ability to interpret the thematic relations of a particular verb. This can be shown in the example 'The mouse chased the cat'. The thematic roles of 'mouse' as agent-subject and 'cat' as theme-object can only be appreciated if the lexical entry 'chased' is understood. It would not be surprising for a person with a sentence-meaning deficit to fall back on knowledge, experience and expectancy and so interpret the sentence as ' The cat chased the mouse'.

The effects of information load and memory span are additional significant factors affecting semantic comprehension. Martin and Feher (1990) have shown that a subject with a memory deficit may be especially impaired in comprehension for sentences containing a large number of content words while variations in syntactic complexity have little effect. In most people with aphasia, however, it is the influence of memory span, information load, semantics and syntax that affects the ability to comprehend.

Syntax

Problems in Language Expression

Agrammatism: This contributes to non-fluent output and is characterised by speech produced in a disconnected manner, function words are omitted to a greater extent than content words, and grammatical inflection is generally lacking. Tissot, Mounin and Lehrmitte (1973) describe agrammatism as speech in which grammatical words are deleted; verb tense inflection may be absent and infinitives are substituted for finite verbs; and agreements, particularly of gender and number, are lost. Gleason, Goodglass, Green, Ackerman and Hyde (1975) identified a hierarchy of difficulty and use of grammatical structures in agrammatic speakers. In order, starting from the easiest to produce, this is as follows:

structure	example
imperative intransitives	'Come here'
imperative transitives	'Close the window'
wh-interrogatives	'What is it?'
declarative transitive	'She draws the picture'
declarative intransitive	'He sleeps'
comparative	'She is smaller'
passive	'The boy was carried'
direct–indirect object	'He gives his mother the flowers'
embedded sentences	'She wanted to be happy'
future	'She will read'

In the severest forms of agrammatism speech consists of isolated words which have the quality of one-word sentences. In other instances the main elements of sentences may be evident and word order is maintained but simplified forms are used, e.g.:

'brush hair...girl'
'mother and boy, girl and jam...there a...lady...tap..oh water'

There is some debate about the nature of this problem which, on the surface, appears to be syntactic. Using the term parallelism, Kolk, van Grunsven and Keyser (1985) propose that agrammatism reflects a central loss of syntax, affecting comprehension and production and even extending to other modalities – a view shared with others (Caplan and Futter, 1986). A further explanation is that it is due to only a partial loss of syntax (Grodinsky, 1986; 1988). Other research suggests that both syntactic and semantic processing play a role (Sherman and Schweichickert, 1989). Yet others believe a syntactic impairment is not a factor (Linebarger, Schwartz and Saffran, 1983). Several recent studies (Jones, 1986; Byng, 1988; Nickels, Byng and Black, 1991; Marshall, Pring and Chiat, 1993) explain agrammatism in terms of difficulties in mapping thematic relations on to the syntactic frame: a 'positional level' deficit, which operates both in sentence comprehension and sentence production. The contribution of this model to the treatment of agrammatism will be shown later.

Paragrammatism: This is speech which has grammatical errors within largely fluent output. Grammatical, or function words, for example 'of'; 'the'; 'and' 'otherwise'; 'may' and morphological elements such as '-ed'; '-ing'; '-s', are incorrectly selected but, unlike agrammatism, are rarely omitted. The problem appears to be due to difficulties in syntactic selection and organisation. Once again, what we hear may deceive our understanding of the true nature of the disorder. Butterworth (1985) describes the errors in paragrammatic speech as 'constructional' and attributes the problem to a lexical selection deficit. He likens the substitutions that occur to semantic-level slips-of-the-tongue that can present in normal speakers. An alternative proposal (Heeschen, 1985) is that agrammatism and paragrammatism arise from a common syntactic processing deficit, and are only behaviourly different because of the monitoring ability of the speaker. In an individual with a lack of awareness of their errors substitutions are not avoided. Where awareness is intact the person recognises the difficulty, and concentrates on the information-giving stressed components (nouns, verbs, adjectives).

Problems of Receptive Language

When a person with aphasia misinterprets or shows a failure to comprehend runs of connected speech it is difficult to tell whether this is caused by a phonological, semantic, syntactic or pragmatic deficit, an attention, memory or other cognitive problem, or a combination of deficits. From evidence at single word and sentence level we can only make tentative proposals about the problems in longer units because the interactions of facets are complex and difficult to disentangle.

Pragmatics

There is plenty of evidence to show that communicative competence, the knowledge of the rules governing language use in context, is retained and pragmatic skills are particularly resilient in aphasia (Holland, 1970; 1991). This means that, in spite of inaccurate phonology, semantics and syntax, messages are often successfully conveyed by the person, and meanings understood from the messages they receive.

Language Expression

Although speech may be unintelligible or absent, many people with aphasia are able to use non-verbal signals such as eye-gaze, pause, gesture, prosody, facial expression, to indicate meanings. They may also engage appropriately in discourse, adopt effective repair strategies, and demonstrate a range of communicative acts including acknowledgement, greeting, request, question and command. Even in severe jargon aphasia (see below) individuals can often convey communicative intent, emotion, question forms and topic change (Dogil, Hilderbrandt and Schurmeier, 1990).

Language Reception

A person with severe verbal comprehension deficits can often make appropriate responses to yes–no or wh- questions, commands etc. because they recognise the meaning implied by prosodic features, visual cues, contextual information and so on. People with aphasia usually have good orientation in time and situation and are well able to recognise props, people and environment. This contextual information directs the person at least to make relevant guesses about a message that could not have been understood out of context. Comprehension and responses are likely to be superior when there is familiarity with the other person(s) involved in the interaction, or when there is personal knowledge of the topic under discussion. In these circumstances it is easier to anticipate the language that will be used. Similarly, if some parts of the preceding linguistic information have been comprehended, later messages will be anticipated more confidently and responses will be more appropriate.

It is not intended to suggest that pragmatic deficits and pragmatically inappropriate behaviours do not occur in aphasia. Particularly where more widespread neurological damage and the right hemisphere is affected, people with aphasia are prone to problems such as failure to recognise situations, feigning understanding, ignoring turn-taking signals, and continuing to jargon in spite of negative feedback from a conversational partner. Other common problems in aphasia are a failure to initiate conversation, change topic or employ a full range of communicative acts. In some instances these problems may be pragmatic in origin; in others they may be secondary to the overall linguistic deficits. As Lesser and Milroy (1993) remind us, difficulty with lexical access or syntactic structure can have pragmatic consequences.

Other Speech Characteristics in Aphasia

To complete this overview of the linguistic problems that arise in aphasia, brief mention has to be made of three other speech behaviours: jargon, automatic responses and repetitive verbal behaviour.

Jargon consists of fluent, generally incomprehensible utterances which may contain any type of paraphasia and neologism, whereas paragrammatism, circumlocution and empty phrases further contribute to the apparently contentless outpouring. Severely impaired monitoring skills usually add to the inability to inhibit jargon. In other cases jargon is accompanied by an awareness of conversational rules and, as indicated earlier, can help convey relevant messages.

Automatic speech may be surprisingly well preserved even in severe cases of aphasia. Serial speech (counting, days of the week), social responses, expletives, familiar overlearned sayings and rhymes may be produced with relative ease. These responses are not dependent on linguistic organisation and have little or no functional use, but sometimes they can be tapped to help access propositional language.

Repetitive verbal behaviour can take several forms. The most common are automatisms and recurrent utterances. Echolalia, perseveration and stereotypy can also occur (Wallesch, 1990) and generally indicate a more severe form of aphasia. Automatisms, recurrent utterences and stereotypy represent different types of meaningful or non-meaningful speech in which a syllable, word, phrase, short sentence, expletive or neologism is fluently and recurrently produced (Code, 1982; 1989; Wallesch, 1990). These may be the sole means of verbal expression. Some individuals show no awareness that the reiteration is inappropriate, whereas others may attempt to inhibit the linguistically inadequate form. When prosodic alterations are applied to the utterance, communicative intent may be conveyed. Echolalia, the repetition of all or part of an utterance just spoken by another person, and perseveration, the reproduction of a previous response in a new situation, similarly indicate that linguistic processing is impaired.

Assessment – a Basis for Treatment

Assessment is used to diagnose, that is to thoroughly analyse all available evidence in order to draw conclusions about (a) the nature and severity of the aphasia and any other contributing disorders; (b) the treatment that would be most appropriate; and (c) the prognosis, or likely outcome. Assessment involves the clinician in making predictions, or hypotheses, about a person's linguistic performance and processing abilities and selecting the appropriate means of testing these hypotheses. By following these principles, a picture is built of the ceiling levels of ability, the points of breakdown, and what helps or impedes performance. From this, treatment goals can be specified in terms of the level of intervention, the processes to be developed, the techniques to be used, and also the achievements or outcomes to expect. In this way, the clinician determines a hierarchy of appropriate treatment tasks and techniques to rehabilitate the linguistic disorder.

In addition, once treatment is under way, ongoing assessment is essential to chart progress in treated and untreated aspects of language, to evaluate treatment effectiveness, and to provide a scientific basis for modifying intervention.

Judgements about receptive and expressive abilities in phonology, semantics, syntax and pragmatics should be drawn from observing responses to, and language behaviour which presents in, a variety of single-word, sentence, paragraph and conversation contexts. Descriptive linguistics and structured analysis help us to decide what linguistic features are available to, and used by, the individual in communication. Interpretations based on psycholinguistic and cognitive neuropsychological principles guide us to identify the processing deficit that is represented by the linguistic performance we have described. To take us further, we also need to carry out conversational or discourse analysis so that we can understand how the linguistic breakdown affects interactions between the person with aphasia and others.

A range of methods of assessment that are appropriate for use with people with aphasia have already been discussed in earlier chapters of this volume. Here only a brief overview of two approaches, conversational analysis and cognitive neuropsychology, will be considered.

Broadly, there are two types of conversational analysis, top-down and bottom-up (Milroy and Perkins, 1992; Lesser and Milroy, 1993). The former takes a deductive approach and identifies whether certain prede-termined features such as speech acts, relevance and turn-taking behav-iours are present or absent. The latter takes a more open and inductive stance in determining how linguistic breakdown affects conversational exchange and what contributes to communicative success and failure as a result of the contributions of both participants.

The following example of a clinician (C) and a woman with aphasia (W) provides a selective account of conversation analysis:

C: Would you like a cup of tea?
W: No, I'll have one before I go...in where I go.
C: When you get home?
W: No, in the /keridɪ/. in the... don't they have a...?
C: In the café?
W: Yes, you should go.

At a structural level the woman appears to have difficulties in lexical access, and at best is able to replace content words with neologism (/keridI/), suggesting there is a phonological lexical access deficit. Grammatical struc-ture is also impaired ('in where I go'). At the same time she demonstrates a significant degree of communicative success through cooperative achieve-ment with the clinician, and their successful use of turn-taking devices, repair strategies and speech acts. Additionally it is clear that linguistic comprehension is unimpaired within this short exchange.

We have already shown that reliance on descriptive linguistics can give an incomplete impression of the underlying processing deficit. The field of cognitive neuropsychology is a major source of help to clinicians. It proposes a range of theoretical models which provide us with a framework for pinpointing the origins of breakdown in processing in an individual. For example, three people who each fail on a task of understanding single printed words may be found to do so for very different reasons. One may have a deficit in recognising the letters, *abstract letter identification*; one a deficit in spelling and associating the form with a dictionary item, thus fail-ing to tell whether it is a real or non-real word, *orthographic input lexicon*; one be unable to interpret the meaning in spite of identifying the target as a real word, *a semantic system deficit* (Kay, Lesser and Coltheart, 1992).

Visual confrontation naming, the production of a target word from a pictured item or activity, is useful to further illustrate the application of the principles of cognitive neuropsychology at single-word level. Lesser (1989) identifies several possible sites of breakdown in processing which cause naming errors:

(i)   *a cognitive or semantic system impairment*: semantic paraphasias present, there will be difficulty in semantic discrimination and comprehension tests in speech and often in reading, and cued phonologically with a semantically-associated word the person often accepts this as the target and reproduces it accordingly;

(ii) *a phonological lexicon impairment*: tip-of-the tongue searching behaviour characterised by phonemic paraphasias and circumlocution is exhibited, demonstrating that the semantic representation is intact, so there is no difficulty in producing the target when the model is given;

(iii) *a phonological assembly impairment*: phonemic paraphasias occur but are more closely associated with that of the target than is evident in phonological lexicon errors, circumlocution is less likely, but there is more difficulty in imitating multisyllabic words;

(iv) *a phonetic planning and realisation impairment*: sequential organisation difficulties in individual and strings of phonemes are manifest in phonetically erroneous attempts. Accuracy is better both on imitation of a model of a target word and in the production of less specific words and speech with less propositional demand;

(v)   *an articulatory impairment*: due to muscle weakness or a movement disorder, that is, the non-linguistic deficit of dysarthria, in which more consistent articulation difficulties are produced.

Careful selection and interpretation of assessments based on psycholinguistic theory can guide the clinician in determining which of these possible levels of breakdown is causing what has been observed as a difficulty in naming.

The Psycholinguistic Assessment of Language Processing in Aphasia (PALPA) (Kay *et al.*, 1992), discussed in Chapters 6, 7 and 8 of this volume, contains tests of auditory processing, reading and spelling, picture and word semantics, and sentence comprehension. These assessments are invaluable when diagnosing the processing difficulties that contribute to the communication problems of the person with aphasia. In addition the clinician can use other observations and individually designed structured assessments to help identify the site of breakdown in processing.

Although cognitive neuropsychology has developed our knowledge of, and ability to identify, processing deficits in single-word and sentence-level contexts it does not explain language above this level, such as narratives and conversation. A combination of assessment procedures has to be conducted to appreciate fully the linguistic deficit of an individual and its impact on communication.

Treatment

A primary aim of aphasia therapy is for the person to achieve their greatest possible independence and success in communication. Improvement in linguistic skills plays a significant part in this process and is aided by therapy which carefully brings together aspects of two broad perspectives of intervention:

1. Treatment which concentrates on specific aspects of language and language processing.
2. Guidance and support of the person and their personal contacts (partners, family, voluntary and paid carers, friends, colleagues), in understanding the linguistic disorder and how linguistic performance can be maximised.

The following discussion of treatment provides some practical examples to illustrate each of these approaches.

Treatment Directed at Specific Aspects of Language and Language Processing

In linguistically orientated approaches, therapy concentrates on a specific impairment of the language system. It involves the application of methods which achieve learning through careful specification and manipulation of the stimuli presented, the type and standard of response required of the person, and the feedback provided by the clinician.

There is a variety of proposals as to how this learning comes about, although perhaps the one most widely accepted is *reorganisation*. The theory behind reorganisation is that, as a result of therapy, a rearrangement of language processing is brought about which achieves a permanent transfer of learning and improved performance in the skill where therapy was directed. Sometimes the treatment might concentrate on the impaired modality, sometimes it is more appropriate to focus on a less impaired modality to bring about a change in behaviour. For example, in a person who has a phonological deficit and is unable to discriminate between spoken words, we might place the emphasis on spoken word to picture-matching tasks, but if reading were superior to speech, written word to picture-matching could be used with a gradual introduction of the spoken counterpart. The ultimate test of the effectiveness of the therapy is whether there is evidence of generalisation to non-treated stimuli and improved performance of the treated skill in more propositional and spontaneous contexts.

A comprehensive programme based on many of the above principles, which covers a wide range of language treatment, is the Language-Oriented approach (LOT) of Shewan and Bandur (1986). Following detailed assessment the clinician directs treatment at a relevant area for the person within one or more of five modalities: *auditory processing;*

visual processing; gestural and gestural-verbal communication; oral expression; graphic expression. For example, in auditory processing the following areas are included: awareness of auditory stimuli; recognition of auditory stimuli; monitoring speech; comprehension of single units; comprehension of short series; comprehension of short meaningful linguistic units; comprehension of sentences; comprehension of paragraphs; comprehension of narratives and discourse. Within the area of each modality a hierarchy of task difficulty is identified. The clinician decides on the stimuli that will be suitable to present, the teaching strategies to use and the response required of the person.

Treatment at Single Word Level

Depending on the nature of the word retrieval or naming disorder that presents, different therapy should be given. To demonstrate this point Nettleton and Lesser (1991) describe the use of two methods to remediate naming disorders, one due to a semantic deficit, the other due to a phonological lexicon deficit:

(i) *Semantic therapy* consists of encouraging semantic processing to help access sufficient semantic information rather than attempting to produce the name of the item. It involves word–picture-matching tasks requiring the appropriate selection of an item from a spoken name, a written label, and a description of its function; yes/no questions, for example 'Is a cat an animal?', 'Does a cat have wings?'; and categorising tasks. Similar therapy is described by Howard, Patterson, Franklin, Orchard-Lisle and Morton (1985) and Mackenzie (1991).

(ii) *Phonological therapy* concentrates on analysing word shapes and practising naming. It involves repeating the names of pictures; making rhyming judgements about words; and naming pictures from a phonemic cue.

A further example of therapy to address word retrieval difficulties which are semantic in origin and to improve descriptive skills is explained by Mackenzie (1991). In this 'verbal expression therapy', in an alternating-turn format with the clinician, the person is encouraged to offer information about common objects based on nine categories: description; size; component parts; composition; shape; colour; associated person; use; and associated item. The clinician reviews the attempt and gives written prompts to help the person's responses.

There are many factors that can influence the ability to access lexical comprehension and word retrieval. These include the effects of individual experience as well as other perceptual, conceptual and linguistic aspects of the lexical item such as frequency of use, familiarity, affective aspects, picturability and abstractness (Buckingham, 1981; Lesser,

1989). For example, 'chair' should be more readily accessed than 'calculus', though a mathematician might find the latter easier. Also semantic category (object, action, colour, letter, number) and grammatical category (noun, verb, adjective) tend to vary in difficulty according to both type of aphasia and individual difference. In therapy it is vital that the clinician not only recognises an appropriate hierarchy of easy and difficult words but ensures that targeted items have a high degree of relevance for the individual.

The purpose of semantic therapy is to stimulate concept and semantic associations and encourage semantic processing skills so that they can be applied in more spontaneous contexts. In more severe cases it may be possible to promote semantic associations through therapy activities using simple categorisation tasks, matching pantomime actions or spoken or written verb phrases to pictured concepts of familiar items, or eliciting spoken words commonly associated with a target word or incomplete common phrase or sentence provided, e.g. 'salt' and ('pepper'); 'the grass is (green)'.

One method which is useful to improve the semantic skills of people with mild or moderate aphasia is *divergent treatment* (Chapey, 1981; 1986). In this creativity and problem-solving skills are developed in association activities requiring a search for a variety of logical and relevant words or ideas, e.g. given a word 'garden' the person has to generate as many wide-ranging words as possible that could be associated with the target. The intention is that this practice in word retrieval through semantic associations will transfer to conversation so that word retrieval is achieved more readily and when a target cannot be recalled a relevant alternative may be offered rather than the person being locked into a failed attempt. The method is also designed to enable a more flexible generation of ideas and better conversational ability. The tasks identified by Chapey not only include listing associated words but also suggesting a variety of uses for an item; imagining problems in a given situation; explaining the differences or similarities between two items; and providing a selection of possible solutions to a problem.

Treatment at Sentence Level

In broad terms, therapy methods at sentence level can be divided into those designed to increase the amount, quality and length of utterances, that is, concentrating on increasing the information or semantic content of speech, and those to improve syntactic use.

An example of the first type is the Programme of Changing Criteria (Rosenbek, La Pointe and Wertz, 1989). This takes the person through up to four levels of utterance length from one or two to nine or more word-length responses, depending on the individual's potential. From realistic action pictures the person is encouraged to elicit responses at the selected level of utterance length, helped by the clinician asking relevant questions and pointing to appropriate aspects of the picture. The questions relate to ideas such as the number of people, what they are wearing, what they are holding, what time it is, what they are doing. When difficulties arise the answer can be guided by cueing with either a model to imitate or a foil, i.e. a contrasting item. If an appropriate sentence were 'Holding a flower' the clinician might help elicit this by either providing this phrase for imitation or asking 'Is he holding a flower, or holding a vase?'

To expand the complexity and range of syntactic structures used by the person the Helm Elicited Language Programme for Syntax Stimulation (HELPSS) (Helm-Estabrooks and Ramsberger, 1986) draws on the sentence structures observed in patients with agrammatism (Gleason, Goodglass, Green, Ackerman and Hyde, 1975), described earlier. There are two stages to this therapy. First the clinician (C) provides a dialogue which includes the target structure demonstrated with a line drawing. The person (P) is then required to respond to a cued question, e.g.:

C: 'Bob's grandchild is bored. He gets a book and reads his grandchild a story. What does he do?'
P: 'He reads his grandchild a story'

The second stage requires the person to complete the utterance given by the clinician, e.g.:

C: 'Bob's grandchild is bored. Bob gets a book and...'
P: 'He reads his grandchild a story'

In any syntax therapy it is important to ensure that treatment introduces as great a range of syntactic structures as possible. An effective and active communicator will use the descriptive and narrative forms that are readily elicited from pictured stimuli but question and command and other forms are also essential. We must also include methods to help the use of syntactic structures in everyday communication.

There are now several detailed accounts of therapy for agrammatism that, instead of retraining specific syntactic structures or sentence types, concentrate on sentence processing and mapping principles to improve the person's appreciation and use of sentence form and meaning (Jones, 1986; Byng, 1988; Nickels *et al.*, 1991; Marshall *et al.*, 1993; Schwartz *et al.*, 1994). Comprehension and production both tend to be affected when agrammatism occurs, and there is evidence to show that by working on language-input skills language-output skills can be improved, so therapy often concentrates on receptive processing. Schwartz *et al.* (1994) describe a sentence processing or mapping therapy in which the person is first given a written sentence to attempt to read aloud, which then is read to him/her by the clinician, e.g. 'The woman is cooking carrots'. Subsequently, three questions are asked relating to the verb ('what is the verb in the sentence?'); the patient/theme ('What is she cooking?'); and the agent ('Which one is doing the cooking?') The person has to underline the appropriate aspect of the written sentence and can then check it against a correct version. The therapy ranges over three phases: action verbs and canonical sentence structures ('The woman is cooking carrots'); state of mind verbs and canonical sentence structures ('The boy hated the sea'); and action verbs with non-canonical sentence structures ('The girl was pushed by the shopkeeper').

Treatment at Discourse Level and Guidance to the Person with Aphasia and His or Her Communicative Partners

Structured, specific treatments have been criticised for not being appropriate for the everyday use of language. Practice of language skills in conversational and other communication contexts is equally, if not more, important. Listening to and producing narratives, role-play and structured conversation are among the activities that might be chosen. As well as encouraging greater linguistic accuracy in these contexts, treatment that heightens awareness of what contributes to effective communication, maximises pragmatic skills, and introduces strategies that compensate for the linguistic impairment are essential. As communication, particularly in conversation, is an interactive process and participant-orientated (Green, 1984; Lesser and Milroy, 1993), both the individual with aphasia and his or her communicative partners should be actively involved in treatment.

People with deficits affecting comprehension are likely to benefit from therapy at discourse level which directs them to determine the topic, extract the key ideas, and anticipate and modify understanding as new information emerges. Treatment might also encourage them to employ verbal or non-verbal methods to request a speaker to slow down, repeat or clarify what they have said (Green, 1982). At the same time their communicative partners should be made familiar with the type of linguistic input that would be most appropriate and with ways to help linguistic processing; for example, slowing the rate of their speech; avoiding ambiguity; pausing; rephrasing; introducing topics carefully; placing key words at the end of sentences; and applying sentence stress which emphasises important words (Green,1984; cf. Chapter 10, this volume).

In many cases when we are dealing with expressive language problems the person has to be guided to accept that linguistic accuracy has to be sacrificed in favour of communication which successfully conveys information. One approach that fosters this and develops ways to compensate for linguistic impairments within communicative partnerships is PACE, Promoting Aphasia Communication Effectiveness (Davis and Wilcox, 1985). In this the person enhances their skills both as an initiator of information as well as a responder to information. They are encouraged to adopt a variety of communication channels (e.g. facial expression; gesture; pointing; drawing; writing; letter, picture or written word selection; speech), and engage in different communicative or speech acts (e.g. acknowledging; requesting; describing; asking) within a turn-taking activity. The approach also gives an opportunity for practising repair strategies to counteract communication breakdown. Although PACE is especially valuable for people with severe linguistic impairments where other methods fail to be functionally useful, it can be adapted to encourage more complex and creative language exchange for those with lesser degrees of deficit. By taking away the pressure of achieving linguistic accuracy it is not uncommon to find that linguistic abilities have developed spontaneously, as well as the achievement of other aspects contributing to effective communication.

Penn (1984) explains a range of compensatory strategies often employed in aphasia including the simplification of messages and prominence of key words; elaboration such as circumlocution to help lexical search; repetition of oneself or the other speaker as aids to clarify or give time to comprehend; using fillers to give time for a search for words; and other devices used to maintain conversational flow. Although every effort must be made to inhibit compensatory strategies that are non-productive, those that are effective should be identified and encouraged in treatment.

As already stressed, personal contacts need support in learning ways to facilitate linguistic performance. The guidance given at a particular point in time will vary. It may concern explanations about reducing fatigue and anxiety; the type of cues that will help linguistic access; encouraging active involvement in communication so that linguistic skills can be realised, practised and developed; fostering positive attitudes; altering the environment; and changing their own communicative behaviour such as giving time to respond.

Conclusion

There is no single method of treating the linguistic deficits in aphasia. An individualised intervention programme must be devised, based on a range of linguistic and non-linguistic information about the particular case and against a background of theoretical and experiential knowledge of aphasia.

Also we must not lose sight of the need to improve communicative effectiveness and provide support to the person and their personal contacts in coping with the effects of the disorder, including its psychosocial effects. Linguistic treatment is core for most individuals with aphasia but will be of limited use without ensuring that it is what the person wants, that the skills involved are applied in everyday situations, and that others on whom the disorder impacts are appropriately incorporated in the programme.

References

Bartlett, C.L. and Pashek, G.V. (1994). Practical implications in aphasia classification. *Aphasiology* 8(2), 103–126.

Buckingham, H.W. (1981). Lexical and semantic aspects of aphasia. In: M.T. Sarno, (Ed.), *Acquired Aphasia*. New York: Academic Press.

Buckingham, H.W. (1992). The mechanisms of phonemic paraphasia. *Clinical Linguistics and Phonetics* 6(1–2), 41–63.

Butterworth, B. (1979). Hesitation and the production of verbal paraphasias and neologisms in jargon aphasia. *Brain and Language* 8, 133–161.

Butterworth, B. (1985). Jargon aphasia: process and strategies. In: S. Newman, and R. Epstein (Eds.), *Current Perspectives in Dysphasia*. Edinburgh: Churchill Livingstone.

Byng, S. (1988). Sentence processing deficits: theory and therapy. *Cognitive Neuropsychology* 5, 629–676.

Caplan, D. (1987). *Neurolinguistics and Linguistic Aphasiology: An Introduction*. Cambridge: Cambridge University Press.

Caplan, D. (1992). *Language; Structure, Processing and Disorders*. London: MIT Press.

Caplan, D. and Futter, C. (1986). *Assignment of thematic roles to positions by an agrammatic aphasic patient*. Brain and Language 27, 117–134.

Chapey, R. (1981). Divergent semantic intervention. In: R. Chapey (Ed.), *Language Intervention Strategies in Adult Aphasia*. London: Williams & Wilkins.

Chapey, R. (1986). Cognitive intervention: stimulation of cognition, memory, convergent thinking, divergent thinking and evaluative thinking. In: R. Chapey (Ed.), *Language Intervention Strategies in Adult Aphasia*, 2nd edn. London/Baltimore: Williams & Wilkins.

Christman, S.S. (1992). Abtruse neologism formation: parallel processing revisited. *Clinical Linguistics and Phonetics* 6(1–2), 65–76.

Code, C. (1982). Neurolinguistic analysis of recurrent utterances in aphasia. *Cortex* 18, 141–152.

Code, C. (1987). *Language, Aphasia and the Right Hemisphere*. Chichester: Wiley.

Code, C. (1989). Recurrent utterances and automatisms in aphasia. In: C. Code (Ed.), *The Characteristics of Aphasia*. London: Taylor & Francis.

Crosson, B.(1985). Subcortical functions of language: a working model. *Brain and Language* 25, 257–292.

Crystal, D. (1987). *The Cambridge Encyclopaedia of Language*. Cambridge: Cambridge University Press.

Davis, G.A. and Wilcox, M.J. (1985). *Adult Aphasia Rehabilitation*. Windsor: NFER-Nelson.

Edwards, M. (1984). *Disorders of Articulation*. New York: Springer-Verlag.

Dogil, G., Hilderbrandt, G. and Shurmeier, K. (1990). The communicative function of prosody in semantic jargon aphasia. *Journal of Neurolinguistics* 5(2–3), 353–369.

Feyereisen, P., Pillon, A. and de Partz, M.-P. (1991). On measures of fluency in the assessment of spontaneous speech production by aphasic subjects. *Aphasiology* 5(1), 1–21.

Garrett, M. (1980). Sentence production. In: B. Butterworth (Ed.), *Language Production*, Vol 1: *Speech and Talk*. New York: Academic Press.

Garrett, M. (1982). Production of speech: observations from normal and pathological use. In: A.W. Ellis (Ed.), *Normality and Pathology in Cognitive Functions*. New York: Academic Press.

Garrett, M.F. (1984). The organization of processing structure for language production: application to aphasic speech. In: D. Caplan, A.R. Lecours and A. Smith (Eds.), *Biological Perspectives on Language*. Cambridge, MA: MIT Press.

Gleason, J.B., Goodglass, H., Green, E., Ackerman, N. and Hyde, M.R. (1975). The retrieval of syntax in Broca's aphasia. *Brain and Language* 2, 451–471.

Goodglass, H. and Kaplan, E. (1983). *The Assessment of Aphasia and Related Disorders*. Philadelphia: Lea & Febiger.

Green, G. (1982). Assessment and treatment of the adult with severe aphasia: aiming for functional generalisation. *Australian Journal of Human Communication Disorders* 10, 11–23.

Green, G. (1984). Communication in aphasia therapy: some of the procedures and issues involved. *British Journal of Disorders of Communication* 16, 35–46.

Grodinsky, Y. (1986). Language deficits and the theory of syntax. *Brain and Language* 27, 137–159.

Grodinsky, Y. (1988). Unifying the various language-related sciences: aphasic syndromes and grammatical theory. In: M. Ball (Ed.), *Theoretical Linguistics and Disordered Language*. Beckenham: Croom Helm.

Heeschen, C. (1985). Agrammatism versus paragrammatism: a fictitious opposition. In: M. Kean (Ed.), *Agrammatism*. London: Academic Press.

Helm-Estabrooks, N. and Ramsberger, G. (1986). Treatment of agrammatism in long-term Broca's aphasia. *British Journal of Disorders of Communication* 21, 39–45.

Holland, A. (1970). Case studies in aphasia rehabilitation using programmed instruction. *Journal of Speech and Language Disorders* 35, 377–390.

Holland, A.L. (1991). Pragmatic aspects of intervention in aphasia. *Journal of Neurolinguistics* 6(2), 197–211.

Howard, D., Patterson, K.E., Franklin, S., Orchard-Lisle, V.M. and Morton, J. (1985). The treatment of word retrieval deficits in aphasia: a comparison of two therapy methods. *Brain* 108, 817–829.

Jones, E. V. (1986). Building the foundation for sentence production in a non-fluent aphasic. *British Journal of Disorders of Communication* 21, 63–82.

Kay, J., Lesser, R. and Coltheart, M. (1992). *Psycholinguistic Assessment of Language Processing in Aphasia*. Hove: Lawrence Erlbaum.

Kirk, A. and Kertesz, A. (1994). Cortical and subcortical aphasias compared. *Aphasiology* 8(1), 65–82.

Kolk, H.H.J., van Grunsven, M.J.F. and Keyser, A. (1985). On parallelism between production and comprehension in agrammatism. In: M. Kean (Ed.), *Agrammatism*. London: Academic Press.

Lesser, R. (1989). *Linguistic Investigations of Aphasia*, 2nd edn. London: Cole & Whurr.

Lesser, R. and Milroy, L. (1993). *Linguistics and Aphasia: Psycholinguistic and Pragmatic Aspects*. London: Longman.

Linebarger, M.C., Schwartz, M.F. and Saffran, E.M. (1983). Sensitivity to grammatical structures in so-called agrammatic aphasics. *Cognition* 13, 361–392.

Mackenzie, C. (1982). Aphasic articulatory defect and aphasic phonological defect. *British Journal of Disorders of Communication* 17, 27–46.

Mackenzie, C. (1991). An aphasia group intensive efficacy study. *British Journal of Disorders of Communication* 26(3), 275–291.

Marshall, J., Pring, T. and Chiat, S. (1993). Sentence processing therapy: working at the level of the event. *Aphasiology* 7(2), 177–199.

Martin, R.C. and Feher, E. (1990). The consequences of reduced memory span for the comprehension of semantic versus syntactic information. *Brain and Language* 30(1), 1–20.

Miller, N. (1992). Variability in speech dyspraxia. *Clinical Linguistics and Phonetics* 6(1–2), 77–85.

Milroy, L. and Perkins, L. (1992). Repair strategies in aphasic discourse: towards a collaborative framework. *Clinical Linguistics and Phonetics* 6(1–2), 27–40.

Myers, P. S. (1986). Right hemisphere communication impairment. In: R. Chapey (Ed.), *Language Intervention Strategies in Adult Aphasia*. Baltimore: Williams & Wilkins.

Nettleton, J. and Lesser, R. (1991). Application of a cognitive neurpsychological model to therapy for naming difficulties. *Journal of Neurolinguistics* 6, 139–157.

Nickels, L., Byng, S. and Black, M. (1991). Sentence processing deficits: a replication of therapy. *British Journal of Disorders of Communication* 26, 175–199.

Penn, C. (1984). Compensation strategies in aphasia: behavioural and neurological correlates. In: K.W. Grieve and R. Griesel (Eds.), *Neuropsychology 11*. Pretoria: Monical.

Pierce, R.S. (1991). Contextual influences during comprehension in aphasia. *Aphasiology* 5(4–5), 374–381.

Rosenbek, J.C., La Pointe, L.L. and Wertz, R.T. (1989). *Aphasia: A Clinical Approach*. Boston: College Hill Press.

Schwartz, M. (1987). Patterns of speech production deficit within and across aphasia syndromes: application of a psycholinguistic model. In: M. Coltheart, G. Sartori and J. Job (Eds.), *The Cognitive Neuropsychology of Language*. Hillsdale, NJ: Lawrence Erlbaum.

Schwartz, M.F., Saffran, E.M., Fink, R.B., Myers, J.L. and Martin, N. (1994). Mapping therapy: a treatment programme for agrammatism. *Aphasiology* 8(1), 19–54.

Shattuck-Hufnagel, S. (1979). Speech errors as evidence of a serial ordering mechanism in speech production. In: W.E. Cooper and E.C.T. Walker (Eds.), *Sentence Processing: Psycholinguistic Studies Presented to Merrill Garrett*. Hillsdale, NJ: Lawrence Erlbaum.

Sherman, J.C. and Schweichickert, J. (1989). Syntactic and semantic contributions to sentence comprehension in agrammatism. *Brain and Language* 37, 419–439.

Shewan, C.M. and Bandur, D.L. (1986). *Treatment of Aphasia: Language-oriented Approach*. London: Taylor & Francis.

Square-Storer, P. (Ed.) (1989). *Acquired Apraxia of Speech in Adults*. London: Taylor & Francis.

Tissot, R.J., Mounin, G. and Lehrmitte, F. (1973). *L'agrammatisme*. Brussels: Dessart.

Wallesch, C.-W. (1990). Repetitive verbal behaviour: functional and neurological considerations. *Aphasiology* 4(2), 133–154.

Wertz, R.T., La Pointe, L.L. and Rosenbek, J.C. (1984). *Apraxia of Speech in Adults*. London: Grune & Stratton.

Chapter 12
Dysfluency and Child Language

FLORENCE L. MYERS

Introduction

The need to take a more broadly based approach to the treatment of certain communication disorders has become salient in recent years. The development of any single aspect of communication does not progress in a vacuum. The pre-eminent variables which feed into the communication system include, minimally, the simultaneous development of the child's speech production, psycholinguistic, cognitive/perceptual and psychosocial skills. Therefore, what may at first glance appear to be an unusual inclusion of a chapter on childhood dysfluency in a text on *Linguistics in Clinical Practice* is not so. A key idea to be developed here is that children during those early formative years need to experience concurrent advances in both the fluency and the linguistic arenas, in the context of simultaneous development in the physiological and psychosocial domains.

Normal development occurs when there is increasing synergy among the various domains as a function of growth and nurture. One perspective on impaired or delayed development is that such delays or disorders occur when there is dyssynergy between two or more domains, or when there is deviant or delayed development within a given domain. It will be seen later in this chapter that there can be an interrelationship between fluency and language and that, in clinical fact, a child can be highly vulnerable to fluency disruptions as a function of attempts at advancing his or her language skills. This chapter has three primary objectives: (1) to summarise briefly our knowledge of the relation between developmental psycholinguistics and dysfluency; (2) to discuss selected theoretical issues and their clinical implications for the treatment of the dysfluent child and the language-delayed child with concomitant fluency disruptions; and (3) to outline principles of diagnosis and treatment. Given the space limitations, the specifics of each of these three sections are selective rather than exhaustive.

Relation between Psycholinguistics and Dysfluency

Language and Fluency

Research has revealed some trends in the relation between developmental psycholinguistics and dysfluency. Over 30 years ago, Andrews and Harris (1964) conducted a large-scale study of children from Newcastle upon Tyne. Although this study had a more general aim of tracing the onset and development of stuttering, it was found that the children who stuttered showed greater delay in speech and language development than the non-stuttering children in the study. Blood and Seider (1981) conducted a survey of 1000 school-aged children who stuttered in the United States: clinicians responding to the questionnaire indicated that 10% of their stuttering children experienced difficulties with language and 11% had articulation problems. St Louis and Hinzman (1988) studied school-aged children with stutters who had varying degrees of deviations in overall communicative competence (i.e. articulation, voice and language). Results indicated that the group of stutterers with more severe overall deviations were more likely to be males and were more likely to have co-occurring speech and language problems than the group with less severe stuttering. Co-occurrence of phonological problems with stuttering was also found by Louko, Edwards and Conture (1990). Using language-sampling techniques, Silverman and Williams (1967) found that stuttering children performed slightly less well in the measures of structural complexity of utterances, mean length of response, and the mean length of the five longest utterances.

Insight into the relation between language and fluency can also be gained by observing the distribution of fluency breakdowns in a child's utterances. For the most part, loci of stuttering seem to cluster at the beginning of utterances (Bloodstein, 1974; Bloodstein and Grossman, 1981; Wall, Starkweather, and Cairns, 1981). More recently, Gaines, Runyan and Meyers (1991) found that incidence of dysfluency exhibited by young stutterers at the beginning of utterances was affected by variations in sentence length during conversational speech. Various interpretations for these findings are plausible, centring on events postulated to occur at clause/phrase boundaries. Events at such junctures include programming of pragmatics, planning of the syntactic and semantic underpinnings of upcoming utterances, and coordination of the speech production system with the rest of the communication system. The common denominator for each of these possible interpretations is the construct of uncertainty and the child's attempt to put into order this state of relative psycholinguistic, psychosocial, and physiological uncertainty.

The conjoining of fluency and language has been exemplified in yet another way. Colburn (1979) observed that preschoolers tend to show a greater degree of non-fluency on syntactic-semantic structures (for example, the *form-content* or *syntactic-semantic* category of locative action in 'I put polo shirt on there') during the time that these structures *were learned and used regularly*, compared with cases in which structures were completely novel to the children, reflecting a so-called *practice effect*. Colburn had originally expected that a rise in non-fluency would be associated with completely novel utterances. The determinants of this co-variation between non-fluency and those syntactic-semantic structures that have not yet been firmly established is yet to be fathomed, but once again we can speculate on the relative contribution of psychosocial, linguistic or physiological variables which influence the non-fluencies exhibited. Further insight into the relation between language and fluency can be gained by observing the non-fluencies of the speech- and language-delayed child. Clinicians and researchers have often observed a rise in dysfluencies in children receiving articulation or language therapy (e.g. Hall, 1977). Colburn (1979) reported that a rise in non-fluencies can be observed in normally developing children during mastery of specific linguistic structures. It is not surprising, therefore, to observe that children experiencing difficulties with articulation and language might also have difficulties in maintaining fluent speech during the acquisition of longer and more complex language structures (Meyers, Ghatak and Woodford, 1989), or even during the acquisition of more intricate coarticulatory sequences. The psycholinguistic, psychosocial, and physiological components of the child's behaviour are all part of one system (Myers and Wall, 1982; Wall and Myers, 1995); resources taken from one part of that system may influence another part of the system. Merits-Patterson and Reed (1981), for example, compared the dysfluency rate during spontaneous speech in three groups of non-stuttering children 4–6 years of age: (a) nine children with language delay receiving language therapy; (b) nine children developing language within normal limits; and (c) nine children with language delay but not receiving therapy. One significant finding is that those language-delayed children receiving therapy exhibited more part-word and whole-word repetitions than the other two groups. This finding might be due to heightened communication pressure accompanying therapy, because the goal of therapy was to increase MLU and syntactic skills.

Pragmatics and Fluency

Parents and clinicians alike have long been intuitively in tune with at least a generic sense of the psychosocial or pragmatic aspects of communication. Davis (1939; 1940a; 1940b) conducted some of the earliest works on the relation between non-fluency and 'certain measures of language maturity and situational factors' through observations of 62 preschoolers during two half-hour sessions of free play. Non-fluencies were noticed most: (a) when the environment contained disruptive and stressful elements; (b) when the child attempted to make demands on others; and (c) when the perceived authority figure made demands on the child.

A major difference between what was available to speech-language clinicians at the time that Davis wrote in the late 1930s and now, is the accessibility of theory (e.g., Halliday, 1975; Bates, 1976) and taxonomies of pragmatics as applied to research and therapy protocols. Pollack, Lubinski and Weitzner-Lin (1986), for example, examined the conversational breakdowns, repairs and resolution strategies used by a mild-to-moderately dysfluent 3-year-old and her mother, during such mother-prepared activities as reading an alphabet book and tracing numerals. A major locus of dysfluency occurred when the child attempted to take control of the discourse situation: by elaborating on a comment, by being more divergent in conversation, by possibly assuming her own agenda rather than following her mother's agenda.

Metacommunicative Awareness and Fluency

Finally, we tap another aspect of the relation between language and fluency by speculating on the influence of metacommunication skills (see Chapter 2, this volume) and degree of fluency. Cognisance of one's speech and language skills or lack thereof can have great impact on one's performance. Wide individual variations exist among children in terms of their awareness of the degree of success with which they convey their intents – ranging from no sensibility at all, to being keenly and painfully sensitive and vulnerable to interpersonal communication breakdowns. Given the importance of feedback in communication, it is entirely likely that the child who is highly sensitive will present a different set of challenges to the clinician from the child who is not as sensitive. The choice of direct or indirect therapy is determined partly by this variable, among others (e.g. degree of physiological involvement in the blocks). If children are aware of their difficulty in outputting a message in a fluent manner, it would seem prudent for the clinician to acknowledge this difficulty in the process of helping them to speak more fluently: either through techniques to enhance fluency (e.g. speaking at slow-normal rate, using shorter and less propositional utterances) or techniques which actually modify their blocks, such as easy onset and loose articulatory contacts.

Selected Issues and Their Clinical Implications

The above discussion summarises some research findings which seem to indicate links between linguistic demands on children and dysfluent behaviours. This section will discuss selected theoretical issues and attempt to draw clinical implications from these issues.

Language/Speech Processing and Fluency

The first issue to be addressed is drawn from a notion that has been coined as a *functionalist model* (Bates and MacWhinney, 1979) or a *limited capacity processor* model (Shatz, 1978; Starkweather, 1987). A basic thesis is that a child – any child, whether normally developing or not – is continually confronted during the communication process with the task of having to encode a highly complex communicative act via the relatively linear modality of speech. The complexity of the communicative act derives from the ongoing need to formulate and integrate the phonological, syntactic, semantic and pragmatic aspects of a given utterance. Furthermore, it can be agreed that not only is the speech modality linear (in the sense that phonemes must be linearly sequenced) but it is also fast, transient, and involves highly complex and overlapping motoric gestures.

Shatz (1978) suggests that we view children as 'limited-capacity processors'. That is, regardless of the degree of linguistic complexity of an utterance, the processing capacities endowed to a child are more or less constant and finite for any given period in time. For example, the child who is at the two-word stage of language development is, by definition, endowed with the capacity to process such semantic notions as *attribution* and *existence*, to conjoin these semantic notions by the most rudimentary of syntactic forms, to convey these semantic/syntactic notions in the context of various egocentric illocutionary intents; and may use reductionary phonological processes such as Final Consonant Deletion and Cluster Reduction. This might be exemplified by the utterance [maI ba] for 'my block' in a situation where the child is trying to convey to his playmates that the block he is holding is his. The point is that a child may experience some momentary breakdown in one part of the system (e.g. syntax) when demands placed on another part of the system (e.g. semantics or pragmatics) exceed the overall capacity (Andrews, Craig, Feyer, Hoddinott, Howie and Neilson, 1983; DeJoy and Gregory, 1985; Starkweather, 1987). These breakdowns may manifest themselves as occasional disruption in fluency, so that the child utters [mm-mm-mmmaI ba] instead of [maI blak] to indicate that 'This is my block' (and don't you take it away from me!). Clinical techniques to gain an optimum blend between the obligations imposed on a child attempting to encode an utterance and his or her capacity will be developed in the following sections, and the theoretical underpinnings of this principle will be discussed again at the close of the chapter.

We have already alluded to a second issue when treating the dysfluent child from a language perspective; that is, the interaction between motoric complexity and linguistic complexity. As linguistic complexity increases, it is often the case that the length of that utterance also increases. Further, as Malecot, Johnston and Kizziar (1972) have shown, at least for adults, utterance length is positively correlated with rate. That is, we speak faster in longer utterances. Rate of speech can have a direct influence on the fluency of speech output. If we consider the child as a system with a finite limited capacity, then we must be mindful of the potency of linguistic and motor interaction in the child's developing communicative system.

Communicative Loading and Fluency

Over the years, as paradigms in the field of linguistics and psycholinguistics have shifted (basically from a very syntactically orientated approach to a more semantic and pragmatic approach), we have come to use the terms *communicative* and *linguistic* with subtle but significantly different connotations. 'Communicative' implies the composite underpinnings of a message, but with particular focus on the pragmatic, intentional, interactional (hence 'communicative') aspects of the message. 'Linguistic' as used in this context has come to imply the more strictly syntactic and formal aspects of language.

The *communicative load* of a message can affect not only the length and syntactic complexity, or the semantic colouration of an utterance, but also the degree of fluency in the speech output of that utterance. At the same time, one should be mindful that increased communicative loading is not always encoded with increased length and complexity of utterances. The utterance which has high 'communicative loading', such as one which is motivated by a great degree of anger, or an attempt to exert one's will upon one's partner, can be conveyed by either a long and complex utterance or a very short utterance (for example, 'Would you mind giving others some consideration and vacate the premises while we deliberate on this issue!' versus 'Leave the room NOW!'). The term 'communicative loading' as used in the previous sentence is reminiscent of the notion of the 'propositionality of an utterance'. Eisenson (1975) defines *propositionality* as a unit of 'intellectually meaningful linguistic content'. Eisenson and Horowitz (1945) and Eisenson (1975) were among the first to use the term 'propositionality' as it relates to stuttering. Eisenson and Wells (1942) also were among the first to observe systematically that stuttering increased when the degree of *communicative responsibility* increased. For example, greater stuttering occurred during solo reading compared with choral reading. Even though the terms 'communicative responsibility' and 'propositionality' were applied to stuttering 50 years ago, when few writers thought of dysfluency in a linguistic context, they continue to hold a high degree of validity as we approach the 21st century. A possible interpretation of 'propositionality' in the late 1990s might be in terms of the pragmatic/semantic complexity and communicative loading of a message. The greater the communicative loading, the greater the possibility of utterance-specific dysfluency. It was this line of thinking which led to the development of the Stocker Probe Technique (Stocker, 1980). A basic principle used in the Probe Technique is the deliberate arrangement of clinician input so as to elicit utterances from the child which are linguistically and communicatively within the child's capabilities. For example, asking a child to identify the colour of a block is less likely to incur a dysfluent response than asking the child why the red block was chosen instead of the blue block. Thus far, we have focused on a synthesis of research findings concerning the relationships between psycholinguistics and dysfluency, and have discussed the clinical relevance of several theoretical issues and constructs. What follows are some principles to consider in diagnosis and therapy, in light of the above research findings.

Principles of Diagnosis and Treatment

Diagnostic Considerations

If we were to dissociate the influence of language from fluency for the moment, and simply consider the fluency behaviour itself, there is some consensus as to which dysfluent behaviours might be considered basic to stuttering, and those which might be considered more accessory. Various taxonomies have appeared in the literature attempting to point to those 'core' behaviours considered essential to stuttering. Bloodstein (1987), Van Riper (1982) and Wall and Myers (1995), for example, consider the behaviours of repetitions, prolongations and tense pauses as core or essential to stuttering. Symptomatology interpreted as a stutterer's reactions to these core behaviours, such as vowel glides or facial tension, exemplify accessory or accompanying behaviours.

Walle (1975) considers the following 'danger sign' behaviours as indicative of possible stuttering, ranging from those of most to those of relatively less concern: avoidance, moment of fear, struggle and tension, pitch rise, tremor, prolongations, schwa vowel, and multiple repetitions. A great deal has been written about considerations of severity of dysfluencies in the diagnosis of stuttering. We should be mindful that severity is governed by both the qualitative as well as the quantitative aspects of dysfluent behaviour. Tense pauses, for example, are often considered qualitatively more serious than word repetitions. At the same time, however, a word which is repeated four times in succession is considered more serious than that same word repeated only once, even though the overt difference between the two sets of repetitions is only a quantitative difference. Given that this chapter is concerned with the psycholinguistic aspects of dysfluency, let us now focus specifically on the relative contributions of syntactic, semantic and pragmatic variables to the assessment of childhood dysfluency.

From time to time, the literature has made reference to the young dysfluent child with articulatory/phonological and language problems. Van Riper, for example, has given us clinical documentation of the so-called 'Track II child', the dysfluent child with concomitant articulatory and language difficulties. This is the child who may show delayed language, who seems to be searching for words, who seems to have 'more back-ups, more retreats, more changes in direction' during utterances. Myers (1992) and St Louis (1992) attempt to capture the essence of a fluency disorder with concomitant speech/language difficulties called cluttering. Cluttering may exist in isolation or in conjunction with stuttering. Regardless, the speech of clutterers seems to be particularly marked by an excessively fast or irregular rate of speaking resulting in poor speech intelligibility, a poor self-monitoring system, and difficulties with aspects of language. When cluttering is exhibited separately from stuttering, the dysfluencies tend to be fillers, incomplete phrases, revisions and word repetitions. The latter behaviours contrast with dysfluencies of pure stuttering which include sound prolongations and repetitions, and tense pauses.

The following are some questions which need to be addressed during assessment, as they relate to the various facets of language and dysfluency:

1. Is there an overall delay or deficit in language development for this child?
2. Does the child have a specific delay in (a) phonological acquisition; (b) syntactic acquisition; (c) semantic acquisition; or (d) pragmatic acquisition?
3. What are the patterns of fluency breakdowns as a function of the linguistic attributes of the child's discourse? Many children, for example, stutter at the beginning of clauses or phrases. Other children become dysfluent when posing wh- questions. Therefore, one needs to identify the loci distribution of the child's dysfluencies.
4. What is the nature of the influence of semantic complexity on the child's dysfluencies?
5. How does syntactic complexity affect the child's stuttering?
6. What types of pragmatic contexts enhance the child's fluency and what types of contexts inhibit fluency?
7. Does the nature and length of the child's narrative affect his or her dysfluencies? German (1987), for example, found a high degree of dysfluencies reflecting word-finding difficulties (e.g. starters and incomplete phrases) when children with word-finding difficulties tried to produce longer compared with shorter narratives.
8. Does the degree of propositionality and communicative loading affect the child's fluency behaviour?
9. How much metacommunicative awareness does the child seem to carry with him or her during moments of fluency breakdown or language breakdown? How does he or she try to repair this communicative/language/fluency breakdown?

10. What are the effects of the parent's language and communication
     styles on the child's fluency?

A major consequence of the pragmatics revolution in the language
sciences has been the evolution of a more precise, and at the same time
more broadly based, analysis of dyadic interactions. We have become
more sensitised to the nature of input and output between discourse
partners, particularly between child and parent as conversational partners. Although dyadic analysis has been applied to normal-speaking children and language-disordered children with their parents (e.g., Snow,
1977), only very recently has there been systematic analysis of
parent–child interactions with reference to children who stutter.
    It is of great theoretical, historical as well as clinical significance that the
earliest theory about childhood stuttering was grounded in the perspective that the nature of parent–child dynamics can influence the onset and
course of stuttering. According to Wendell Johnson's (1955) diagnosogenic theory, the onset of stuttering occurs when parents react emotion-
ally to a child's dysfluencies, or label the types of non-fluent speech they
hear as 'stuttering' (hence also called the *semantogenic* theory of stuttering). Intrinsic to this theory is an 'interactive' component, because it is the
child's absorption of this affective reaction from the parent that eventually
leads him or her to try not to 'stutter'. However, the very act of trying not
to be dysfluent incurs further aggravation of the initial dysfluencies,
according to the diagnosogenic theory as well as Bloodstein's *anticipatory struggle hypothesis* (1987). The primary focus of Johnson's theory has
been on the nature of parental interactions and reactions as a specific
function of the child's dysfluencies. Owing largely to advances in the
theory and practice of pragmatics, we have come to be more broadly
scoped in our examination of parent–child interactions. That is, we are
not necessarily only examining the 'emotional reactions' of parents during
interaction with their child but also many of the other parameters of
dyadic exchanges (e.g. adjacency effects, speech rate, pause time between
turns, non-verbal behaviours, intents). Moreover, we are now able to be
more finely tuned in the analysis of each of these verbal, paralinguistic and
non-verbal parameters. The prospect of learning more about the nature of
parent–child interactions and their effects on the subsequent course of
development of a child's fluency behaviours is most welcome. Ultimately,
of course, we wish to apply these advances in linguistics and fluency to
clinical practices, as will be detailed in the next sections.

Therapy Considerations

Parent Education and Counselling

With the importance of the nature of parent–child interactions in mind, let us now look at therapeutic considerations as they relate to parental counselling. To analogise an old adage that 'Charity begins at home', let us consider the possibility that 'Fluency behaviours begin at home'. Granted, the latter is too simplistic if interpreted literally, but a great many therapeutic gains can be made if parents are aware of discourse variables at home which can either facilitate/maintain or mitigate the fluency gains made in the clinic.

At this point, I am reminded of a point once made by Beatrice Stocker, developer of the Stocker Probe Technique (Stocker, 1980). During an intermission respite at a New York State Speech–Language–Hearing Association presentation on therapy strategies to improve parent–child pragmatics for young stutterers (Myers, 1987), Stocker remarked that perhaps the term 'parent education' (rather than 'parent counselling') might be a more appropriate term to use when we are referring to many of the parent–clinician conferences that take place. In many cases, these conferences consist of the imparting of information (hence, 'parent education') on how parents can help facilitate fluency in their child and how parents themselves can modulate their own speech and language behaviours in order to provide effective modelling for their child. It might be that to many parents the term 'counselling' connotes the need to resolve deep psychological problems either on the part of their child or perhaps themselves. This is a point well taken, if our intent during any given conference is primarily to impart information to parents on those communicative behaviours which have been found to facilitate fluency in youngsters. What follows, then, is a set of fluency-enhancing principles to be tried out at home.

1. Monitor and modulate parental rate of speech

The rate of parental utterances, much less the pragmatic coloration of parental communication (for example, parents making a request of the child versus rebuking the child), can have a powerful effect on the child's rate and fluency of speech. It would be impractical, of course, to suggest that parents maintain a specific rate for each and every utterance, especially as maintaining a precisely even cadence would sound unnatural. The ideal would be to maintain natural cadence and interaction patterns with a 'fundamental discourse frequency' which can be easily processed by the child and generally thought of as a slow-normal rate. Several rationales underlie the need to modulate a too-fast rate of parental speech. First, as with other aspects of human behaviour, parents' own behaviours represent a potent source of direct and indirect modelling for their offspring. A household in which the significant adults' speech is very rapid, particularly if this is coupled with a household pace which is fast and abrupt, is likely to engender a sense of 'rush' in the child's speech and non-speech activities. Using a single-subject design on the effect of adult rate of speech on 4-year-old non-stuttering children, Newman and Smit (1989) found that the children adjusted on-line to the conversational pace (i.e. pause time between turns) set by adults. At this point, it should be mentioned that the rate at which the parent speaks may be 'fast' only with respect to what the child's own system can handle. If the parents are not aware of the effects of their own speech rate on the child and do not modulate the fast rate, then it may be the case that the child will take it upon him or herself to quicken his or her speech rate. When our speech apparatus is going faster than we can handle, we are usually in a state of heightened muscular tension. Muscular tension reduces coordination, and discoordination reduces fluidity of movement – in this case, the fluidity of speech movement.

2. Use simple, short utterances

Particularly when interacting with preschoolers, it is often wise to talk with them using utterance complexity and length which are appropriate to the child's level of linguistic development. Let us analyse a hypothetical scenario in which a 5-year-old child is being admonished by his parent, and the parent utters in a rushed and angry tone: 'Given the situation this family faces, I'm quite surprised that you did do such a thing and I want an explanation'. Several possible sources of difficulty exist in this utterance. First of all, the rushed and angry tone generates a sense of tension in the child. Second, the utterance carries with it a rather complex syntactic structure, consisting of a complex-compound sentence. Third, some of the words (e.g. 'situation,' 'explanation') may not be in the child's reper-toire. These words may give pause to the child for another reason. Even if the child were familiar with the meaning of these words, lexical items such as 'situation' and 'explanation' are none the less generic enough to make it difficult for the child to decide quickly which particular 'situation' the parent is angry about, and what type of 'explanation' would be stra-tegic or valid enough to pacify the parent's anger.

The sheer length of the utterance can overtax the child's processing constraints. Gordon and Luper (1989), for example, observed an interac-tion between aspects of language and fluency disruptions in children of 3, 5 and 7 years of age. They found that (1) utterances produced fluently were also those produced with syntactic accuracy; (2) later-developing syntactic structures were more likely to contain dysfluencies; and (3) the children showed fewer dysfluencies during a sentence imitation task compared with elicitation and sentence modelling. Finally, in the parent–child scenerio cited above, the overall propositionality or com-municative load placed on the child by the parent's previous turn is taxing: the child needs to muster all of his or her cognitive/perceptual/affective resources to provide a pragmatically convincing solution to this predica-ment. Further research is necessary to examine more closely the specific effects of length and complexity of adult utterances on child language. However, one can speculate that children who are surrounded by adult input which far exceeds their own language abilities might themselves attempt to approximate, or at least come closer to, the adult model. Research has shown that we tend to speak faster when generating a longer utterance compared with a shorter utterance. A possible scenario is that not only is the child trying to model utterances from parents that are too long or too complex, but also that the rate at which the utterance is being attempted is too fast for fluency to occur. For all the above reasons, then, parents should be educated as to the efficacy of modulating length/complexity of utterances (as well as speech rate) appropriate to their child's ability.

3. Heighten sensitivity to pragmatic variables

Yet another principle to convey to parents is the wisdom of modulating pragmatic variables in the home and school. The fact that this is much easier said than done becomes readily apparent if we simply reflect on our own longstanding and at times subliminal pragmatics used with a good friend or with family, and how difficult it is to modify such habits of pragmatics. A great deal of marital or family counselling, for example, consists of talking about and 'undoing' undesirable and longstanding psychosocial patterns among family members. It is no coincidence that pragmatics has been closely linked with 'social knowledge' (Ervin-Tripp and Gordon, 1986) and with affect (Dore, 1986).

The modulation of affect and psychosocial dynamics does not rest exclusively within the realm of the intellect. Not only must we be prepared to impart information (in this sense 'educate') but we must also be prepared to heighten parents' sensitivity (in this sense 'counsel') to the effects of their 'affect' (vis-à-vis their pragmatic behaviours) on their dysfluent child, and vice versa. For example, the pragmatic behaviour of frowning exhibited by a parent following the child's block can reflect the affect of disapproval or alarm to the child. Not all aspects of the pragmatic domain are necessarily intimately tied to the affective domains of discourse; they vary in degree. The pragmatic device of presupposition (see Chapter 9, this volume), for example, necessitates an ability to take the listener's perspective, so that we convey neither too little nor too much information to our listener. This particular pragmatic skill is less 'affective' in nature than, for example, the pragmatics of disapproval or rebuke. In a very real sense, the domain of pragmatics seems almost too broad to capture in one sitting. Nearly all that we do verbally and non-verbally, indeed even what we choose not to exhibit, is rooted in pragmatics. Parents may exhibit subtle, and at times not so subtle, non-verbal behaviours during the child's dysfluencies, including stiffening of bodily movements, momentary arrest of breathing, turning away, or averting gaze (Starkweather, Gottwald and Halfond, 1990). The bottom-line thesis during these parent education/counselling sessions should be to heighten the parents' sensitivity to those pragmatic variables which are disruptive or stressful to the child, or which are conducive to conversational and fluency breakdowns for either the child or the parents. Facilitation of pragmatic behaviours which are conducive to fluency might then follow the heightening of sensitivity. One way to gain a grasp of the plethora of pragmatic behaviours available to us is to organise them on the basis of Grice's (1975) Conversational Postulates. These postulates essentially stress that during conversation we should remain truthful, relevant, clear or perspicuous (i.e. easy to understand), sincere, and give neither too much nor too little information. Violation of any one of these postulates can result in momentary conversational breakdown and interpersonal stress. The parent whose conversational style is pervasively not easy to understand (due, for example, to use of overly complex syntax/semantics) or who shows a lack of interest and sincerity (e.g. abrupt changes from child's chosen topic of conversation), or who provides too much information at a time to the child, is likely to incur a heavy conversational toll. Coping with this load even as the child is trying to cope with his or her own developing speech and language system may result in fluency breakdowns. Typically we speak in order to exchange or share information and feelings. However, it is often the case that children are asked to speak for 'display' of their knowledge or skill. The pragmatic purpose of 'display' in itself can incur stress, because the child is essentially asked to 'perform' in front of an important audience such as grandparents or adult family friends. The types of interactive styles which parents might be encouraged to strengthen instead include the following:

(a) Be a patient and attentive listener.
(b) Allow children the time they need to express their ideas and feelings.
(c) Speak in a slow-normal rate, using appropriate and frequent pauses between thought or language units.
(d) Do not continuously interrogate the child.
(e) Talk about topics which are commensurate with the child's cognitive level (e.g. talk more about the here and now with very young children).
(f) Use language structures and vocabulary words which are commensurate with the child's linguistic capacity.
(g) Avoid a preponderance of 'display' talk.
(h) Pay particular heed to the above strategies if the child is observed to be tired, anxious, overly excited.

Therapy Strategies

Although the previous section relates to principles of parent education and counselling, the above principles can also be applied to the clinician's own communication style during therapy. The above are aspects of the interactions which 'impinge' upon the child. What follows are some points which need to be considered when attempting to modulate the child's own utterances in order to enhance fluency. As has already been mentioned, the kinds of communication behaviours which adults exhibit have a direct influence on those of the child. It is not surprising, therefore, that the following principles, applied to the output of the child, parallel (and, in fact, interact with) those which were discussed in terms of parental input to the child.

1. Encourage the child to use short, simple utterances

A very important principle of therapy is to create a discourse environment in which the length of the child's utterances is appropriate to his or her language skills. This notion of demands and capacity has become very useful in recent years, as applied to a child's language (Slobin, 1977) and fluency (Andrews, Craig, Feyer, Hoddinott, Howie and Neilson, 1983; DeJoy and Gregory, 1985; Starkweather, 1987). Increased length can lead to increased rate of speech as well as the possibility of increased motor complexity. The chapters on language assessment have discussed length of utterance (MLU) for children at various phases of language development. Although it is not always the case, increased utterance length does often co-occur with more syntactically/semantically complex utterances.

2. Gradually extend and vary the range of structures included in therapy

This leads us to the next principle, that of the need to vary the degree of syntactic/semantic complexity of the child's utterances. A good way to attempt to control length and complexity of utterance is to put careful thought into the clinical and linguistic milieu of the therapy session. Structure the therapy session to ensure that the materials and activities are not so open-ended that the length and complexity of utterances are completely unreined. If necessary, the clinician might consider using elicited imitation over modelling of extemporaneous utterances as a means to minimise dysfluencies. Gordon (1991), for example, found that both young stuttering children (ages 3–7 years) and non-stuttering children showed more dysfluencies when asked to model sentences of varying syntactic structures (i.e. encoding one's own utterances following a model) than when asked simply to imitate an adult's sentences.

3. Use therapy activities which create ambience of calmness

Level of excitement of the speech activity should also be monitored, and tempered if necessary. It is often the case that heightened emotions compound the task of formulating and executing speech and language. It is also often the case that topics which have a high degree of excitability also are topics which necessitate relatively more convoluted narratives requiring more complex thought, syntax/semantics, as well as perhaps more stressful pragmatics.

4. As the child develops fluency, gradually increase communicative loading of utterances

This brings us to the principle of developing a hierarchy of pragmatic contexts to desensitise the child to fluency breakdowns. Two key words underlie this principle, the words 'hierarchy' and 'desensitise'. As with the learning of any life skill, including communicative fluency, mastery and learning are achieved through a series of stages rather than an all-or-none proposition. A child first learns bicycle riding on very short stretches of a flat surface. At first there are bound to be false starts and various kinds of disruptions to a 'fluent' ride. As the child gains more confidence with motor skills, bicycle riding succeeds with less effort and, indeed, becomes a seemingly semi-automatic motoric act. The child remains proficient in increasingly complex riding contexts – whether he or she is talking to another child who is riding along, or carrying a little bundle of groceries with one arm as the other steers the handlebar, or careering down a slope at a precarious rate. This bicycle-riding analogy was chosen to draw parallels between the motor act of biking and that of speaking, as both sets of skills can be influenced by complexity, rate and interference from distractions if the child is 'overloaded'.

To apply this analogy to stuttering therapy, the clinician must first observe and isolate pragmatic variables which appear to induce fluency breakdowns. These might include the following examples: situations in which the child has to talk fast in order to get in a turn, if the topic of conversation is highly exciting, if the discourse partner (particularly if it is an important adult, such as a parent) is likely to become pragmatically demanding, if the adult presupposes too much on the part of the child in terms of the latter's cognitive/perceptual or language abilities. After isolating those pragmatic variables which appear to be disruptive to fluency, they are then arranged in a hierarchical fashion from least to most pragmatically taxing. Using the principles of desensitisation therapy as discussed by Van Riper, for example, one then systematically helps the child to maintain fluency in increasingly more challenging situations.

5. Attend to the physiological aspects of fluency in speech

Another principle of therapy which may be necessary is to monitor and modulate the child's physiological system in tandem with his or her linguistic system. Recall the notions subsumed under the functionalist model by Bates and MacWhinney (1979), that the child has to encode a very complex non-linear message using the very linear and rapid single-channel medium of speech. In the end, speech is reduced to a physiological phenomenon. This motor act, in large part because it is so intricately sequenced and so fleeting, does not have a great deal of tolerance for error. Moreover, included in a fluent motor act is the coordination of respiration and phonation with the coarticulatory gestures. If we typically speak at our upper limits to begin with, either as children or as adults, then the tolerance for error is further reduced.

Some therapy strategies which may facilitate greater coordination between the physiological and the linguistic systems include: (1) adopting a somewhat slower speech rate; (2) reducing the length of the linguistic unit to afford a better match between the linguistic unit and the breath unit; (3) using 'easier' or 'softer' speech to alleviate tension and discoordination of the speech musculature; and (4) modulating the types of utterances (e.g. responding to questions vs. making assertions) expected from the dysfluent child (see Weiss and Zebrowski, 1992). In the end, the ideal communication act is one in which there is a high degree of synergy between the linguistic/pragmatic system and the physiological or speech production system (Myers, 1992).

Concluding Remarks

We have become accustomed to looking at the various aspects of speech production (i.e. respiration, phonation, articulation, resonation) from a systems approach. The prevailing theme of a systems approach is that the various subcomponents of that system should work together as a synergistic whole. Synergism implies cohesiveness and synchrony. Phonatory gestures, for example, should be coordinated with the articulatory gestures. Likewise, as part of the overall communication system, the various subcomponents of the language system should be cohesive with the speech production system. Especially with a developing system such as that of a child, delay or deficits in one part of the system may influence another aspect of that system.

The varying degrees of synergism should be considered within the broader perspective of the capacity versus demands placed on that system. Slobin (1977), Shatz (1978) and Starkweather (1987) discuss the notion of constraints of a child's system, constraints which affect the capacities of that system. We need to bear in mind that this capacity versus demands ratio is not a constant, but fluctuates from moment to moment. The fluctuations come about from changes stemming from a number of sources. At any given moment, a rather unique set of linguistic, communicative, psychosocial and physiological variables impinge upon the child. The demands requisite for talking with one's mother about a squabble with another child down the street, just as she is in the middle of redecorating her study or rewiring the word processor, are quite different from the demands of calling the family dog for its daily meal.

The discourse context might be considered to be the macrostructure of this talking task, especially if one looks at communication from a top-down model. The context sets the intents, the motives and the motif, the affect and the effects. Once the child has assessed the psychosocial dynamics of the situation, she or he needs to find an appropriate syntactic/semantic means to encode the intent. It is in this sense that Bates (1976) postulates that pragmatics is the deep structure of language – our pragmatic intents dictate the words we choose and the syntax we use to encode our meaning; in turn, the syntax/semantics chosen may dictate the degree of fluency achieved. Moreover, children need to coordinate their speech production system, largely a physiologically based enterprise, such that the intent, the meaning, the syntax and the articulatory gestures of that utterance are so well-tuned that the syllables, the sounds, the voice onset times, and the breath stream all come out smoothly, naturally and seemingly effortlessly. Given that a kindergartener speaks slightly above two syllables per second (Starkweather, 1980), all of the above 'calculations' must take place at an awesome pace. Even if the speech production skills become somewhat semi-automatic over time, the cognitive/perceptual processes requisite for discourse are, by definition, not so automatic. Moreover, even as we are in the act of encoding our own thoughts, we are engaged in a continuous process of decoding the verbal, paralinguistic and non-verbal feedback from our partner. The following are some considerations in the most demanding of discourse scenarios: the child is functioning at his or her upper limits both for the speech and for the language systems; society is making ever-increasing demands on the child with rising expectations and standards; the child perceives this escalation of demands; and, at the same time, is increasingly aware of a need for parental and peer love and approval. When examining the speech- and language-developing child in this light, one almost wonders why more dysfluencies are not observed in normally developing youngsters. At-risk children carry several additional burdens. They may have the sense that speaking is not always an easy task and that others may also be reacting to the speaking difficulties. At-risk children may also be experiencing other speech and language problems, and possibly even some learning difficulties. Further, such children may experience greater variability for any given domain of endeavour, reflecting a general state of instability. With all this in mind, it would not be unreasonable to surmise that the dysfluent child's communicative system is in a continual state of tension and flux – a give-and-take between one part of the system and another, between the constraints placed on the system and its ability to 'give'. The dysfluent child is in a state of greater 'torque' (Myers, 1987), capable of releasing energy but not always assured if his or her ability can match the task in an adequate and evenly modulated way. The child might experience a momentary breakdown in one part of the system (for example, in fluency) as a function of extra loading imposed on another part of the system (such as the linguistic system).

This chapter started with the proposition of treating the dysfluent child from a psycholinguistic perspective within an overall more broadly based context. I have attempted to summarise some pertinent research on childhood language and fluency; discuss some issues pertinent to this relationship; and apply the research and theory to therapy. This chapter concludes by reiterating the need to look at a child who is at risk for dysfluency in the larger scope of a 'system', with its unique and fluctuating set of skills and the equally unique and ever-changing set of constraints imposed on this system. Neither diagnosis nor therapy can proceed without a close examination of the interaction between the psycholinguistic, psychosocial and physiological variables that go into the make-up of this system.

References

Andrews, G., Craig, A., Feyer, A., Hoddinott, S., Howie, P. and Neilson, M. (1983). Stuttering: a review of research findings and theories circa 1982. *Journal of Speech and Hearing Disorders* 48, 226–246.

Andrews, G. and Harris, M. (1964). The syndrome of stuttering. *Clinics in Developmental Medicine*, 17. London: Spastics Society Medical Education and Information Unit, in association with William Heinemann Medical Books.

Bates, E. (1976). *Language and context*. New York: Academic Press.

Bates, E. and MacWhinney, B. (1979). A functionalist approach to the acquisition of grammar. In: E. Ochs and B. Schieffelin (Eds.), *Developmental Pragmatics*. New York: Academic Press.

Blood, G. and Seider, R. (1981). The concomitant problems of young stutterers. *Journal of Speech and Hearing Disorders* 46, 31–33.

Bloodstein, O. (1974). The rules of early stuttering. *Journal of Speech and Hearing Disorders* 39, 379–394.

Bloodstein, O. (1987). *A Handbook on Stuttering*. Chicago, IL: National Easter Seal Society for Crippled Children and Adults.

Bloodstein, O. and Grossman, M. (1981). Early stutterings: some aspects of their form and distribution. *Journal of Speech and Hearing Disorders* 24, 298–302.

Colburn, N. (1979). Disfluency behaviour and emerging linguistic structures in preschool children. Doctoral dissertation, Columbia University, New York.

Davis, D. (1939). The relation of repetitions in the speech of young children to certain measures of language maturity and situational factors: Part I. *Journal of Speech Disorders* 4, 303–318.

Davis, D. (1940a). The relation of repetitions in the speech of young children to certain measures of language maturity and situational factors: Part II. *Journal of Speech Disorders* 5, 235–241.

Davis, D. (1940b). The relation of repetitions in the speech of young children to certain measures of language maturity and situational factors: Part III. *Journal of Speech Disorders* 5, 242–246.

Dejoy, D. and Gregory, H. (1985). The relationship between age and frequency of disfluency in preschool children. Journal of Fluency Disorders 10, 107–122.

Dore, J. (1986). The development of conversational competence. In: R.L. Schiefelbusch (Ed.), *Language Competence: Assessment and Intervention*. San Diego, CA: College Hill Press.

Eisenson, J. (1975). Stuttering as perseverative behavior. In: J. Eisenson (Ed.), *Stuttering: A Second Symposium*. New York: Harper & Row.

Eisenson, J. and Horowitz, E. (1945). The influence of propositionality on stuttering. *Journal of Speech Disorders* 10, 193–197.

Eisenson, J. and Wells, C. (1942). A study of the influence of communicative responsibility in choral speech situation for stutterers. *Journal of Speech Disorders* 7, 259–262.

Ervin-Tripp, S. and Gordon, D. (1986). The development of requests. In: R. Schiefelbusch, (Ed.), *Language Competence: Assessment and Intervention*. San Diego: College Hill Press.

Gaines, N., Runyan, C. and Meyers, S. (1991). A comparison of young stutterers' fluent versus stuttered utterances in measures of length and complexity. *Journal of Speech and Hearing Research* 34, 37–42.

German, D. (1987). Spontaneous language profiles of children with wordfinding difficulties. *Language–Speech–Hearing Services in Schools* 18, 217–230.

Gordon, P.A. (1991). Language task effects: a comparison of stuttering and nonstuttering children. *Journal of Fluency Disorders* 16, 275–287.

Gordon, P.A. and Luper, H. (1989). Speech disfluencies in nonstutterers: syntactic complexity and production task effects. *Journal of Fluency Disorders* 14, 429–445.

Grice, P. (1975). Logic and conversation. In: P. Cole and J. L. Morgan (Eds.), *Syntax and Semantics*, Vol. 3: *Speech Acts*. New York: Academic Press.

Hall, P. (1977). The occurrence of disfluency in language-disorderd school-age children. *Journal of Speech and Hearing Disorders* 42, 364–369.

Halliday, M.A.K. (1975). Learning how to mean. In: E. Lenneberg and E. Lenneberg (Eds.), *Foundations of Language Development*, Vol. 1, pp. 17–32. New York: Academic Press.

Johnson, W. (1955). A study of the onset and development of stuttering. In: W. Johnson and R. Leutenegger (Eds.), *Stuttering in Children and Adults*, pp. 37–73. Minneapolis: University of Minnesota Press.

Louko, L., Edwards, M. L. and Conture, E. (1990). Phonological characteristics of young stutterers and their normally fluent peers: preliminary observations. *Journal of Fluency Disorders* 15, 191–210.

Malecot, A., Johnston, R. and Kizziar, P. (1972). Syllabic rate and utterance length in French. *Phonetica* 26, 235–251.

Merits-Patterson, R. and Reed, C. (1981). Disfluencies in the speech of language-delayed children. *Journal of Speech and Hearing Research* 24, 55–58.

Myers, F.L. (1987). Focus on stuttering in young children. Paper presented at the New York Speech–Language–Hearing Association Convention, Lake Kiamesha, New York.

Myers, F.L. (1992). Cluttering: A synergistic framework. In: F.L. Myers and K. St Louis, (Eds.), *Cluttering: A Clinical Perspective*. Kibworth, UK: Far Communications.

Myers, F . and Wall, M. (1982). Toward an integrated approach to early childhood stuttering. *Journal of Fluency Disorders* 7, 47–54.

Myers, F. and Wall, M. (1983). Language-based therapy for young child stutterers: rationale and techniques. Paper presented at the American Speech–Language–Hearing Association Convention, Cincinnati, Ohio.

Meyers, S., Ghatak, L. and Woodford, L. (1989). Case descriptions of nonfluency and loci: Initial and followup conversations with three preschool children. *Journal of Fluency Disorders* 14, 383–397.

Newman, L. and Smit, A. (1989). Some effects of variations in response time latency on speech rate, interruptions, and fluency in children's speech. *Journal of Speech and Hearing Research* 32, 635–644.

Pollack, J., Lubinski, R. and Weitzner-Lin, B. (1986). A pragmatic study of child dysfluency. Journal of Fluency Disorders 11, 231–239.

Shatz, M. (1978). The relationship between cognitive processes and the development of communication skills. In: B. Keasey (Ed.), *Nebraska Symposium on Motivation, 1977*. Lincoln, Nebraska: University of Nebraska Press.

Silverman, E.-M. and Williams, D. (1967). A comparison of stuttering and nonstuttering children in terms of five measures of oral language development. *Journal of Communication Disorders* 1, 305–309.

Slobin, D. (1977). Language change in childhood and in history. In: J. MacNamara (Ed.), *Language Learning and Thought*. New York: Academic Press.

Snow, C. (1977). Mother's speech research: from input to interaction. In: C. Ferguson and C. Snow (Eds.), *Talking to Children*. Cambridge: Cambridge University Press.

St Louis, K.O. (1992). On defining cluttering. In: F.L. Myers and K.O. St Louis (Eds.), *Cluttering: A Clinical Perspective*. Kibworth, UK: Far Communications.

St Louis, K.O. and Hinzman, A. (1988). A descriptive study of speech, language and hearing characteristics of school-aged stutterers. *Journal of Fluency Disorders* 13, 331–355.

Starkweather, C.W. (1980). Speech fluency and its development in normal children. In: N. Lass (Ed.), *Speech and Language: Advances in Basic Research and Practice*, Vol. 4. New York: Academic Press.

Starkweather, C.W. (1987). *Fluency and Stuttering*. Englewood Cliffs, NJ: Prentice Hall.

Starkweather, C.W., Gottwald, S. and Halfond, M. (1990). *Stuttering Prevention: A Clinical Method*. Englewood Cliffs, NJ: Prentice Hall.

Stocker, B. (1980). *Stocker Probe Technique: For Diagnosis and Treatment of Stuttering in Young Children*. Tulsa, OK: Modern Education Corporation.

Van Riper, (1982). *The Nature of Stuttering*. Englewood Cliffs, NJ: Prentice Hall.

Wall, M. and Myers, F.L. (1995). *Clinical Management of Childhood Stuttering*, 2nd edn. Austin, TX: Pro-Ed.

Wall, M., Starkweather, C. and Cairns, H. (1981). Syntactic influences on stuttering in young child stutterers. *Journal of Fluency Disorders* 6, 283–298.

Walle, G. (1975). *The Prevention of Stuttering* (film). Memphis, TN: Speech Foundation of America.

Weiss, A. and Zebrowski, P. (1992). Disfluencies in the conversations of young children who stutter: some answers about questions. *Journal of Speech and Hearing Research* 35, 1230–1238.

Chapter 13
Developmental Language Disorders

CATHERINE ADAMS AND GINA CONTI-RAMSDEN

The order of authors is alphabetical as the work represents the equal contribution of both co-authors.

Introduction

The group of children who fall into the category of developmental language disorders forms a vastly heterogeneous population. The unifying theme is that every child in this group demonstrates a linguistic system which, in certain aspects, is different from that of their normally developing language-learning peers (Friel-Patti and Conti-Ramsden, 1984). Clinically, this broad criterion is translated into a definition by exclusion: that is, developmental language disorders are characterised by the late appearance and/or slow development of expression and/or comprehension of spoken language which cannot be explained in terms of mental retardation, hearing loss, or social-emotional difficulties (Leonard, 1979; Stark and Tallal, 1981; Bishop 1992). Historically, various terms have been used to refer to this group of children, including 'delayed language' (Lee, 1966), 'congenital aphasia' (Eisenson, 1972), 'deviant language' (Leonard, 1979), 'language disordered' (Rees, 1973) and 'specific language deficit' (Stark and Tallal, 1981). For the purpose of this chapter, the broad term 'developmental language disorders' will be used and assumed to reflect the fact that a large diversity of individuals belong to this group. Phonological disorders will not be included here as this area is covered by Chapter 14, this volume.

Clinicians working with children with developmental language disorders may well feel overwhelmed by the lack of homogeneity of this group. It is very difficult to draw uniform guidelines for diagnosis and intervention when the variation within the group is so great. Included within this group, for instance, according to our present understanding, are children with obvious deficits in the form of language, but with reasonable comprehension and conversational competence given their restricted output. Also included within this very broad group, however, are very different children with fluent, verbose language, and additional problems of conversational interaction and word meaning (Bishop and Adams, 1989). This diversity within a clinical population presents the language clinician with a remarkable challenge in directing intervention approaches appropriately. To complicate matters further, clinicians are not just being asked to pinpoint the child's language problem but also to explain how this specific difficulty interacts with other aspects of the child, for example, hearing and cognitive skills (Van Kleeck and Richardson, 1988). Thus, the field of developmental language disorders has to borrow from a variety of areas and theories, each providing a particular set of answers on specific aspects of assessment and intervention. Unfortunately, no one theory can successfully address all the critical questions at once. The present chapter aims to provide an eclectic view of developmental language disorders, emphasising individual needs of children.

Planning Assessment and Intervention for the Individual Child

The Child as an Individual

Peter is a 4-year-old boy who attends regular speech and language therapy. Peter has an uneventful birth history and developed fairly normally; he sat at 7 months and walked at 18 months. But language was delayed, single words did not appear until after two years of age and he did not put two words together until he was 3 years of age. Peter has normal hearing and performs within the normal range in non-verbal tests of ability and tests of verbal comprehension. Peter is cooperative and uses a lot of gestures to try to get his needs and desires understood.

John is a 4 ½-year-old boy who attends a language unit within an ordinary school. John was born one month prematurely and was a breech birth. He then developed slowly, sitting at 11 months and walking at 24 months. Language was non-existent until he was over 3 years when he developed some single words to refer to familiar objects and events. John performed within the low but normal range of non-verbal abilities and although he suffered recurrent otitis media, had hearing within normal limits when he was not congested. His range of performance in comprehension tests ranged from the 30 months level to age appropriate as John has a particularly good receptive vocabulary which his parents greatly encourage. John is an active, aggressive and difficult child who has frequent temper tantrums.

Sandra is a 4-year-old girl who has just been referred to the speech and language therapy services. Sandra is adopted and thus no birth history was available. Parents report that she appeared to develop physically like all children do. From age 2 ½ to 3 ½ years the most striking characteristic of Sandra's language was her echolalia and inability to combine words into sentences. From age 3 ½ years echolalia decreased but Sandra's utterances are currently mainly jargon with the occasional stereotypic sentence. Symbolic play skills appear poor and she has marked comprehension problems. She fails to respond to anything but simple questions and directives.

The above three children, although all of pre-school age, have different aspects of their communication system failing. Peter is a healthy boy who enjoys interaction and uses gesture to make up for his verbal deficiencies whilst Sandra is a little girl who repeats what other people say and is in her own world (she uses a lot of jargon) without attempting to interact. John, on the other hand, had a difficult start in life and is not a well child. He has had slow motor development, constant ear infections and behavioural problems. His hyperactivity makes it difficult for him to pay attention and concentrate on the objects, events and people around him. The wide-ranging picture presented by the three developmental language-disordered 4-year-olds described above underscores the importance of focusing on the child's individual characteristics and profile as opposed to concentrating on whether or not the child shares certain key features with a particular labelled group of children.

The publication of the Warnock Report (Warnock, 1982) epitomises a new wave of thought in the Special Needs field: labels and group characteristics are not useful in assessment intervention, it is the individual child that we have to concentrate on. Developmental language disorders are no exception to this rule. To say a child has 'comprehension problems' is as sweeping as to say that John and Sandra are similar children; to say a child has expressive problems is as sweeping as to say that Peter and John are similar children. The emphasis suggests that clinicians need to be aware of many variables, such as particular aspects of comprehension, expression and others, which they need to integrate into a cohesive framework and apply this framework in addressing the individual characteristics and needs of each developmental language-disordered child. The onus of our work is now on individual needs and differences and away from group characteristics and similarities. Interestingly it is the addition of linguistic knowledge which has largely supported the language clinician's ability accurately to map out individual abilities in terms of strength and weaknesses of a particular child's language. Thus linguistic theory may yet provide us with an accurate compass to find our way through the minefield of heterogeneity.

The concept of the child as an individual has further implications. In assessment and intervention, there needs to be a constant interaction between looking at the individual as a whole (as development is unified) and looking at specific aspects of the individual's development (be it cognitive, social, language or others). This back-and-forth process is referred to as 'zooming in and zooming out' by Van Kleeck and Richardson (1988). These clinician-researchers use the analogy of camera lenses to illustrate the above point. They conceptualise the process of assessment and intervention as one of viewing the child with successive levels of magnification. The levels are like lenses which allow one to zoom in more and more specifically to the child's weaknesses and strengths and then zoom back out as one considers how the specific identified problems affect each other and the functioning of the whole child. It is to this process that we now turn in more detail.

Looking at the Whole Child

The assessment intervention process begins with the clinician's attempt to obtain an overview of the whole child and the child's environment. This process has the aim of identifying those aspects of the child that require further evaluation. After all, language difficulties may well be the first sign that *anything* is wrong with the child. Thus, clinicians need to investigate the reasons for the language problem, its implications for other areas of the child's functioning and for the child's development as a whole. Four key aspects have been identified by Van Kleeck and Richardson (1988) in this respect: the *physical*, the *cognitive*, the *social* and the *linguistic*. In the physical system, key areas such as hearing, vision, motor development, sensory integration and neurological integration need to be investigated. As for the cognitive system, clinicians should ask: What is the level of functioning of the child? At what level is the child's concept formation? How does the child reason, problem solve and process information? Does the child have a preferred learning style and if so, what is it? What is the child's current level of achievement? In the social system, the clinician needs to explore the child's self-help skills, non-verbal communication, interaction and play. Also within this realm emotional, behavioural and environmental factors ought to be evaluated. The linguistic system will be described in the next section so no details will be given here.

With the exception of the linguistic area, clinicians may need to collaborate with several other professionals to gather information; examine the status of each system; and further evaluate the relationships among them. In many cases it is clinicians who act as coordinators, who gather all the necessary information and who attempt to get the whole picture of the child. It is this important role of the language clinician that needs to be recognised, emphasised and developed, otherwise we may be in the difficult situation where different people have different pieces of the puzzle and each is trying to determine what the picture is all about.

Looking at Aspects of the Child

The previous section sketched the very basic questions concerning three of the major aspects of the individual child's development: the physical, the social and the cognitive. Each of these aspects deserves at least a chapter, but space considerations restrict their evaluation to a bare outline. In this section, it is the linguistic aspect that will be examined in more detail.

To begin with we need to identify the role that linguistics has played in aiding our understanding of developmental language disorders. Linguistics provides the basis of a developmental-descriptive approach to language disorders. In the 1970s, clinicians reacted against the medical and processing models for understanding developmental language disorders as they were dissatisfied with the inability of these models to provide guidelines for therapy. The medical model (Myklebust, 1954; McCormick and Schiefelbusch, 1984) with its emphasis on categorisation and aetiology, and the processing model (Rudel and Denckla, 1974; Cromer, 1978; Johnson, Stark, Melitts and Tallal, 1981) with its emphasis on specific mental processes, both focus on the *causes* of developmental language disorders but do little to point us towards intervention. Stark *et al.* (1988) attempt to extrapolate from the auditory processing deficits model to intervention, but find implications limited to discussion of children with rare deficits (e.g. Landau–Kleffner syndrome). The other legacy of the abandonment of the medical model and adoption of a clinical-linguistic one was the dispensing with the old notion of language disorder as a unitary construct. In contrast, the linguistic-descriptive approach underscores the importance of describing the observable communication skills of the child. It underscores the need to know how the child's language system works and places less emphasis on explanations for the disorders. This approach affords us with a general framework for assessment and intervention.

What is the nature of the data gathered by the linguistic approach? In assessment as well as in intervention there are two types of data available to us: reported data and observation data. Reported data include all information about the language system of the child presented to the clinician by other people. Parents are a well-known example and their contribution is often useful to clinicians (Warner, Byers-Brown and McCartney, 1984) and researchers (Barrett, 1986) alike. Observational data are the major source of information for clinician-researchers interested in developmental language disorders. These data can be divided into three types: standardised tests, informal elicitations and spontaneous language samples (Van Kleeck and Richardson, 1988). Each data type provides us with different information and, thus, each is useful for answering different questions. Descriptions can focus on expressive versus receptive skills and each of these can in turn focus on specific aspects of language, traditionally phonology, syntax, semantics and pragmatics. It is no coincidence that these same areas constitute headings of chapters in Section II of this book. In that section, authors attempt to describe and evaluate some of the multitude of tests available for assessing the specific component of language they are examining (see, for example, Chapter 6 for expressive syntax and Chapter 8 for semantics, this volume), they also discuss the types of informal tasks we can use to elicit information as to the specific language behaviours being considered (see for example Chapter 7 on receptive syntax, this volume), and, finally, they also discuss the numerous analysis procedures for examining spontaneous language samples (see for example Chapter 9, this volume). The reader is referred to Sections I and II of the volume for detailed discussion of each of the components of language.

Developmental language-disordered children can have difficulties with any combination of areas of the linguistic system (phonology, syntax, semantics and pragmatics) and these problems can be manifested in various degrees of severity either expressively and/or receptively. Deficits in a single linguistic level are rare. At a more micro level, there exists the possibility within any one language-impaired child at any one linguistic level of *within-level asynchronies* (Miller, 1991) – the typical gaps and patchy profiles of ability which become evident under linguistic analysis. The task of the clinician-researcher at this level is to obtain a fine-grained picture of each of the components of the child's language system and identify those which require intervention. These identified areas of intervention then need to be reconsidered within the larger view of the system to which they belong (the zooming out process described by Van Kleeck and Richardson, 1988). For example, how does a difficulty in receptive verb vocabulary interact with other aspects of the linguistic system? To mention just a few of the possible considerations: how does this difficulty in receptive verb vocabulary interact with other areas of lexical development, with syntactic clause development, with the way in which the child gets his or her needs and desires known with language? As well as making sound clinical sense, these are very pertinent questions, as recent studies, e.g. Prelock and Panagos (1989), Masterson and Kamhi (1992), provide evidence for the existence and importance of interaction of linguistic levels in developing language. As Van Kleeck and Richardson (1988) put it: 'the anguish that is sometimes experienced at the intrasystem analysis level with trying to neatly segment complex behaviours into component areas is somewhat alleviated at this level where the interaction among areas is explored'. This exploration of the interaction among areas needs to continue within the linguistic system, then across systems (the linguistic, physical, cognitive and social) and finally the child as a whole needs to be considered.

Let us take a specific example to illustrate the zooming in and out approach to assessment and intervention. We start at the micro-analytic level looking at specific aspects of the linguistic system in order to identify particular areas of impairment. We will take the case of Paul who is 4 years of age and is only using single words. The first area of impairment is that of grammar or syntax, that is, Paul is not using word combinations at all, unlike normally developing children. We might wish at this stage to sample Paul's speech in various settings and map out the vocabulary available to him. Therapeutic assessment would also tell us whether Paul is able to access any word combinations given a fairly constrained and repetitive encouragement for these, and this in turn would feed into therapy decision-making. But before we proceed to this stage the question arises as to the aspects of the system such as phonology, semantics and pragmatics. Considering phonology first, what is Paul's phonology like? Is it related to his language production difficulties? Paul has problems with the pronunciation of the fricatives in this system (s, sh, ch). As a matter of fact, Paul has very few words which contain the aforementioned fricatives, thus he does not appear very unintelligible. Ingram (1987) has pointed out that the extent of a child's phonological disorder is the consequence of an inverse relationship between the child's phonological difficulty and the size of his or her vocabulary. Thus, in the case of Paul, he does not appear phonologically disordered because he only has a few words containing fricatives. If, as part of our intervention, we work on his grammar by teaching him new words and word combinations without regard to his particular phonological difficulty with the fricatives, we may be improving his grammar but worsening his phonological difficulty, or alternatively his grammar may not improve because of the fricatives involved in the therapeutic plan. We need to take into consideration the relationship between the different aspects of the linguistic system before we can target our intervention. Paul needs to start putting words together and he has a weakness with fricatives which alerts us to treat words with such sounds carefully in therapy. At first, the clinician may well want to avoid words with fricatives so that Paul can concentrate on the job of developing his grammar by attempting to put two words together. This does not mean we should not work on phonology. What we need to understand is that working on one aspect of the linguistic system may lead to deterioration in others (Crystal, 1987; see also Chapters 1 and 12). In the case of Paul, we know he has an existing problem with the fricative system so why 'overload' him by working on the grammar plus working on the fricatives *at the same time*. Our awareness of the intra-system interactions allows us to see the relationship between the linguistic subsystems and, thus, to come to a more informed therapy plan than we would otherwise. But we also need to consider other possible relationships.

How about syntax and semantics? As it turns out, Paul has a very restricted semantic system in that his vocabulary consists of words from two major lexical categories: foods and toys. He is particularly lacking on action words such as *come, go, put,* and interpersonal-relational words such as *hello, bye, no,* more. This information enables the clinician to understand Paul's grammatical system in relationship to his semantic system. Paul does not have a wide enough semantic basis from which he can encode relationships syntactically. Before Paul can begin to put words together such as 'no doggy', 'more milk', he needs to have the necessary lexical categories at his disposal. It is important that therapeutically the clinician builds Paul's semantic system, so that the grammatical encoding of basic semantic relations can begin to occur.

Finally, at the intra-system level we need to take into consideration the relationship of semantics, syntax and phonology to pragmatics. This latter interaction was, until fairly recently, neglected, but it is now clear that many pragmatic abilities rely on competence at other linguistic levels (Leonard and Fey, 1991). The key issue in pragmatics is that language is used and learned in social interaction. For this reason our therapy programme for Paul needs to be carried out in planned but natural contexts where Paul *needs* to communicate the semantic-syntactic relationships we want him to learn. A more detailed discussion of this interactive approach follows in the pragmatic perspective section.

There is little doubt that the linguistic-developmental approach is an invaluable tool in the assessment and intervention of language disorders. But, like all tools, it has its limitations. The contribution of linguistics in clinical intervention for developmental language disorders is considerable, but now perhaps somewhat taken for granted. Excellent models of the way in which expressive grammar and phonology emerge in the developing child have nurtured a developmental approach to treatment. Where theoretical models are less well defined, or are still in a process of evolution (e.g. semantics, pragmatics), one can witness a corresponding wavering confidence regarding clinical management. There are large gaps in our knowledge of how normal children develop language, especially during the school years, thus leaving us with few data with which to compare older language-disordered children (Prather, 1984; Snyder, 1984). This is especially true of vocabulary and semantics, sometimes described as the 'Cinderella' of language therapies (Haynes, 1992 after Crystal, 1987). Second, when the knowledge is available on normal development, assessment procedures have not always been developed to apply that knowledge to the disordered population (see for an exception Wetherby, 1991). Third, there is little information as to the variation among normal language-learning and language-disordered children in the amount of time it takes for them to learn specific aspects of language, therefore there is not a sense of what is the 'average time to learn this or that'. Fourth, there is a constant danger of simplistic application of developmental linguistic data to language disorders. That is, to assume that language-disordered children go through the same patterns and sequences of language learning as normally developing children is not always warranted (Blank, Gessner and Esposito, 1980; Conti-Ramsden and Gunn, 1986), nor indeed can it be taken for granted that normal children go through stages in the same manner or style. Language-disordered children may well find certain aspects of language to be major hurdles whilst normal language-learning children do not. It must also be attested that there are aspects of developmental language disorders such as word-finding deficits, which do not lend themselves neatly to the linguistic-development approach, and which might find more hope of an explanation in terms of a cognitive neuropsychological model (see Chapters 2, 6, 7, 8 and 11).

Continued research into the nature of within-level asynchronies as pioneered, for example, by Fletcher and colleagues (Fletcher, 1990; King and Fletcher, 1993) and Miller (1991), should provide the language clinicians of the future with more detailed descriptions of the way in which language develops and changes over time in language-impaired children. Recent advances in developmental psycholinguistics may also directly avail the language clinician of support for clinical intervention strategies. Those advances which emphasise *how* children learn language and not so much *what* they learn would be especially applicable to this field. For instance, in *learnability theory* (Pinker, 1989) and its subsequent offshoots the child is seen as a deductive language learner, deriving syntactic and semantic information and rules from the input by so-called 'bootstrapping' processes driven by an innate linguistic capacity. In a paper discussing therapeutic implications of such a theory, Van der Lely (1992) outlines how specific intervention strategies might be designed by manipulating semantic/syntactic features of the *input* to facilitate the derivation of linguistic rules by the language-impaired child.

The Process of Intervention

The clinician new to working with developmental language disorders might be forgiven for wondering what the process of 'language intervention' is. It is a curious fact that the management procedures and contexts for developmental language disorder are not as well documented or even agreed upon as are therapeutic procedures for other conditions. Within the confines of this chapter there is only room to give a brief outline of the current major conceptual themes in language intervention in developmental language disorder, and some indication of how these are currently moulded into an integrated approach to therapy.

For want of a better description one might describe two approaches to intervention as being 'bottom up' or data driven, and 'top down'. The latter focuses mainly on the communicative context of the individual, and as such represents a pragmatic perspective on language intervention.

Bottom-up or Analytical Approaches

The bottom-up approach to language intervention assumes that children with developmental language disorders will progress in language learning if taken through a series of learning goals, starting with small steps at a low level, and then progressing upwards to more advanced structures or meanings, according (usually) to the accepted model of normal development. This approach is the natural complement of linguistic profiling approaches such as those available for syntactic and phonological development and disorders. Two recent examples of published intervention procedures which might be included under this heading are those of Jacklin (1993) and Lewis and Penn (1990). Jacklin describes the implementation of individual therapy programmes derived from linguistic profiling and standardised testing in a small classroom setting. Lewis and Penn describe a programme of activities based on the levels of grammatical development in LARSP (Crystal, Fletcher and Garman, 1976). These sorts of approaches have the advantage that they bear resemblance to the sorts of linguistic theory and linguistic skills which are most clearly defined and are therefore relatively tangible in terms of describing goals of therapy. Levels of development may be broken down into goals, then into subgoals and then into special activities chosen to exemplify a particular structure. There is scope for individualising intervention. Moreover, the efficacy of direct training of grammar, particularly, has been investigated many times, Leonard concluding in 1981 that a 'number of training approaches appear effective in teaching the use of linguistic forms to children with specific language impairment'. It will be seen, however, that these approaches can exist happily together with pragmatic approaches in a symbiotic relationship.

The Pragmatic Perspective

As Conti-Ramsden and McTear point out (Chapter 9), a broad view of pragmatics encompasses much more than just another set of linguistic skills. It provides us with an integrative view of the child's development where the child is inextricably linked to the social environment. In this sense, the question: 'In what contexts, and under what conditions, should assessment and intervention take place?' becomes crucially important.

Corsaro (1981) points to the well-known fact that language is acquired and used in social contexts. Furthermore, the aim of learning language is to be able to share communicative functions with others. Developmentally, children are linked to significant people with whom they interact and learn. Figure 13.1 illustrates this developmental progression.

Early in the child's life the caregiver and the child are a closely knit dyad. The routines shared by mother and infant form the basis for children's early language learning and understanding of social interaction (Bruner, 1983). As children grow older, caregivers (usually parents)

1. CAREGIVER(S)–INFANT
2. CAREGIVER-MEDIATED INTERACTION:
    (a) CHILD–ADULT
        ↑

        Caregiver
    (b) CHILD–CHILD
        ↑

        Caregiver
3. CHILD–CHILD (peer interaction)
4. ADULT–CHILD (teacher–pupil interaction is particularly relevant at this stage)
5. ADULT–ADULT

Figure 13.1: Significant social contexts in the child's development

continue to be the major agents of the child's socialisation as they continue to interact with the child and act as mediators between the child and others. Thus, the context within which the child can interact grows to include *adult–child* mediated interactions and *child–child* mediated interactions (Corsaro, 1981). As time passes and children attend nurseries and pre-school provision, the child is more frequently engaged in peer interaction. Corsaro (1981) points out that this context is particularly important as children interact with other children of the same status and this interactive alignment provides social experiences which are different from those provided by the family unit. At this time other adults enter the social scene of the child. Of these, one of the most important is the teacher and, for the language-disordered child, the therapist. *Teacher–child* and *therapist–child* interactions provide a new field of experiences and learning for the young and growing child. As children grow into young adults, peer and adult–child interactions become more important. We then reach the bottom of Figure 13.1 and may return to the top again but this time as caregivers, not infants.

This developmental progression of interactive alignments from *caregiver–child* to *adult–child* provides us with a pragmatic model for the contexts in which assessment-intervention need to occur. The social importance of language directs us to the dyad as the minimum unit of assessment and intervention, and the above developmental framework gives us information as to who the significant others are in the child's life. Clinicians are thus able not only to look in detail at the child's linguistic and other systems, but also to collect that information in ecologically valid and socially significant contexts. These contexts need to continue and expand in the intervention process. The idea of parents as agents of change in the *parent–child* dyad is not new (Weistuch and Byers-Brown, 1987; Conti-Ramsden, 1993) and peers as agents of change in the child–child dyad is currently a reality (Cooper and Cooper, 1984; Muma, 1984).

The pragmatic perspective on language intervention is, and will undoubtedly remain, elusive of exact characterisation and description. This is inherent in the nature of pragmatics – that we are not able to organise its rules neatly into profiles and developmental charts, and it would be inappropriate to do so (Gallagher, 1991). Rather the pragmatic perspective provides us with an emphasis, and that is on the *communicative context*, and the motivation behind communication in terms of exchange of information and other purposes. The pragmatic perspective implies that language clinicians should avoid at all costs the temptation to set up a new and separate communicative context which the child only experiences during a language remediation programme. This does not mean that we cannot set up games or plan and organise the child's experience, but all the games and plans we share with the children in our daily workload need to respect what pragmatically occurs in natural interaction between two individuals.

An Integrated Interactionist Approach

The good language clinician knows that the pragmatic approach to intervention must be incorporated into a management strategy. Gone are the days of language drills, endless imitation and repetitions. Instead there is a tendency now to try to blend the pragmatic approach with focused stimulation and elicitation. The contributions that the advent of pragmatics have made to intervention are outlined by Gallagher (1991) as:

(a) expanding the range of language goals that might be included in intervention;
(b) increasing the number of agents or participants in the intervention;
(c) promoting communicative strategies as compensatory devices for the linguistically impaired.

This chapter has used case examples from a relatively young group of language-impaired children. Aspects of caregiver–child interaction are particularly pertinent to this group. But it is essential to recognise that there are some children, especially of school age, who will need explicit instruction in some aspects of language, particularly those individuals whose linguistic profiles show major gaps or imbalances. This is not to say that the pragmatic back-up for that sort of fairly direct teaching has to be abandoned. (In fact, Lewis and Penn, *op. cit.*, incorporate aspects of the pragmatic approach in their descriptions of therapy.) There is far more likelihood of a particular structure or meaning being retained and incorporated into the child's future language if the teaching is carried out in a context which is meaningful and natural for the acquisition of that part of language, as part of adult–child interactions or child–child interactions.

The blending of the pragmatic and aualytical approaches might be best illustrated by a short example from a therapy session. In this extract the objective is to have the child use word combinations to express the construction, subject + verb, as being an appropriate developmental goal for this child. Rather than merely exposing the child to pictures and asking him or her to repeat what the adult says (a rather passive atypical interaction), the therapist takes into account the individual child's interest and motivation for using this kind of grammatical construction in real interactions. The child and therapist play a posting game. They sit at opposite ends of a desk with a cardboard screen between them which has one posting slit in it to post cards to each other. They both have a set of cards of dogs, cats and other animals doing different things. The child and clinician take turns asking each other to post a particular picture card. The clinician can then say 'the dog is jumping' and the child should pass that particular picture card. Then it is the child's turn. The child may first say 'sitting' and then the clinician can then say 'well, I don't know which one you mean. I've got lots of animals sitting. Tell me some more.' The child may say 'dog sitting' and the clinician can then model 'the dog is sitting'. Thus criteria of the pragmatic perspective are fulfilled in terms of naturalness of the interaction and the word combination goal is achieved.

This chapter has emphasised the importance of interaction amongst linguistic levels. In the same way that aspects of linguistic development act synergistically during the learning phase, it is possible for the analytical and pragmatic approaches to language intervention to provide substance and support for each other. With careful blending these approaches can both be seen as important tools in achieving the optimal strategy for intervention for any one individual. That said, there is still an urgent need for further studies to investigate the efficacy of the pragmatic and integrated approaches. Readers are referred to Law (1994) for practical ideas and discussions about specific approaches to intervention with language-impaired children.

Concluding Remarks

Within a generation the study of child language development and disorders has experienced a broadening of perspective from an emphasis on form to a concern with function. There has also been a move from the analysis of the speaker to an analysis of the communicative dyad and from viewing group characteristics to focusing on the child as an individual. And, last but not least, the realisation that language always occurs in a context has come home to clinicians and researchers alike. These changes of focus have brought about new methodologies, issues and problems which directly affect how we plan and carry out the assessment and intervention of developmentally language-disordered children.

The aim of this chapter has been to illustrate the methodologies and

issues for the clinician interested in assessment and intervention, not to
provide a method for either. The eclectic position taken by the authors
leaves clinicians with the complex task of translating these general principles to specific approaches for each individual language-disordered
child. It is hoped that this chapter, along with the information provided
in Section II of this book, will together go a long way towards making
this task easier.

References

Barrett, D.M. (1986). Early semantic representations of early word usage. In: S.A.
    Kuczaj and D.M. Barrett, *The Development of Word Meaning*. New York:
    Springer-Verlag.
Bishop, D.V.M. and Adams, C. (1989). Conversational characteristics of children
    with semantic-pragmatic language disorder, II: What features lead to a judge-
    ment of inappropriacy? *British Journal of Disorders of Communication* 24,
    241–263.
Bishop, D.V.M. (1992). The underlying nature of language impairment. *Journal of
    Child Psychology and Psychiatry* 33, 3–66.
Blank, M., Gessner, M. and Esposito, A. (1980). Language without communication: a
    case study. *Journal of Child Language* 6, 329–352.
Bruner, J. (1983). *Child's Talk: Learning to Use Language*. Oxford: Oxford University
    Press.
Conti-Ramsden, G. (1993). Using parents to foster communicably impaired chil-
    dren's language development. *Seminars in Speech and Language* 14, 289–295.
Conti-Ramsden, G. and Gunn, M. (1986). The development of conversational dis-
    ability. *British Journal of Disorders of Communication* 21, 339–351.
Cooper, C.R. and Cooper, R.G. (1984). Skill in peer learning discourse: What de-
    velops. In: S.A. Kuczaj (Ed.), *Discourse Development*, pp. 77–98. New York:
    Springer-Verlag.
Corsaro, W.A. (1981). The development of social cognition in pre-school children:
    implications for language learning. *Topics in Language Disorders* 2, 77–95.
Cromer, R. (1978). The basis of childhood aphasia: a linguistic approach. In: M. Syke
    (Ed.), *Developmental Dysphasia*. New York: Academic Press.
Crystal, D. (1987). Comments on the plenary session. In: *Proceedings of the First
    International Symposium on Specific Speech and Language Disorders in
    Children*, pp. 147–157. Brentford, UK: HGA Printing Company.
Crystal, D. (1987). Teaching vocabulary: the case of a semantic curriculum. *Child
    Language Teaching and Therapy* 3, 40–56.
Crystal, D., Fletcher, P. and Garman, P. (1976). *The Grammatical Analysis of
    Language Disability*. London: Edward Arnold.
Eisenson, J. (1972). *Aphasia in Children*. New York: Harper & Row.
Fletcher, P. (1990). Subgroups of school-age language-impaired children. *Child
    Language Teaching and Therapy* 6, 47–58.
Friel-Patti, S. and Conti-Ramsden, G. (1984). Discourse development in atypical
    language learners. In: S.A. Kuczaj (Ed.), *Discourse Development*. New York:
    Springer-Verlag.
Gallagher, T.M. (1991). A retrospective look at clinical pragmatics. In: T.M. Gallagher
    (Ed.), *Pragmatics of Language: Clinical Practice Issues*. London: Chapman &
    Hall.

Haynes, C. (1992). Vocabulary deficit – one problem or many. *Child Language Teaching and Therapy* 8, 1–17.

Ingram, D. (1987). Categories of phonological disorder. In: *Proceedings of the First International Symposium on Specific Speech and Language Disorders in Children*, pp.148–160. Brentford, UK: HGA Printing Company.

Jacklin, A. (1993). Approaches to the development of language and communication with children who have speech and language disorders. *Child Language Teaching and Therapy* 9, 116–132.

Johnson, R., Stark, R., Melitts, E. and Tallal, P. (1981). Neurological status of language impaired and normal children. *Annals of Neurology* 10, 159–163.

King, G. and Fletcher, P. (1993). Grammatical problems in school-age children with specific language impairment. *Clinical Linguistics and Phonetics* 7, 339–352.

Law, J. (1994). *Before School: A Handbook of Approaches to Intervention with Preschool Language Impaired Children*. London: AFASIC.

Lee, L. (1966). Development of sentence types: a method of comparing normal and deviant syntactic development. *Journal of Speech and Hearing Disorders* 31, 311–330.

Leonard, L.B. and Fey, M.E. (1991). Facilitating grammatical development: the contribution of pragmatics. In: T.M. Gallagher (Ed.), *Pragmatics of Language: Clinical Practice Issues*. London: Chapman & Hall.

Leonard, L.B. (1979a). What is deviant language? *Journal of Speech and Hearing Disorders* 37, 427–446.

Leonard, L.B. (1979b). Language impairment in children. *Merill-Palmer Quarterly* 25, 205–232.

Leonard, L.B. (1981). Facilitating linguistic skills in children with specific language impairment. *Applied Psycholinguistics* 2, 89–118.

Lewis, R.E. and Penn, C. (1990). *Language Therapy: a Programme to Teach English*. London: Whurr Publishers.

Masterson, J.J. and Kahmi, A.G. (1992). Linguistic trade-offs in school-age children with and without language disorders. *Journal of Speech and Hearing Research* 35, 1064–1075.

McCormick, L. and Schiefelbusch, R. (1984). *Early Language Intervention*. Columbus, OH: Charles E. Merrill.

Miller, J.F. (1991). *Research on Child Language Disorders*. Austin, TX: Pro-ed.

Miller, J. (1981). *Assessing Language Production in Children*. Baltimore: University Park Press.

Muma, J.R. (1984). Speech–language pathology: emerging clinical expertise in language. In: T.M. Gallagher and C.A. Prutting (Eds.), *Pragmatic Assessment and Intervention Issues in Language*. London: Taylor & Francis.

Myklebust, H. (1954). *Auditory Disorders in Children*. New York: Grune & Stratton.

Pinker, S. (1989). *Learnability and Cognition: the Acquisition of Argument Structure*. Cambridge, MA: MIT Press.

Prather, E.M. (1984). Developmental language disorders: adolescents. In: A. Holland (Ed.), *Language Disorders in Children*. London: Taylor & Francis.

Prelock, P. and Pahagos, J. (1989). The influence of processing mode on the sentence productions of language-disordered and normal children. *Clinical Linguistics and Phonetics* 3, 251–263.

Rees, N. (1973). Auditory processing factors in language disorders: The view from Procrustes bed. *Journal of Speech and Hearing Disorders* 38, 304–315.

Rudel, R. and Denckla, M. (1974). Relation of forward and backward digit repetition to neurological impairment in children with learning disabilities. *Neuropsychologia* 12, 109–118.

Snyder, L.S. (1984). Developmental language disorders: elementary school children. In: A. Holland (Ed.), *Language Disorders in Children*. London: Taylor & Francis.

Stark, R.E. and Tallal, P. (1981). Selection of children with specific language defects. *Journal of Speech and Hearing Disorders* 46, 114–122.

Stark, R.E., Tallal, P. and McCauley, R.J. (1988). *Language, Speech and Reading disorders in children: neuropsychological studies*. Boston: College Hill Press.

Van der Lely, H. (1992). Theory meets therapy. *Bulletin of the College of Speech and Language Therapists*, November.

Van Kleeck, A. and Richardson, A. (1988). Language delay in children. In N. Lass, I. McReynolds, J. Riothern and D. Yoder (Eds.), *Handbook of Speech–Language Pathology and Audiology*. Toronto, Canada: B.C. Decker.

Wetherby, A.M. (1991). Profiling pragmatic abilities in the emerging language of young children. In: T.M. Gallagher (Ed.), *Pragmatics of Language: Clinical Practice Issues*. London: Chapman & Hall.

Warner, J.A.W., Byers-Brown, B. and McCartney, E. (1984). *Speech Therapy: A Clinical Comparison*. Manchester: Manchester University Press.

Warnock, H.M. (1982). *Special Educational Needs: Report of the Committee of Enquiry into the Education of Handicapped Children and Young People*. London: HMSO.

Weistuch, L. and Byers-Brown, B. (1987). Motherese as therapy: a programme and its dissemination. *Child Language Teaching and Therapy* 3, 57–71.

Chapter 14
Developmental Speech Disorders

KIM GRUNDY AND ANNE HARDING

Introduction

The major contribution of linguistics to the field of developmental speech disorders is that it has provided clinicians with a framework of analysis which enables the important distinction to be drawn between articulation disorder and phonological disorder. Recent research by linguists, psycholinguists and clinician-researchers has furthered our understanding of phonological disorder. This chapter will outline current knowledge of the development of the speech sound system and discuss issues relating to differential diagnosis within the population of children with developmental speech disorders. Current approaches to intervention will be evaluated in the light of these discussions.

The Whole Child

Adams and Conti-Ramsden state in the previous chapter that 'the assessment and intervention process begins by the clinician's attempt to obtain an overview of the whole child and the child's environment'. The same applies to children with developmental speech disorders, not least because intelligibility breakdown may be part of a more general developmental language disorder. Thus, evaluation of the four key areas identified by Van Kleek and Richardson (1988) – linguistic, cognitive, social and physical – is equally valid for children with developmental speech disorders.

Particularly relevant to speech development is information about any complications in pregnancy or birth, about feeding patterns and any difficulties with sucking or coping with solids. Communicativeness and responsiveness in infancy may indicate the relative needs of the child for speech. Some babies are very vocal, engage adults in smiling games and shout when unattended. Other babies observe their world closely but in a more passive manner. A history of particularly quiet infancy should be regarded as a potential symptom of hearing loss and investigated with further questioning and observation. With hearing in mind, information about colds, ear infections, sleeping and eating patterns is essential. Chronic nasal obstruction by day and/or by night might precipitate open mouth posture which may have a marked effect on habitual tongue posture and may diminish both growth of the midface (Oblak and Kozelj, 1984) and use of the tongue tip in early speech. Visual problems which might have affected visual perception of speech, extended or repeated hospitalisations, and family details such as the child's position in the family and the family's communicative style are all important clinical considerations.

In addition to this overview of the child's general level of functioning we suggest it is important to investigate the carer's and child's view of the speech problem. It may be assumed that children referred with speech disorders are aware of having difficulty communicating and are therefore aware of the words that cannot be understood by other people. Clinical experience indicates that although children may be aware of failed interaction, they may not be aware of the cause of the communication failure. That is, they may not have recognised that the problem lies in the quality of the message that they themselves have sent. Parents too may be unaware or only partially aware of mispronunciations and may need to be helped to recognise the aspects of speech judged by the clinician to require intervention. Intervention is likely to be more successful if it takes into account both parental and child perception of the child's speech.

Development of the Speech Sound System (Phonology)

Speech development begins rather earlier than is commonly thought. First words might be identified as the point at which speech starts to develop, but vocalisations as a form of communication begin at birth as the child vocalises with the first intake of breath. From this time on the baby explores ways of changing her or his voice to indicate different meanings. Meanwhile all the muscles that will later be used for speech are exercised in feeding and in vocal play. Where structural or functional orofacial anomalies, or neurological impairment, are diagnosed in infancy, speech development is considered to be at risk. Specialist speech and language therapists contribute to the early management of children with diagnoses such as cleft palate, Down's syndrome, hearing impairment and cerebral palsy. Feeding advice is given and early interactive skills are often discussed with parents in the child's first year of life. Thus, normal vocal and communicative development needs to be considered in the context of cognitive and physical progress.

More commonly, children are referred to speech and language therapy in the second or third year of life and present with no associated medical diagnosis. In these cases early vocal and communicative development is routinely investigated during the process of speech and language differential diagnosis. The following paragraphs describe normal development of the speech mechanism and early vocal behaviour.

In the first six months, the primary functions of the 'articulatory' mechanisms are breathing and eating; however, articulatory potential may even be influenced prenatally by lingual posturing and movement in relation to the palate (Morley, 1970). Trost-Cardamone (1990) describes early oromuscular development. At birth the vocal folds are immediately exercised in the reflexive first cry. Neonatally the larynx sits high in the vocal tract and the epiglottis nearly touches the palate; the tongue is large and fills the oral cavity, only able to rock and thrust, and as a result breathing is exclusively nasal. Infant vocalisations are vegetative sounds which are universally produced with high lingual postures and back lingual contacts, that is, nasalised high vowels, velar stops and velar/uvular fricatives. By six months the larynx has lowered and the breathing pattern is more adult-like, allowing alternation between mouth and nose breathing. Emergence of nasal/oral [m b] distinction and experimentation with oral pressure in vocal play such as blowing raspberries demonstrates development of velopharyngeal sphincteric control. As articulatory control develops so lung capacity increases facilitating longer utterances on greater air support.

As physical changes occur, so the nature of vocalisations also develops. Lewis (1951) hypothesised that early back consonants [ç g x k] were produced in association with comfortable states whereas [m n] are associated with a distressed state and other sounds were associated with emotional/physical states, e.g. feeding associated with [p b]. In addition to native (mother-tongue) consonant-like sounds, babble also contains phonetic elements which are non-native.

Initially, vocalisations are to some extent involuntary and random but during the first four months the child will begin to vocalise in response to adult vocalisation. There is some evidence that adult imitation of a child's productions encourages further child vocalisations (Locke and Pearson, 1992). Kent (1992) summarises early vocalisations in relation to physical development:

0–3 months: mostly vowels with some velar consonants;
2–4 months: vocal tract is remodelled and goes on changing throughout the first year;
4–6 months: increased articulatory control and emergence of supraglottal contacts.

Kent (1992) suggests that the increased range of articulatory contacts results from structural remodelling of the vocal tract and development of velopharyngeal valving. The timing of these periods of development also coincides with neurological maturation (Bever 1961).

Putting early vocalisations into the context of gross motor development, Ingram (1976) has observed a correlation between Piaget's model of physical development in which Piaget (1962) emphasised the importance of imitation. His stages of development are summarised as:

Piaget's sensori-motor stages		
II	0–0;4m	sporadic imitation of body movements by visible body parts
III	0;4–0;8m	systematic imitation of movements child has already seen and made
IV	0;8m–1;0yr	imitation of movements previously made by the child but not visible
V	1;0–1;4	systematic imitation of new models not previously made by the child
VI	1;4–1;6	deferred imitation of models seen earlier

Ingram (1976) demonstrates the relationship between these stages of development and development of pre-speech vocalisations:

Ingram's application of Piaget's stages to pre-speech vocalisations		
II	0–0;4m	vocal contagion – vocalises at the sound of the human voice imitating the child
III	0;4–0;8m	imitates those sounds he or she can make spontaneously
IV	0;8m–1;0yr	first attempts at new sounds not previously made
V	1;0–1;4	first attempts to imitate whole words through trial and error
VI	1;4–1;6	deferred imitation of adult words heard earlier

The relationship between physical and vocal development is evident as babble develops into repetitive syllable sequences /bə bə bə bə / referred to as *reduplicated babble*. As similar physical rhythmic stereotypes occur, for example, in the limbs and fingers, Ingram (*op. cit.*) hypothesised that reduplicated babble might be a vocal manifestation of a general tendency towards repetitive movement patterns (6–8 months).

Progression out of reduplicated babble pattern into a period of non-reduplicated (or *variegated*) babble occurs at approximately 8–10 months. The non-reduplicated babble period is thought to be one of the most important stages in development of motor speech patterns (Trost-Cardamone, 1990). The child develops ability both to alternate between consonant types in any one syllabic sequence and to produce an increased range of consonant types, some of which are non-native. The first attempts to imitate adult words, at around 12 months, are considered vital to the development of language.

Development of Infant Feedback Mechanisms

As the child makes involuntary and/or reflex movements, receptors in the moving muscles send messages back to the brain. This is termed *intrapersonal neuromuscular feedback*. Neuromuscular feedback facilitates the development of *proprioceptive* and *kinaesthetic* awareness. Proprioception is the sensory awareness of (a) the precise position of body parts, and (b) the direction of movement of any body part. For example, without looking you can tell whether or not your lips are apart or together and, also without looking, you can change their position. Kinaesthesis is the sense of muscular effort that accompanies a voluntary movement of the body. The fact that we do not crash our teeth together when closing our mouths or completely flatten a straw between our lips when drinking provide examples of oral kinaesthetic sense. Oral proprioceptive and kinaesthetic awareness are considered to be prerequisites for speech development. These senses are enhanced during the babbling period. Any difficulties experienced during the development of feeding and/or any impedance to natural 'babble' (for example, the permanent dummy [US comforter]) may inhibit appropriate development of these senses.

When the child vocalises a sound-wave is produced which is heard and perceived not only by others but by the child itself. The sound-wave thus provides the child with *auditory* feedback. As this type of auditory feedback involves only the child – it occurs whether or not anyone is listening – it is referred to as *intrapersonal auditory feedback*. Integration of intrapersonal auditory and neuromuscular feedback begins to develop during the babbling period. Adult speech provides babies with auditory patterns which they may attempt to match during babble. When adults engage in vocal play with babies they tend to imitate and model babble patterns closest to native speech patterns thus reinforcing those particular patterns. The sensory feedback (auditory, visual, tactile, etc.) available to the child from another person is termed *interpersonal feedback*. Thus the synthesis of intrapersonal auditory and neuromuscular feedback and interpersonal feedback can be seen as essential to the development of native speech patterns.

Consonant Acquisition

Glottal and pharyngeal consonant-like sounds characterise earliest vocalisations from the underdeveloped speech musculature. Consonant-like sounds move from the back anteriorly during the first six months of life. As babble becomes proto-words and proto-words lead to early words so consonants take their place in first words. The pattern of back contacts has been replaced by more forward placements so that consonant development is generally described as beginning with bilabials and gradually moving backwards. This pattern is shown in Grunwell's (1985) consonant development which is outlined in Figure 14.1.

		Labial		Lingual					
Stage I (0;9 – 1;6)	Nasal								
	Plosive								
	Fricative								
	Approximant								
Stage II (1;6 – 2;0)		m		n					
		p	b	t	d				
		w							
Stage III (2;0 – 2;6)		m		n				(ŋ)	
		p	b	t	d			(k)	(g)
		w							(h)
Stage IV (2;6 – 3;0)		m		n				ŋ	
		p	b	t	d			k	g
		f			s				
		w		(l)			j		h
Stage V (3;0 – 3;6)		m		n				ŋ	
		p	b	t	d	(tʃ)		k	g
		f			s			(ʃ)	
		w		l			j		h
Stage VI (3;6 – 4;6)		m		n				ŋ	
		p	b	t	d	tʃ	dʒ	k	g
		f	v		s		z	ʃ	
		w		l		(r)	j		h
Stage VII (4;6 <)		m		n				ŋ	
		p	b	t	d	tʃ	dʒ	k	g
		f	v	θ	s	ð	z	ʃ	(ʒ)
		w		l		r	j		h

Figure 14.1: PACS Developmental Profile: Consonant Acquisition. Reproduced by kind permission of Pamela Grunwell

It has been thought that consonant acquisition was universal across different languages but Ingram's (1986) cross-linguistic study indicates that each language has its own basic inventory that characterises the child's first phonemes. *Functional load* is a factor in this. The more a particular sound occurs in the native language, the more a child is likely to hear it. The more the child hears the sound, the more likely he or she is to produce it and the more he or she produces it in babble the more likely it is to be used in early speech. So the sounds most frequently heard in early babble (in English [h w j p b m t d n k g] also occur in the first fifty words (Locke, 1989). There is evidence that unusual babble patterns result in atypical early speech patterns (Stoel-Gammon, 1992). From the first words, development of articulation occurs synchronously with phonological development, hence it is difficult to isolate a pure articulatory disorder (cf. Chapter 3, this volume).

Differential Diagnosis between Articulation and Phonological Disorders

An articulation disorder is a speech production disorder. Children with an articulation disorder are thought to be physiologically unable to articulate one or more of their native speech sounds. They are therefore unable to produce correct target sound(s) in single words, longer utterances, or *in isolation*. So, for example, the child who is misarticulating /s/ as [ç] will produce [ç] at every place that /s/ should occur in normal speech and when asked to imitate [s] in isolation will say [ç].

In a strict linguistic sense, phonological breakdown occurs when there is a reduction in the ability to signal differences in meaning. In this example one speech sound is being substituted for only one other: /s/ is replaced by [ç]. As this is the only substitution used by the child, the ability to signal meaning differences remains intact. Theoretically, it is possible for a child to represent the entire target adult phonological system with non-native speech sounds. Where there is a one-to-one correspondence between non-native sounds and target adult sounds, the child may be described as having a *pure articulation disorder*.

The nature of phonological disorder is less easily defined and is discussed in more detail below. In contrast with children who have an articulation disorder, those with a 'pure' phonological disorder *are* able to imitate sounds uttered in isolation but 'mispronounce' them in their everyday speech. When asked to produce or imitate the sound [s] in isolation they say [s] but when asked to say *soup* they say [tup] or [dup] or [hup], for example. Phonological analysis of the speech of children with 'pure' phonological disorders reveals that these sound substitutions occur in patterns. It is likely that the child who says [tup] for *soup* will also say [tok] for *sock*, [ti] for *sea* and so on. These patterns are referred to as *systemic phonological processes*; examples are *Stopping of Fricatives* (the replacement of fricatives by stops or plosives); *Fronting of Velars* (velar sounds are replaced by alveolars). Systematic phonotactic differences may also be identified and are referred to as *structural phonological processes*, for example *Cluster Reduction* (where target clusters are produced by the child as singleton consonants). For full discussion of phonological processes see Grunwell (1987).

Linguistic Classification of Developmental Speech Disorders

We have said that a distinction can be drawn between *pure articulation disorders* and *pure phonological disorders*. With the former, children substitute non-native speech sounds in a one-to-one correspondence with target adult sounds. More often, children with physiological speech production difficulties tend to substitute a non-native sound for more than one target adult phoneme. For example, let's say a child is physically unable to articulate the sounds /s/ and /ʃ/, which are very similar, and resolves this articulatory difficulty by substituting [ç] as the closest approximation for both. This child has an articulation disorder but also has a reduced ability to signal meaning differences: *sell* and *shell* would both be produced as [çɛl]. For clinical diagnostic purposes, then, we may wish to describe such children as having an *articulation disorder with phonological consequences*. Children with a structural defect who substitute native phones for a range of phonemes in response to their structural difficulties (for example, [h] for /p t k/ in cleft palate) may also be included in this category.

Children with physiological pathology have traditionally been diagnosed as having articulation disorders. However, analysis of their speech patterns may reveal that the misarticulations they are using are systematically distributed to signal meaning differences (see also Hewlett, 1985). For example, one 8-year-old child (E), with velopharyngeal insufficiency, had the word initial plosive system of:

/p/ → [p˭]   /t/ and /k/ → [t˭]

/b/ → [ʘ]   /d/ and /g/ → [ǃ]

These patterns may be accounted for by E's velopharyngeal insufficiency. That is, it may be that E had adequate velopharyngeal closure to produce weak, unaspirated, voiceless plosives but insufficient velopharyngeal closure to produce voiced plosives. The clicks may thus be explained by E utilising an alternative breath stream mechanism in order to maintain the voiced/voiceless contrast. We may be tempted to describe this child as having an articulation disorder with phonological consequences. However, further analysis of her speech patterns revealed the processes of *Stopping of Fricatives, Word Medial and Word Final Glottal Realisations, Cluster Reduction* and *Final Consonant Deletion*. Because these processes cannot necessarily be accounted for by E's velopharyngeal insufficiency, there would appear to be a co-occuring phonological disorder. Thus, it is suggested here that this type of difficulty should be described as *mixed articulation and phonological disorder*.

In summary then, clinically we have now four potential linguistic-based diagnostic categories for a child presenting with reduced intelligibility:

1. **pure articulation disorder** where a child substitutes non-native speech sounds for one or more of their native phonemes but in one-to-one correspondence with their native phonological system and therefore with no disruption to their ability to signal meaning differences;

2. **pure phonological disorder** where the child is physically able to articulate all of their native speech sounds but does not use these sounds appropriately in their speech, resulting in reduced ability to signal meaning differences. Systemic and structural phonological processes are evident;

3. **articulation disorder with phonological consequences** where the non-native substitution of speech sounds crosses phonological boundaries and reduces the child's ability to signal meaning differences; and/or native substitutions occur as a direct result of reduced physiological abilities;

4. **mixed articulation and phonological disorder** where a child is unable physiologically to articulate some of their native speech sounds and substitutes non-native speech sounds for these. In addition, systemic and/or structural processes may be identified in the child's speech patterns.

Within the classification of phonological disorder, further categories have been suggested. Grunwell (1988) identifies three groups:

delayed – where children appear to be following the normal pattern of development but at a slower rate than is expected for their chronological age;

uneven development – where processes from one stage of development are observed to co-exist with processes from a later stage in development; for example a child may be observed to be *Fronting Velar Consonants* (normally not evident after age 2;6) when *Clusters* (normally emerging from age 3;0) are well developed.

deviant development – where some of the processes identified in the child's speech are unusual or idiosyncratic. Grunwell (*op. cit.*) advocates caution in referring to these processes as deviant because similarly unusual processes evident in the speech of normally developing younger children have been referred to as creative.

Bradford and Dodd (1994) also identify three subgroups:

delayed – all processes evident in speech are developmental. Use of at least two processes that are not age-appropriate;

deviant consistent – use of at least two deviant phonological processes applied consistently so that errors are consistent. (See Appendix for examples of developmental and deviant processes suggested by Bradford and Dodd [*op. cit.*].)

deviant inconsistent – use of deviant errors with no observable error pattern. Inconsistencies in production exist in the absence of articulatory groping on volitional phoneme production or any other potential characteristics of dyspraxia. (See Chapter 3 for characteristics of dyspraxia.)

We suggest that by combining the Grunwell and Dodd groupings, four subgroups of *pure phonological disorder* (category 2. above) emerge:

2. (i)   **delayed phonological development;**
2. (ii)   **uneven phonological development;**
2. (iii) **deviant consistent phonological development;**
2. (iv)   **deviant inconsistent phonological development.**

It is important to note that the diagnostic categories suggested above are descriptive in nature rather than explanatory. That is, they are arrived at through observing, analysing and describing the child's speech patterns (data orientated, Hewlett 1985). These diagnoses make no attempt to explain why the child is observed to use these speech patterns.

From these descriptive diagnoses we could make the following clinical decisions:

- children who have articulatory difficulties need articulation therapy;
- children with pure phonological difficulties need phonological therapy;
- children with a combination of difficulties need articulation therapy within a firmly established phonological framework.

However, to decide on the most appropriate approach to articulation or phonological therapy we may wish to go further than description and to try to explain the disorder.

Aetiology of Articulation Disorders

Articulation disorders are not a homogeneous group but the fundamental cause of any articulation disorder is a breakdown in one or more of the physiological processes of speech production. The breakdown may be due to a structural malformation, such as cleft palate; or to a neurological malfunction, as in dyspraxia or dysarthria. In the absence of any clear pathology, it is assumed that the child has simply mislearned the production of certain speech sounds (*learned misarticulation*).

Children with congenital organic disorders affecting the speech mechanism will not have produced a full range of early vocalisations, babble may have been limited and their potential as communicators will be different from their peer group. They may have attempted normal interactive babble and, having failed to engage adult attention, they may respond to articulatory difficulties by lapsing into silence before language development is formally under way. Other children might adapt to early awareness of production difficulties and seek alternative methods of producing a wide range of babble sounds. For example, some children with cleft palate develop characteristic compensatory articulations which are evident in babble.

The most common organic causes of articulation disorders are listed in Table 14.1, with the most likely articulatory consequences. Hearing loss is listed in this table as a cause for articulation disorder. However, as Parker (1986) points out, whilst children with a profound hearing loss (and no other physiological or anatomical deficit) do lack a requisite

Table 14.1: Common organic causes of articulatory disorders with articulatory consequences

Organic cause	*Articulatory consequences*
Neuromuscular disorder, e.g. cerebral palsy	weak or nasal articulation of obstruents with possible lack of nasal/oral contrast; limited articulatory accuracy
Cleft palate, velopharyngeal insufficiency and related disorders	*resonance disorders*: predominantly hypernasality; nasal emission and turbulence; *articulatory difficulties*: pressure consonants most affected; *phonological consequences* may affect entire consonant system
Structural imperfections: (a) dental/occlusal irregularities (b) lingual: short frenum; micro/macroglossia (c) enlarged tonsils/adenoids (d) nasal obstruction	(a) and (b) relatively minor articulatory variations (c) nasal resonance disturbances (d) hyponasal target nasal consonants; possible backing of alveolar targets; nasal fricatives may develop during a period of nasal obstruction
Hearing impairment	labial articulation most reliably acquired; non-labial targets tend to be backed; glottal articulation may be prevalent; timing of voicing can be problematic; stopping of fricatives; vowel distortions, e.g. vowel lengthening and intrusion of schwa [ə]; prosodic disturbances (Ball, 1993)

part of their *speech-reception mechanisms,* their speech-production mechanisms are normal (see also, Grunwell, 1987). Nevertheless, the inclusion of hearing impairment emphasises the importance of hearing and/or speech perception to the development of articulation. For differential diagnosis of the varying pathologies in Table 14.1 the reader is referred to Bamford and Saunders (1985); Grunwell (1990); Milloy (1991).

As stated above, it is often not possible to identify a specific organic aetiology for the individual child. In these instances, non-organic explanations have been hypothesised to account for *learned misarticulations*. These are listed in Table 14.2.

Aetiology of Phonological Disorders

As phonology is part of language it exists in the psychological part of Saussure's speech circuit (see Chapter 1, this volume). As such, phonological processing is not open to direct scrutiny. Determining the cause of phonological disorder involves drawing inferences from observed behaviours. Research over the past few years has fine-tuned the elicitation of observed behaviours so that inferences have become more sophisticated. The next few paragraphs offer an overview of the development of hypotheses on the nature of phonological disorder.

To begin with, in a gross simplification of the suggested process of phonological acquisition, we will consider acquisition of the word *cat*. Suppose that the adult points to a cat and says /kat/. The child sees the animal, perceives the sound pattern [kʰat] and forms an association between the two. The concept *cat* and a 'template' for the sound pattern [kʰat] (hereafter referred to as SPT-sound pattern template) are stored in the child's brain. When the normally developing child attempts to say cat he or she tends to go through stages (over a period of time) during which their production is (variously) unlike the adult target, but eventually they produce the word accurately.

Table 14.2: Non-organic explanations of articulatory disorders with articulatory consequences

Non-organic explanations	Articulatory consequences
Auditory perceptual difficulties	articulatory mismatches which are frequently inconsistent
Articulatory play	whilst exploring articulatory possibilities, idiosyncratic, physically satisfying consonants can be discovered which persist and stabilise in the phonological system, e.g. nasal fricatives
Family member with atypical consonant productions	child develops consonant production similar to family member

For the purposes of this example we will assume that the child with a 'pure' phonological disorder has not yet reached the stage of being able to say /kat/. The question to be answered is why not? There are several possible explanations, all of which centre on the storage of the SPT.

First, it may be postulated that the child has stored the SPT accurately, but fails to produce the correct form. There are at least two possible reasons for this:

(i) the connections between the stored SPT and the child's speech production centre are faulty and therefore the instructions to the articulators are wrong; or

(ii) the instructions to the articulators are correct, but the combination of phonemes is too complex for the child's current articulatory skills. The child therefore produces a form that is not beyond his or her articulatory skills, for example, [tʰa].

Either of these hypotheses implies that phonological disorder is productive in nature.

Alternatively, it may be hypothesised that the child has stored the SPT inaccurately. Again, there are at least two possible reasons for this:

(i) the child has misperceived the adult utterance, i.e. when the adult says /kat/ the child perceives [tʰa] and therefore stores the SPT [tʰa]. If this was the case, then phonological disorder would be the result of a speech perception breakdown.

(ii) the child perceives the adult form correctly, but has no place in his or her current storage system for (in this example) CVC words or words which begin with /k/. The child therefore accommodates the SPT to his or her current system and stores [tʰa]. The resultant explanation of phonological disorder would be that it is organisational in nature.

Thinking in the late 1980s, initiated by Ingram (1976) and expounded by Leonard (1985), was that phonological disorder may be the result of processes operating on either the productive, or the perceptual or the organisational mechanisms of speech.

A third possibility is that the child *is* in fact making a phonological distinction but one which is not perceptible to the adult who perceives *categorically* (see Chapter 4). In this instance the child who is perceived to say [tʰa] for /kat/ is saying neither /ta/ nor /kat/ but something between the two. This possibility would provide an alternative explanation to the *fis-phenomenon* (Berko and Brown, 1960). The fis-phenomenon is so called because the original hypothesis was based on a child's mispronunciation of *fish* as [fis]. In this example, an adult used the child's form [fis] and the child responded 'not [fis]...[fis]!' This response has been interpreted to indicate that the child did not have inter-personal auditory perception difficulties because he perceived accurately the adult's mispronunciation, but did have intra-personal perception difficulties because he did not perceive his own mispronunciation. If, however, the child was making a subphonemic distinction then his response 'not [fis]...[fis]!' would indicate that he has neither inter-personal nor intra-personal speech perception difficulties because he has perceived that the adult is not producing the same utterance as himself. Indeed, this explanation may account for the observation that parents frequently understand their child's 'unintelligible' speech (see also Priestly, 1980). One could say that it is the 'untuned' adult, rather than the child, who has the perception difficulty. The Macken and Barton (1979) study of the acquisition of the voicing contrast offers support to the possibility that children perceived as producing homophones are producing subphonemic cues. The results of their study show that full acquisition takes approximately 18 months and that the gradual acquisition includes periods where consistent subphonemic distinctions are made. Spectrographic analysis of the speech of a child perceived to be backing alveolar plosives revealed that there was a statistically significant difference in Voice Onset Time between productions of the two phonemes (Grundy, 1985).

It may be argued that in such cases the child does not have a phonological disorder because she or he is making a distinction between the two phonemes. The cause could be characterised as a phonetic disorder (Hewlett, 1985, 1990). That is, the child is aiming for the correct target and the difficulty lies in phonetic implementation. Support for this hypothesis may be drawn from Gibbon and Hardcastle (1991) who demonstrated through electropalatography that a child perceived to be backing alveolar plosives was in fact making consistently distinct articulatory gestures for alveolar and velar targets.

However, it may also be hypothesised that the phonetic implementation is based on an inaccurate sound pattern template. Taking the /kat/ vs [tʰa] example, the child could be perceiving Voice Onset Time differences between /k/ and /t/ and vowel differences between CV and CVC structures; the SPT includes these acoustic characteristics (but excludes other perceptually more salient cues) and the phonetic implementation reflects the stored pattern. When the adult says [tʰa] the acoustic characteristics registered by the child in perception and utilised in production of /kat/ are not evident and the child rejects the adult form as dissimilar to his or her own. In this case we could postulate a phonological explanation because the child has not yet identified and assimilated *all* the salient acoustic characteristics which distinguish /k/ from /t/ and CV from CVC words. Bird and Bishop (1992) identified phonologically disordered children who had difficulty with phoneme identification tasks across different word contexts. These children also had difficulty in rhyme judgement and rhyme generation tasks and Bird and Bishop concluded that they were failing to analyse words at the level of phonemic segments. Such a failure could result in the scenario outlined above.

Is Phonological Disorder Due to Perceptual, Cognitive or Productive Deficits?

Linguistically, phonological breakdown is a unitary phenomenon. That is, when we are describing phonological breakdown there is only one characteristic: the loss of contrast in speech. The loss of contrast may fall on a scale from mild to severe but nevertheless phonological breakdown may be described simply as loss of contrast in speech. This unitary description may have led to the tendency in the literature to look for a unitary explanation. In fact, research over the last decade lends support to the view that the phonologically disordered population is 'probably clinically heterogeneous' (Grunwell (1981, p. 35)).

Dodd provides evidence to indicate that the subgroups identified by her on the basis of observed speech patterns may have different underlying causes. She suggests that delayed phonology may arise through impoverished language environment or immature maturation (Dodd, 1987, cited in Dodd, Leahy and Hambly, 1989). The deviant consistent group, she suggests, have deficits at the organisational level (Dodd *et al.*, 1989); whilst the deviant inconsistent group appear to have motor programming deficits (Bradford and Dodd, 1994).

Other recent research has highlighted the fact that studies which evaluate groups of children and present group results may mask important individual differences (Bird and Bishop, 1992; Stackhouse and Wells, 1993). Researchers approaching developmental speech disorders from a psycholinguistic perspective suggest that individual children may have a range of underlying deficits which result in phonological disorder. That is, any individual child may have underlying perceptual deficits and/or underlying cognitive deficits and/or underlying phonetic implementation deficits. In a very accessible paper Stackhouse and Wells (1993) describe how clinicians may attempt to pinpoint the specific abilities and deficits in individual children, largely utilising assessments currently used in clinic. They advocate the use of single case studies in future research suggesting that by collating information from individual psycholinguistic profiles it may be possible in the future to identify subgroups of children.

In summary, it has been recognised that the search for a single explanation of phonological disorder is inappropriate and there has been a move in favour of a search for different underlying causes for different subgroups of phonologically disordered children. More recently, this approach has been modified and the indications are that any individual child may present with a mixture of abilities and deficits in any of three modalities: perception/cognition/phonetic implementation. Thus, current researchers suggest that in addition to detailed phonological assessment, it is essential to identify as far as possible the specific profile of abilities and deficits for each individual child. This profile may then guide the clinician towards the most effective therapy for the individual child.

Treatment Planning for Children with Developmental Speech Disorders

The first sections of this chapter suggest that linguistic analysis enables us to distinguish between speech production patterns which are articulatory in nature and those which are phonological in nature. Linguistic analysis also provides a means of identifying subgroups of phonological disorder. Hewlett (1985, 1990) asserts that a third distinction should be drawn which is that of *phonetic implementation deficit*. He suggests that the term articulation disorder may be used to characterise organic-based speech impairments, such as cleft palate. The term phonetic implementation deficit might then be used to characterise less obviously identified articulatory difficulties, the most tangible of which would be dyspraxia. We consider that this tripartite characterisation of developmental speech disorders (*articulation disorder; phonetic implementation deficit; phonological disorder*) is important in treatment planning. Nevertheless, we would suggest that with the gross distinction between articulation disorder and phonological disorder in mind, it is possible to identify some simple underlying principles for therapy.

Underlying Principles of Articulation Therapy

• the child 'has' a demonstrably intact internal phonological system;
• the aim of therapy is correct pronunciation of target consonants in spontaneous continuous speech;
• individual sounds are worked on in isolation until correct articulation is achieved.

Underlying Principles of Pure Phonological Therapy

• the child may not 'have' an intact internal phonological system;
• the aim of therapy is for the child to develop an intact internal phonological system and/or to differentiate between all phonemes in speech output – precisely correct articulation of each phoneme is not essential to establish phonological contrasts;
• phonemes are worked on contrastively in whole words.

Current Approaches to Intervention

Traditional Articulation Therapy

Traditional articulation therapy has been based on the work of Van Riper and Irwin (1958) and Morley (1972). Morley recommended auditory discrimination as a preliminary to all articulation work. She divided her production procedures into four stages:

1. practice and facilitation of the sound in isolation;
2. introduction of the new sound into the simplest phonetic sequences, preferably nonsense syllables;
3. the newly acquired syllable would be introduced into a simple non-linguistic 'phrase' of CV CV CV as in [pa pa pa]; and
4. the consonant vowel sequences would be modified to become meaningful units.

To this day, Morley's facilitative and adaptive articulation treatment suggestions remain relevant and helpful as a basis for individually tailored therapeutic programmes. For example, to undermine substitution of [x] for /s/, she recommends overly fronting /s/ which might be practised as [θ] at first. In general, Morley recommends following a developmental pattern of consonant selection for articulation therapy but she also suggests that clinicians explore which are the most stimulable consonants and work on those that are most easily produced. Further consonants might be elicited through the first in a consonant group to be acquired, e.g. in the absence of any fricatives, a first fricative might be [ʃ] from which /s/ might be developed by modifying [ʃ].

Pure articulation work is probably most applied in the field of cleft palate. Whilst current understanding of cleft palate speech contends that there are phonological consequences of the structural imperfections, much of the articulation work described in the cleft palate literature can usefully be applied and modified to any articulatory problem. Bzoch (1979) described a very accessible programme which he called 'multiple sound articulation therapy'. At each session selected targets are produced first in isolation, a week later in CV, the next week in words and finally in phrases. New targets are added to the game so that some targets are being produced in isolation whilst others have reached production in phrases. In the same volume, Hahn (1979) describes a 'directed home programme for children with cleft palate' and Philips (1979) gives specific therapeutic strategies for stimulating verbal communication with specific phonetic targets embedded into language stimulation. Whilst these programmes have all been developed with cleft palate populations they could all be individually adapted within a phonological framework and might progress from exclusively input modelling to output production practice.

More recent approaches to articulation therapy as outlined by Lancaster and Pope (1989) extend traditional approaches to therapy by highlighting the need for flexibility of any given target production to the phonetic context in spontaneous speech. For example, productions of [t] in 'Put two tickets in the post' vary phonetically according to the surrounding consonants and vowels, the stress, pace and emphasis with which the phrase is spoken. Given this model of articulation learning, particular care should be taken, not only with the selection of target words in therapy but with the gradual increase in the complexity of the phonetic context into which targets sounds are produced. Work on [t] might be introduced in VC before CV because final [t] does not need the additional aspiration component. A long vowel preceding [t] as in [ɑt] *art* [it] *eat* allows fractionally longer preparation for the final plosive. A close vowel, such as [i], might provide better preparation for the alveolar placement of the following [t] than the more open [ɑ]. Subsequent stages might be to select CVC words without initial stops, e.g. *'heart, heat, wait, rate'*, so that production of syllable initial consonants is unlikely to disturb the SPT for final [t]; then words with stops in initial position which are in the same or near places of articulation such as 'dart, chart, late, night', and finally a varied selection of stops with different places of articulation could be elicited in phrases and sentences. An appropriate progression of this kind can be developed for all children with articulation problems and may reduce or avoid potential confusions. In the absence of confusions there will be rapid strengthening of sensorimotor patterns facilitating the desired modification of the child's Sound Pattern Template with minimal conscious effort by the child.

An important point to note with regard to articulation therapy is that it is possible for different individuals to make different articulatory gestures to produce a sound which is perceptually the same. For example, some people produce the alveolar fricative /s/ with their tongue tip pointed up towards the alveolar ridge, whereas others produce /s/ with their tongue tip pointed down behind their lower front teeth. Either of these articulatory postures results in a sound perceived by the listener as /s/. Thus we suggest that the primary aim of articulation therapy is to establish movements for articulation which result in an auditory match with the consonant target. This may be achieved by encouraging the child to experiment with different articulatory gestures in his or her attempts to imitate models of the target sound. This represents a slight shift in emphasis from the traditional approach which utilises articulatory phonetic knowledge to achieve 'correct' placement for target consonants using instruction and/or physical manipulation. Instead we are suggesting that the child should be presented with repeated opportunities to attempt an auditory match with the adult target. Given such opportunities we suggest that the child is more likely to develop an awareness of mismatches between his or her own productions and target productions; and may be more likely to take an active role in eliminating the discrepancy.

Babble-play

Our own clinical experiences are that children who appear unable to produce consonant sounds or postures following a model and visual-tactile cues sometimes manage to produce the sound during unfocused babble-play. By this we mean literally pretending to be babies (maybe even lying on the floor with the child) and producing CVCV... babble strings, with a range of native and non-native sounds, for each other to imitate. This provides the child with opportunities to experiment with and develop new motor patterns. As clinician and child become competent at imitating one another's strings, clinician-babble can become more focused and target sounds can be introduced to the strings. It may be that this type of input may be particularly effective for children with Hewlett's (1985, 1990) phonetic implementation deficits.

Phonological Approaches

Dean and Howell (1990): Metaphon

As indicated by its name, Metaphon introduces the concept of meta-linguistic awareness (see Terminology chapter, this volume) to phonological therapy. Dean and Howell cite research which indicates that some children with phonological disorder have poorer metalinguistic skills than some normally developing children. They therefore advocate that working on metalinguistic awareness is a valid aim for phonological intervention. This is the first of two key theoretical principles underlying this approach.

The second theoretical basis is rooted in learning theory. Dean and Howell assert that the Piagetian model of cognitive development (disequilibrium, assimilation, accommodation) can and should be applied to phonological intervention. That is, Piaget indicates that children are active participants in their own cognitive development. Phonological processing is a cognitive activity. Phonological intervention should therefore facilitate children's development of their own solutions to their phonological difficulties.

Metaphon has two phases. Phase 1 is regarded by Dean and Howell as the most important phase and that which is most radically different from other published approaches. Phase 1 aims to develop metalinguistic awareness of speech sounds and their properties. Children are introduced to a vocabulary of concepts which is then used throughout phases

1 and 2 to talk about specific speech sounds. The concepts *long* and *short*, for example, are taught using various means such as playing long and short notes on musical instruments. Long and short are then applied to sounds – fricatives being taught as long sounds and plosives as short sounds. Minimal pair words are subsequently introduced and discussed in relation to their distinctive features using the established vocabulary. Phase 2 then uses minimal pairs in 'secret message' games and again utilises the learned vocabulary to discuss productions of the pairs.

Dean and Howell state that, in their experience, phonologically disordered children who have articulatory difficulties are in the minority. Thus the Metaphon approach would appear to be directed at those children categorised above as having a pure phonological disorder.

In our view a major concern with this approach is the vocabulary of concepts associated with target sounds which is developed in Phase 1. Setting aside the fact that children with phonological disorder often have associated semantic deficits and may therefore experience difficulty in acquiring the vocabulary, the lexical items chosen to associate with each sound should be carefully considered. The potential confusions arising from this suggested vocabulary raise several issues worthy of discussion in the light of increased scientific understanding of consonant production and recognition.

Long and *short*: in natural conversation, *all* speech sounds are fleeting, lasting only fractions of a second and, in certain phonetic contexts, *some plosives are of longer duration than some fricatives*. Fricative sounds may be *made* long but this is a *phonetic* or articulatory activity rather than phonemic. Teaching a child to appreciate the continuous nature of fricatives by unnaturally extending the length of a sound in a word (*shhhoe*, *washhh*, for example), may not help them to pick out fricative sounds in everyday speech. After all, one would not teach a child to write capital letters and expect them to work out lower case symbols for themselves.

Mr Noisy and *Mr Quiet* are used to discuss the contrast between voiced and voiceless sounds. Voiced sounds are taught as noisy and voiceless as quiet, yet perceived voicing distinctions are not necessarily dependent upon the presence or absence of vocal fold vibration during production of the sound. In English, the contrast between word-initial voiced and voiceless plosives is not dependent upon the existence or non-existence of voicing during the closure phase of the sound, but on *voice onset time*, the point at which vocal fold vibration begins *after* release of the closure. So, in word initial voiced plosives, voicing begins immediately after release of the closure, whereas in word initial voiceless plosives, voicing begins between approximately 40 and 80 milliseconds after release. Thus, if the minimal pair *pa* and *bar* were recorded and the vowel cut out from the recording, *both* the [p] and the [b] would be voiceless.

In word final position, phonemic transcription of the two words, (the) *use*: /jus/ and (to) *use*: /juz/, may lead one to assume that the difference between these two words is that the word final fricative of (the) *use* is voiceless, whereas the word final fricative of (to) *use* is voiced. In some phonetic environments this may be the case, but even then *voicing* will not be the only acoustic difference. Denes (1955) demonstrated that, in English, 'the relative durations [lengths] of vowel and final consonant can be used as a cue for hearing the final sound as voiced or unvoiced' (p. 761). For example, if you extend the length of the vowel (but do not change production of /s/) in /jus/, the word produced will sound more like /juz/.

In fact, any two speech sounds may differ by a variety of phonetic cues (Lisker, 1978). We suggest that using terms such as *long* and *short* to differentiate between fricatives and plosives and *noisy* and *quiet* to differentiate voiced and voiceless sounds may elevate the prominence of *one* acoustic cue and make it more difficult for the child to acquire the full range of cues that are necessary for discriminating between sounds in words.

Dean and Howell advocate that the concepts *front* and *back* should be used when discussing alveolar (front) and velar (back) contrasts. Children are taught to recognise the front and back of objects (trains, people, houses etc.) and Mr F (front) and Mr B (back) are suggested as pictorial referents. Unfortunately, as [b] is a front sound Mr B can cause considerable confusion in some children. It would seem simpler to acknowledge the articulatory nature of this approach and to develop awareness of front and back of mouth using more traditional methods such as visual and tactile senses to develop awareness of the front/back of the child's own mouth.

Thus, whilst Metaphon is described as a phonological approach directed at phonologically disordered children who have no articulatory deficits, Phase 1 is in fact a *metaphonetic* approach (Grundy, 1995). That is, the metalanguage used in Phase 1 is directed at phonetic (or articulatory) activities rather than at phonological processing. It is suggested here that long/short; noisy/quiet are acoustically inaccurate terms to distinguish fricatives/plosives, voiced/voiceless sounds, and may be semantically unhelpful. Traditional articulation therapy terms such as 'snake sound' for [s]; 'dripping tap sound' for [t] are more appropriate.

Despite these concerns with the treatment suggestions included in the Metaphon package Dean and Howell's assertion that development of metaphonological skills should be a target for phonological therapy is not disputed. It has long been known that children with phonological disorders may be at risk for developing later reading and writing difficulties. Research into dyslexia indicates that children at age five with persisting speech disorders who have poor phonological awareness and poor letter-sound knowledge are at greatest risk for developing reading difficulties, particularly if there is a history of dyslexia in the family

(Snowling, 1995). Reading researchers suggest that phonological awareness training should begin with sound localisation activities, move on to
syllable segmentation tasks, rhyme awareness and onset and rhyme tasks
prior to phoneme segmentation tasks (Lundberg, Frost and Petersen,
1988; Stackhouse, 1991). For details of such activities see Hatcher
(1994). Letter–sound associations are also important to develop. We
would therefore suggest that all pictorial referents used in therapy activities should include the written word or a letter symbol ('s' with the
snake picture for example). Letterland (Wendon, 1985) is used in many
schools to develop letter–sound associations and could also be used in
clinic.

Like Dean and Howell, we would advocate that children should be
active in finding their own solutions to their phonological problems. Use
of minimal pairs in therapy seems to us to provide children with opportunities to generate such solutions. When presented with a minimal pair
and required to produce the target word, the child is thrown into a state
of disequilibrium when the adult misunderstands his or her utterance.
The child then needs opportunity to assimilate this information and to
try out a few solutions to the problem, eventually finding his or her own
solution. Potentially we interfere with this generation of solutions by the
child if we provide our own solutions to the problem. Whilst this may
help the child at that particular instant and with that particular contrast,
it may not help them to generate solutions to their difficulties when
someone is not there to guide them, or to generalise this new problem-
solving skill to other contrasts.

An alternative, then, to offering solutions is to ensure that the child
has opportunities to identify pertinent acoustic cues through presention
of minimal pairs (and sets) in perception activities. When production of
minimal pairs is attempted by the child, research indicates that better
attempts to alter an incorrect production are made when the adult indicates that they have understood the child to say a word which is unrelated to the target. Weiner and Ostrowski (1979) set up an experiment
where the child's utterance was met with one of three types of response:

1.   using the correct form, e.g. 'did you say sail?';
2.   using the child's form, e.g. 'did you say tail?';
3.   using an incorrect, unrelated form, e.g. 'did you say whale?'.

They found that children were best able to alter their production in situation 3. This may be because using such a form immediately indicates to
the child *which* phoneme in the word needs adjustment. That is, when
children have difficulty in discriminating between /s/ and /t/, for example, words like *tail* and *sail* may sound very similar to them and they
may be unable to decide how to change production of the *whole word*
in order to meet the adult's requirements. By using an unrelated form,

such as *whale*, the adult is providing the child with the information that it is the first sound of the word that needs changing.

Hodson and Paden (1991): Targeting Intelligible Speech

Hodson and Paden have developed an approach to phonological therapy through working with severely unintelligible children over a period of 15 years. Based on nine underlying principles, this programme has three key elements: cyclical planning; auditory bombardment and production practice.

Cyclical Planning is based on the principle that phonological acquisition is a gradual process. A cycle will address a number of different phonological patterns focusing on each for a minimum of two hours before moving on to the next. Hodson and Paden use a 12-week cycle. They indicate that although this is an arbitrary time-scale to fit in with school semesters it is also close to the length of time thought to be necessary for a child to acquire a new phoneme (three–four months). At the end of Cycle 1 the child is reassessed and phonological patterns identified for the next cycle. Hodson and Paden have found that children find target patterns easier to produce when they return to them in the second cycle.

Auditory Bombardment is based on the premise that children with normal hearing typically acquire the adult sound system primarily by listening. They cite research which indicates that phonologically disordered children benefit from low-level amplification of target sounds in words. Thus this part of their programme involves the child listening to a list of 15 words containing the target phoneme through earphones at slightly amplified volume for two minutes at the beginning and end of each session. Carers are required to read the list to their child daily whilst he or she plays quietly. They are instructed to speak clearly but not to over-emphasise the target phoneme.

Production Practice is based on the principle that as the child acquires new speech patterns he or she associates kinaesthetic with auditory sensations which enables later self-monitoring. This part of the programme constitutes the major part of each session. Hodson and Paden advocate the use of tactile and visual means to help the child to achieve accurate production of the target phoneme in three to five target words which have been carefully chosen to promote phonetic facilitation. They consider accurate production of the target is essential to ensure that appropriate kinaesethetic sensations develop. The child is thus engaged in several different games which provide opportunities for accurate practice of the target words. The child is also required to practise the target words once a day at home.

As its title suggests, this approach is directed at children with unintelligible speech. Hodson and Paden use the term non-phonemic alterations to describe speech patterns that we would suggest fall into the category *articulation disorder* (e.g. tongue protrusion, lateralisation, nasalisation) (1991, pp. 48–50). It would seem, then, that this approach may be suitable for children falling into any of the diagnostic categories outlined earlier in this chapter. Ingram's (1986) finding that children develop first those phonemes which occur most frequently in their native language provides theoretical justification for the approach of auditory bombardment: what they hear most they will use first. However, the heavy emphasis on production in this programme may not suit all children, or indeed all clinicians. Indeed, in some cases, the strict requirement for correct articulation may preclude the possibility of the child experimenting with sound production and gradually achieving accurate productions for him or herself.

Lancaster and Pope (1989): Working with Children's Phonology

Lancaster and Pope advocate the use of an eclectic approach. They suggest that as children develop their phonological skills through hearing speech, processing speech and producing speech all three modalities should be addressed in the remediation of unintelligible speech. Thus their book has chapters on an auditory approach, meaningful minimal contrast therapy and articulation therapy.

The Auditory Approach: Lancaster and Pope suggest that auditory input should always be included in therapy, even if it is not the predominant mode. They promote use of Hodson and Paden's auditory bombardment technique and extend the principle of auditory bombardment to *Auditory Input Therapy*. Auditory Input Therapy involves engaging the child in games which allow the clinician to make frequent use of words containing the target phoneme. They outline several innovative activities as well as simple suggestions such as modifying 'Simon says' to utilise the target phoneme, e.g. George says 'jump, jiggle, jog...'. The child responds as is appropriate to the game and there is no requirement for her or him to speak. All the suggested activities emphasise the importance of fun and of using the chosen input vocabulary in a meaningful way for the child.

Meaningful Minimal Contrast Therapy: This is a natural extension of homophony confrontation (Weiner, 1981). In homophony confrontation the child is presented with minimal pairs which are perceived as homophonous in the child's production. For example, a child who is stopping fricatives may be confronted with pictures depicting *tea* and *sea*. The child is required to say *sea* and when she or he says [ti] is understood to have said *tea*. It is anticipated in this approach that the child will then alter his or her production to become more *sea*-like. Lancaster and Pope develop this technique by suggesting a more pragmatic approach to the use of minimal pairs and sets. They offer many suggestions for entertaining games which utilise minimal pairs and can be used to work on both perception and production of the words. One of the most important aspects of MMCT is that it is meaningful. The games suggested always ensure that it is the production of the target word that will have the most appealing outcome. For example, in a *stick/tick/sick* set where the production target is *stick*, three chairs are placed in front of the children, on one is placed a picture of a clock (*tick*) on another a picture of an ill person (*sick*) on the third goodly quantities of sticky tape (*stick*). If the child is heard to say *tick* the clinician sits on the tick chair and says 'tick, tick, tick', on the sick chair the clinician sits and looks ill but on the stick chair the clinician sticks to the chair and makes humourous unsuccessful attempts to get unstuck.

Articulation Therapy: Lancaster and Pope acknowledge that some phonological disorders may have an articulatory component. Thus they present a chapter which discusses the development of articulation; the relationship between articulation and phonology; articulatory disorders; and articulatory approaches to remediation. (It is interesting to note that they refer to Metaphon within this chapter on articulation indicating that they had interpreted the Metaphon programme as articulatory in nature.) Practical suggestions for eliciting sounds and fun games for production practice are also included in the chapter.

This three-way approach may be used with children falling into any of the diagnostic categories described earlier in this chapter. Lancaster and Pope advocate that an individually tailored 'cocktail' of the three modes of therapy should be developed for use with children who have reduced intelligibility. The proportions of each mode will vary depending on the child's individual and changing needs.

All three of the above pairs of authors emphasise that intervention should be based on thorough phonological assessment and evaluation. However, none of the above approaches is supported by unequivocal research. Dean and Howell and Hodson and Paden present case studies indicating successful use of their respective approaches but there is a lack of comparative research to guide us towards the best approach for any individual child or group of children. In their own ways, all three approaches advocate simultaneous work on perception and production which appears to dispense with the necessity of deciding which to work on first. It seems appropriate to conclude that in the absence of comparative efficacy research clinicians may safely select aspects of any of these approaches. The theory presented in this chapter and personal clinical experience lead us to favour the eclectic approach of Lancaster and Pope, perhaps with the greatest emphasis on auditory input therapy.

A relatively new linguistic approach for treating children with *phonological delay* has been proposed by Hoffman (1992). He draws attention to the interrelation between different language levels citing research which suggests that phonological disorders do not simply create higher level language disorders but that there is an interdependence between the two. For example, it has been suggested that *Final Consonant Deletion* will prevent the child from indicating morphological markers such as plurality, past tense etc. Hoffman suggests that this phenomenon is not unidirectional but bidirectional. In other words, lack of grammatical knowledge (in this instance plurality and tense markers) may contribute to phonological disability (in this case final consonant deletion). Hoffman suggests that this is a more appropriate characterisation of language acquisition. The child starts with whole utterances and parses them down to smaller units rather than starting with the smallest units (speech sounds) and building up into utterances, a top-down rather than a bottom-up approach (see futher Chapter 1). This view lead Hoffman to use a whole-language approach when treating a child with a phonological delay who also had higher level language difficulties. The whole-language approach was compared with a more traditional single-word minimal-pair approach and results indicated that the phonological gains were similar for both subjects. In addition, the child who had participated in whole-language therapy had made greater gains in other language skills (Hoffman, Norris and Montjure, 1990). The success of this approach to treating phonological delay would seem to lend support to Dodd's (1987) suggestion that phonological delay may arise through an impoverished language environment. It would be interesting to evaluate this approach with children who have other types of phonological impairment.

Summary

Evershed Martin (this volume) has pointed out that the nature of developmental speech disorders has not changed. The symptoms remain the same; the child's speech will fall somewhere within the range of unclear to totally unintelligible. The causes remain the same. What has changed over recent years is our understanding of the nature of phonological disorders. Subgroups of phonologically disordered children have been identified on the basis of observed speech behaviours. Individual differences amongst children within subgroups have led researchers to focus on the individual child and to suggest that each child may have an idiosyncratic profile of abilities and deficits which contribute to their phonological disability. As Stackhouse and Wells (1994) suggest, it may be that through collating information on individual children, subgroups of phonological disorder will emerge. In the meantime, it is important to attempt to identify the specific skills and deficits in each individual child in order to create a tailored therapy programme which most effectively and efficiently facilitates changes in speech patterns.

Acknowledgements

Our thanks to Pam Grunwell for helpful comments on the final draft of this chapter.

References

Ball, M.J. (1993) *Phonetics for speech pathology*. London: Whurr.

Bamford, J. and Saunders, E. (1985). *Hearing Impairment, Auditory Perception and Language Disability*. London: Edward Arnold.

Bever, T. (1961) Prelinguistic Behaviors: A systematic analysis and comparison of early vocal and general development. Honors thesis. Cambridge: Harvard University.

Berko, J. and Brown, R. (1960). Psycholinguistic research methods. In: P. Mussen (Ed.), *Handbook of Research Methods in Child Development*. New York: Wiley.

Bird, J. and Bishop, D. (1992). Perception and awareness of phonemes in phonologically impaired children. *European Journal of Disorders of Communication* 27, 289–311.

Bradford, A. and Dodd, B. (1994). The motor-planning abilities of phonologically disordered children. *European Journal of Disorders of Communication* 29, 4, 349–370.

Bzoch, K.R. (1979). Rationale, methods and techniques of cleft palate speech therapy. In: K.R. Bzoch (Ed.), *Communicative Disorders related to Cleft Lip and Palate*. Boston: Little, Brown.

Dean, E., Howell, J., Hill, A. and Waters, D. (1990). *Metaphon Resource Pack*. Windsor: NFER-Nelson.

Denes, P. (1955). Effect of duration on the perception of voicing. *Journal of the Acoustical Society of America* 27(4), 761–764.

Dodd, B., Leahy, J. and Hambly, G. (1989). Phonological disorders in children: underlying cognitive deficits. *British Journal of Developmental Psychology* 7, 55–71.

Gibbon, F. and Hardcastle, B. (1991). Visual display of tongue-palate contact: electropalatography in the assessment and remediation of speech disorders. *British Journal of Disorders of Communication* 26(1), 41–74.

Grundy, K. (1985). *Childhood homophony: in the mouth of the child or the ear of the adult?* Unpublished MA dissertation, Leeds University.

Grundy, K. (1995). Metaphon: unique and effective? *Clinical Linguistics and Phonetics* 9(1), 20–24.

Grunwell, P. (1981). *The Nature of Phonological Disability in Children*. London: Academic Press.

Grunwell, P. (1985). *Phonological Assessment of Child Speech*. Oxford: NFER-Nelson.

Grunwell, P. (1987). *Clinical Phonology*, 2nd edn. London: Croom Helm.

Grunwell, P. (1988). Phonological assessment, evaluation and explanation of speech disorders in children. *Clinical Linguistics and Phonetics* 2(3), 221–252.

Grunwell, P. (Ed.) (1990). *Developmental Speech Disorders*. London: Churchill Livingstone.

Hahn, E. (1979). Directed home training. In: K.R. Bzoch (Ed.), *Communicative Disorders related to Cleft Lip and Palate*. Boston: Little, Brown.

Hatcher, P. (1994). *Sound Linkage: an Integrated Programme for Overcoming Reading Difficulties*. London: Whurr Publishers.

Hewlett, N. (1985). Phonological versus phonetic disorders: some suggested modifications to the current use of the distinction. *British Journal of Disorders of Communication* 20, 155–164.

Hewlett, N. (1990). Processes of development and production. In: P. Grunwell (Ed.), *Developmental Speech Disorders*. London: Churchill Livingstone.

Hodson, B.W. and Paden, E.P. (1991). *Targeting Intelligible Speech*, 2nd edn. Texas 78758: Pro-ed.

Hoffman, P.R. (1992). Synergistic development of phonetic skill. *Language, Speech and Hearing Services in Schools* 23, 254–260.

Hoffman, P.R., Norris, J.A. and Montjure, J. (1990). Comparison of process targeting and whole language treatments for phonologically delayed preschool children. *Language, Speech and Hearing Services in Schools* 21, 102–109.

Ingram, D. (1976). *Phonological Disability in Children*. London: Edward Arnold.

Ingram, D. (1986). Explanation and phonological remediation. *Child Language Teaching and Therapy* 2, 1–19.

Kent, R.D. (1992). The biology of phonological development. In: C.A. Ferguson, L. Menn and C. Stoel-Gammon (Eds), *Phonological Development*. Maryland: York Press.

Lancaster, G. and Pope, L. (1989). *Working with Children's Phonology*. Oxford: Winslow Press.

Leonard, L.D. (1985). Unusual and subtle phonological behaviour in the speech of phonologically disordered children. *Journal of Speech and Hearing Disorders* 50, 4–13.

Lewis, M.M. (1951). *Infant Speech: a Study of the Beginnings of Language*, 2nd edn. London: Routledge & Kegan Paul.

Lisker, L. (1978). Rapid vs rabid: a catalogue of acoustic features that may cue the distinction. *Haskins Laboratories Status on Speech Research* (SR-54). New Haven, CT: Haskins Laboratories.

Locke, J.L. (1989). Babbling and early speech: continuity and individual differences. *First Language* 15, 663–668.

Locke, J.L. and Pearson D.M. (1992). Vocal learning and the emergence of phonological capacity. In: C.A. Ferguson, L. Menn and C. Stoel-Gammon (Eds), *Phonological Development*. Maryland: York Press.

Lundberg, I., Frost, J. and Petersen, O.P. (1988). Effects of an extensive program for stimulating phonological awareness in preschool children. *Reading Research Quarterly* 23, 263–284.

Macken, M.A. and Barton, D. (1979). The acquisition of the voicing contrast in English: a study of voice onset time in word-initial stop consonants. *Journal of Child Language* 7, 41–74.

Milloy, N. (1991). *Breakdown of Speech*. London: Chapman & Hall.

Morley, M.E. (1970). *Cleft Palate and Speech*, 7th edn. Edinburgh: Churchill Livingstone.

Morley, M.E. (1972). *The Development and Disorders of Speech in Childhood*, 3rd edn. Edinburgh: Churchill Livingstone.

Oblak, P. and Kozelj, V. (1984). Basic principles in the treatment of cleft at the university clinic for maxillofacial surgery in Llubljana and their evolution in thirty years. In M. Hotz, W.M. Gnoinski, M.A. Perko, H. Nussbaumer and E. Hof (Eds), *Early Treatment of Cleft Lip and Palate*, Proceedings of the Third International Symposium. Zurich: Hans Huber.

Parker, A .(1986). *Phonological assessment and speech therapy for hearing-impaired people*. Paper presented at 1986 BAAL Seminar, Leicester Polytechnic.

Phillips, B.J.W. (1979). Stimulating syntactic and phonological development in infants with cleft palate. In: K.R. Bzoch (Ed.), *Communicative Disorders related to Cleft Lip and Palate*. Boston: Little, Brown.

Piaget, J. (1962). *Play, Dreams, and Imitation in Childhood*. New York: Norton.

Priestly, T. (1980). Homonymy in childhood. *Journal of Child Language* 7(2), 413–427.

Snowling, M. (1995). *Identifying specific learning difficulties (dyslexia) in the early years*. Paper presented at Literacy Development and Difficulties in the Early Years: a day conference on specific learning difficulties (dyslexia), Leicester University.

Stackhouse, J. (1991). Promoting reading and spelling skills through speech therapy. In: P. Fletcher and D. Hall (Eds), *Specific Speech and Language Disorders in Children*. London: Whurr Publishers.

Stackhouse, J. and Wells, B. (1993). Psycholinguistic assessment of developmental speech disorders. *European Journal of Disorders of Communication* 28(4), 331–348.

Stampe, D. (1979). *A Dissertation on Natural Phonology*, Ed. I. Hankamer. New York: Garland.

Stark, R. (1980). Stages of speech development in the first year of life. In: G. Yeni-Komshian, J.F. Kavanagh and C.A. Ferguson (Eds), *Child Phonology, Vol. 1: Production*. New York: Academic Press.

Stoel-Gammon, C. (1992). Prelinguistic vocal development. In: C.A. Ferguson, L. Menn and C. Stoel-Gammon, *Phonological Development, Models, Research, Implications*. Maryland: York Press.

Trost-Cardamone, J.E. (1990). Speech in the first year of life: a perspective of early speech acquisition. In: D.A. Kernahan and S.N. Rosenstein, *Cleft Lip and Palate: A System of Management*. Baltimore: Williams & Wilkins.

Van Riper, C. and Irwin, J.V. (1958). *Voice and Articulation*. Englewood Cliffs, NJ: Prentice-Hall.

Van Kleek, A. and Richardson, A. (1988). Language delay in children. In: N. Lass, L. McReynolds, L. Riothern and D. Yoder (Eds), *Handbook of Speech–Language Pathology and Audiology*. Toronto: B.C. Decker.

Weiner, F.F. and Ostrowski, A.A. (1979). Effects of listener uncertainty on articulatory inconsistency. Journal of Speech and Hearing Disorders, 44, 4, 487–493.

Weiner, F.F. (1981). 'Treatment of phonological disability using the method of mean-ingful minimal contrast: two case studies. *Journal of Speech and Hearing Disorders* 46, 97–103.

Wendon, L. (1985) Letterland. Dorking, Surrey: Templar Publishing Limited.

Appendix

Example of Developmental and Deviant Phonological Processes (Bradford and Dodd, 1994)

Developmental Processes	*Deviant Processes*
Final consonant deletion	Initial consonant deletion of a class of phonemes
Cluster reduction	
Weak syllable deletion	Medial consonant deletion
Reduplication	Intrusive consonants
Prevocalic voicing	Backing
Final consonant devoicing	Medial consonant substitutions
Fronting of fricatives and velars	Denasalisation
Stopping of fricatives and affricates	Devoicing of a class of phonemes
Gliding	Sound preference substitutions
Deaffrication	Use of non-native language phonemes
Assimilation	

Chapter 15
Acquired Neurogenic Speech Disorders: Applying Linguistics to Treatment

NIKLAS MILLER AND GERRY DOCHERTY

A fast-expanding literature incorporating detailed speech and language analyses of normal and disordered performance has brought great advances over recent years in our understanding of *how* language and movement relate to produce normal and atypical speech, *what* is happening in disordered speech and *why* it might be happening.

Clinicians specialising in the field of acquired speech disorders have benefited greatly from this literature. An exposition of the theoretical and practical questions raised by these trends is, however, beyond the scope of this chapter. The aim here is more modest: to outline the contribution of linguistic insights to the treatment of these disorders. The linguistic perspective is examined in terms of: (a) the theoretical framework that it provides for looking at issues related to speech treatment; (b) the implications of this for assessment and the link between assessment and therapy; and (c) what indications are suggested for targets and techniques in therapy from a linguistic perspective.

A Theoretical Framework

The classification and differential diagnosis of motor speech disorders has been beset by theoretical and practical arguments probably more than any other area of patho-linguistics. Clinicians have felt justified in ignoring theoretical issues related to assessment and treatment because, they claim, theoreticians have not considered day-to-day clinical factors and what patients really do or don't do. Theoreticians have rebuked some clinicians for applying bits of theory in a piecemeal, haphazard fashion and failing to take cognisance of well-established experimental facts. It is important for theory builders not to forget the real-life situations that their theories are meant to account for. At the same time it is important that clinicians have insight into what package of assumptions they are buying when they pick a particular taxonomy of disorders, method of assessment or path to treatment. This first section highlights some assumptions behind current views of acquired neurogenic speech disorders, and looks at some consequences they have for applying linguistics in this area.

Speech, like writing, manual signing and typing is a medium, composed of physical movements. Its function, however, is to convey meaning. One argument runs that extracting meaning from speech rests first on the ability to identify structures, word boundaries and sounds within the words. Linguists analyse speech in this way and many assessments reflect this segmental perspective. It is important to remember, though, that speech (as you are sure to testify if you have tried to understand a foreign language you do not know well) consists of a continuous stream of interweaved movement and corresponding overlapping sounds. Instrumental recordings do not display a string of separate segments, either at phoneme, word or phrase level. This already hints at a principle to follow in therapy: whilst many assessment approaches might deal in discrete units and static postures, therapy must aim for connectivity, contrast and dynamism.

The interweaving of these continuous speech movements, however, is not arbitrary. It grows out of a complex interaction between the properties of moving systems and the organisation of the language being spoken (Lindblom, 1990b). This gives an immediate problem in the description and explanation of normal and disordered speech. How are language and movement related? How can one reconcile mental units (phonemes, words etc.) with physical units – e.g. the mechanical forces of moving masses, gravity, inertia, elasticity, acceleration, velocity; the electrochemical reactions of nerve impulses? Numerous solutions answer this in quite different manners. It is important to understand these as they offer quite different explanations for the aetiology of disorders and how they should be assessed and treated.

Hierarchical Models of Speech Production

A central feature of these models (there are several versions) is that there is some kind of central command or programme for a (set of) movement(s), which once initiated is unfolded level by level from the top of the hierarchy to the bottom. The central programme contains all information that is required for the command to drive execution. Successive levels simply translate elements of the command from one set of units into another until they are realised as sounds (Buckingham, 1986; Abbs, 1988; Miller, 1989a for overview). These models present a strict demarcation between syntactic-semantic and phonological processing on the one hand and motor planing and control on the other.

Within those broad divisions a further split exists between syntax and semantics and phonology and between so-called higher cortical aspects of action planning (praxis) and more 'peripheral' aspects of sensori-motor functioning. The general scheme for producing a spoken word involves a semantic 'module', which passes information to a phonological component that 'looks up' phonemes and the associated abstract sound specifications required for the word. This information in turn is passed down to a motor speech 'module' where the previously looked-up abstract phonological strings are 'mapped' on to or translated into motor commands for the movements to produce the sounds. These commands, finally, are directed to muscles to produce the target sounds.

This view is reflected in the traditional demarcation between dysphasia, phonemic paraphasia, speech dyspraxia and the dysarthrias. These are seen as linked to breakdown in the different modules and can be differentially diagnosed according to the characteristic 'errors' associated with dysfunction at the particular level – e.g. selection and ordering of phonemes, undershooting of articulators owing to articulator weakness. Different therapeutic strategies are deemed appropriate according to which underlying process is believed to be at fault.

Such perspectives have been criticised on several grounds (Fowler, 1985; Wilson and Morton, 1990; Weismer and Liss, 1991; Miller, 1989a for overview). For the purposes of this chapter – the diagnosis of motor speech disorders and the choice of intervention strategies – the main problem centres around the relationship between the planning and execution of sound strings, i.e. traditional phonology, and the planning and execution of the motor commands to produce the sounds. The hierarchical view just sketched saw the sound and motor components as strictly segregated. The 'sleight of hand' (Fowler, 1985, p.195) by which the phonological specifications are translated into movement specifications hides, however, a theoretical flaw. As Jackson long ago summarised in his famous footnote (1878), 'physical units cannot fine away into mental units'.

This raises important questions: amongst them, is it possible to maintain theories where abstract units become concrete, physical entities, and if so how? If not, how can one couch units of description and/or explanation in equivalent terms that do not need translation across a whole process? How does one describe how the acoustic signal and its perception by the listener emerges from the total effect of simultaneous operations (neuropsychological, physiological, mechanical, etc.) each with its own degree of autonomy?

None of these conundrums is solved by traditional hierarchical accounts. Nor are they felt by many to be able to cope adequately in a descriptive or explanatory way with much of the behaviour observed in speech. For example, without abandoning the tenets of fixed top-down translation from one module to another, hierarchical models have difficulty accounting for the apparent source of semantic errors in the phonological component or vice versa (Caramazza and Hillis, 1990;

Caramazza and Miceli, 1990). The finding of apparent 'motor'-based errors in what is considered an abstract phonological sphere (e.g. McNeil, Liss, Tseng and Kent, 1990) would also pose problems. Further, the notion that broader syntactic and semantic context can influence speech and its intelligibility (Hammen, Yorkston and Dowden, 1991) sits uncomfortably in such a model. These observations suggest at least a degree of bottom-up (i.e. peripheral influencing more central) as well as top-down interaction between putative components, if not hinting at a wholly different organisation.

Coalitional Models of Speech Production

Attempts to form an interactive, unified (that is of phonology with action, movement) description of speech production have taken, and are taking, several forms. Fowler (1985, 1986) has been associated with moves towards a solution of the psychological–physiological divide by developing a physical description of perception and production of speech. The articulatory phonology of Browman and Goldstein (1990) and the task-dynamic approaches of Saltzman and Munhall (1989) – see Hawkins (1992) for review – have developed notions of phonology in which sound production is described in terms of physical parameters, such as, for instance, the gestures of articulatory phonology. Workers such as Stevens (1989), or Ohala (1990) have moved in a similar direction, but on a different path, premising their accounts of speech production on the properties and functioning of the vocal tract as an integrated physical instrument for producing sound. Lindblom (1990a) begins from another point on this path, asking what it is about the properties of a speech production–perception system that results in there being a finite set of sounds/contrasts used in human speech despite a vastly greater perceptual-motor capacity. If these properties could be identified (Stevens, 1989, is one possible answer) then it could serve as a basis for a unified explanation of speech production–perception, with its implications for speech pathology and therapy. This chapter is not the place to discuss these directions in detail (see Hardcastle and Marchal, 1990; Docherty and Ladd, 1992; Docherty and Miller, in preparation). Suffice it to say that, in shaping linguistic contributions to the treatment of acquired speech disorders, they dictate a quite different rationale from hierarchical approaches where operations happen in a strict sequence of separate steps.

In particular, coalitional models stress an interactive, integrative perspective on description, diagnosis and treatment. Phonology without movement is mute; but action without phonology would be amorphous. Language variables interact with speech variables; phonological variables integrate with motor factors; emergence of the acoustic signal is subject to influence from speaker–listener interaction. A target sound is no longer viewed as the inevitable outcome of a fixed programme run off in a predetermined fashion through an invariant line of commands. There is not a straightforward reductionist-style retrievability or explanation of units at one 'level' of programming from another by simple translation of features. There is no one-to-one, simple linear correspondence between neuropsychological, physiological, kinesic, acoustic or perceptual variables. Rather, sound is an emergent phenomenon: it arises from the total interaction (e.g. of airflow through the interlocking, moving parts of the whole vocal tract; of acoustic signal with listener perception and awareness of the surrounding syntactic-semantic context) of all the contributory variables, rather than residing in any one level independently. No supposed 'level' is necessarily a prime locus of control, the source of the whole command. Control grows out of concerted action, or the locus shifts according to the demands of the internal and external (to the speaker) demands of the environment.

Such a perspective makes it pointless to speak of phonemic versus phonetic in any orthodox sense of the distinction; it is misleading to separate language from motor influences on sound production and perception. Recognition of this has brought a re-examination of assessment and treatment approaches. These changes are reflected in the work of, for instance, Folkins and Bleile (1990) who examined these implications for a taxonomy of speech disorders; Crary (1993) who emphasised the interaction in his motolinguistic model of assessment and intervention; Weismer and Liss (1991) who stressed qualitative and non-reductionist approaches to the analysis of disordered speech; or Vogel and Miller (1992) whose treatment approach stresses a top-down direction in tandem with the more traditional bottom-up departure.

The lack of a one-to-one relationship between units of perception, acoustics and so on, and the non-fixed nature of where dominant control lies in production and perception, both complicates and simplifies the assessment and treatment task. It complicates it in so far as it becomes very difficult to extricate (consciously or unconsciously applied) compensatory strategies from what might be considered primary loci of breakdowns. For example, is a perceived speech error the result of a correct specification of production parameters distorted by peripheral problems of muscle tone, or is it the outcome of faulty specification with a later attempt at correction? On the other hand, the therapist's task is simplified because (a) there is not necessarily a prime node of breakdown (e.g. so-called phonological stores, or mapping processes), so it becomes more important to describe how manipulation of variables influences speaker-productive outcome or listener-perceptual reaction/success; and (b) the same adaptability of the system overall can be exploited in therapy to shift the locus of control away from problem areas of production (see below).

Linking Assessment and Therapy: Functional Features

What kind of indications does this approach have for questions one might ask of assessment and the shape and direction therapy might take? This section establishes some markers for the direction.

The strength of linguistic and phonetic input to management is that it can provide the knowledge and descriptive framework for describing the components of communicative acts from their broad social setting down to the millisecond minutiae of vowel duration variation. This enables clinicians to identify the key factors in the person's behaviour leading to communication breakdown and to define the goals and subgoals required to restore effective intelligibility. It also provides a principled and reliable system of description to monitor change.

As indicated in the last section, clinicians should not be misled into assuming that the link between motor disorder and language disorder is a one-way, one-to-one relationship. Because the vocal tract operates as an integrated unit, breakdown in one structure or function is not automatically predictive of impairment overall. A deficit in one (linguistic and/or motor) component can negatively influence a coupled but unimpaired component. Conversely, intact components may cover up disability in the impaired area. As Ludlow and Bassich (1983, p. 122) neatly summarise, 'walking is no more the direct result of the strength of the biceps femoris than speech impairment can be directly reflected by the strength of contraction of the orbicularis oris'. The data of Abbs, Hunker and Barlow (1983) highlighted the hazards of taking a one-to-one cause–effect view and inferring from the acoustic or perceptual judgements to underlying pathophysiology in a particular speech–language subsystem. The cerebral palsied speaker, they report, demonstrated how different speech subsystems (tongue and lips in this case) can be subject to different degrees and type of impairment. Dworkin and Aronson (1986) illustrate how articulator strength, alternate motion rates and intelligibility are not necessarily predictive of each other.

Some more examples help illustrate this further. What are heard or seen as similar characteristics arise from varying underlying pathologies. Imprecise consonants could stem from reduced range or mistiming of movements (themselves of multiple aetiology) or poorly fitting dentures, or a combination of these and other factors. Breakdowns in some dimensions will have more effect on intelligibility than others. Loss of /θ~t/ from English, for example, does not have a drastic effect on communication, but the loss, especially inconsistent loss, of /k~t/ would be quite different. Excessive but equal stress can be detrimental to listeners' motivation to continue attending, even though it may not unduly alter intelligibility, whereas unpredictable changes in speech rhythm might impair the speaker much more (see also Chapter 10). Mild to moderately imprecise consonants across the board could still serve as a basis for effective speech. However, if in addition there were poor breath support and incompetent velum, either of the latter two could seriously tip the balance towards non-intelligibility.

Hence, two people with what sounds like the same disorder and apparently identical physical deficits might nevertheless vary in what has brought about their speech disorder and unintelligibility. This is why it is important to carry out not only a physical (oral) examination and linguistic analysis, but also an assessment of intelligibility (below) and a functional assessment to ascertain what the person actually can and does do with the means at his or her disposal. Such procedures would preferably be conducted in the person's habitual environment – with a hearing-impaired spouse and noisy background, for example.

Assessment I

The technique of diagnostic intelligibility testing (Weismer and Martin, 1992) is one way of achieving this. Instead of giving coarse estimations of the overall severity of speech impairment, this technique seeks to establish – through controlled elicitation and responses to minimal pair utterances – which speech variables contribute, and to what degree, to the loss of intelligibility. This might be the effects of syllable complexity; of the loss/impairment of syllable or word initial consonants versus syllable/word final sounds. From an articulatory angle it might examine the effects of impairment to particular articulatory positions or manners of articulation. The effects of altered phonation, resonance, rate and loudness can also be looked at. One can contrast success in conveying information in single words versus sentences. Other potentially potent factors looked at might include the correlation between inconsistency of realisation of sounds, or the extent of preparatory struggle, and the degree of intelligibility. Attempts have been made to develop measures that quantify the effects of different losses on intelligibility overall (Leinonen-Davies, 1988; Connolly, 1989) and these might be gainfully adapted to choosing and prioritising targets for therapy.

In the context of diagnostic assessment, instrumental acoustic and articulatory techniques for speech analysis offer the possibility of a fine-grained account of which speech variables are implicated in a reduction in intelligibility. In addition they provide a quantitative base-line against which to measure any change in a speaker's performance. Almost every aspect of impaired speech production can be investigated by making use of a diversity of 'physiological' techniques for studying aspects of articulation. These range from respiratory activity (Till and Alp, 1991; Solomon and Hixon, 1993), through to laryngeal functioning (Olson Ramig, 1992), articulatory kinematics (Hunker, Abbs and Barlow, 1982; Schönle *et al.*, 1987; Forrest, Weismer and Turner, 1989; Forrest *et al.*,

1991; Svensson, Henningsow and Karlsson, 1993), linguo-palatal contact (Hardcastle and Edwards, 1992), velopharyngeal function (Netsell, 1969), and even the firing patterns of individual muscles (Forrest *et al.*, 1991, Hartman and Abbs, 1992).

Whilst these 'physiological' techniques offer an analysis resolution beyond that achievable by even the well-trained auditory system, a disadvantage associated with their use is that they are, in some cases, invasive, resulting in difficult-to-quantify compensatory activity by the speaker which degrades the quality of the data which are provided. Equally problematic is the fact that the data which these techniques provide are often extremely complex and difficult to interpret (see, for example, Ladefoged and Fromkin,1969, on interpreting EMG signals, or Solomon and Hixon, 1993, and Hoit, 1994, on the interpretation of respiratory traces). In recent years, acoustic techniques have been used increasingly in studies of clinical speech, partly because of their non-invasive nature, and the reasonably well-understood relationship between acoustic characteristics of speech and underlying articulatory parameters (Kent and Rosenbek, 1983; Weismer *et al.*, 1988; Ackerman and Ziegler, 1991; Forrest *et al.*, 1991; Seikel, Wilcox and Davis, 1991; Square-Storer and Apeldoorn, 1991; Ansel and Kent, 1992; Kent *et al.*, 1992, Le Dorze *et al.*, 1992, Weismer *et al.*, 1992; Hertrich and Ackermann, 1993; Schlenk, Bettrich and Willmes, 1993; Ziegler, Hartmann and Hoole, 1993; Leuschel and Docherty, 1995).

To a certain extent clinicians have always striven towards pinpointing key factors affecting a speaker's communication, but diagnostic intelligibility testing and the added detail of instrumental assessments offer a structured, reliable way of measuring speech status at any point and across time which was not realised by earlier methods. However, although diagnostic intelligibility testing can potentially offer important insights into the nature of a speaker's impairment, it is important to bear in mind that speech perception, and consequently speech intelligibility and understanding, is a function of what Lindblom (1990b) refers to as *signal-dependent* and *signal-independent* information.

Signal dependent refers to all of the information present in the acoustic waveform which impinges on the listener's peripheral auditory system. Signal independent refers to the huge amount of 'top-down' processing carried out by the listener during speech perception. In normal speech communication, the listener does not blindly attempt to parse the incoming signal in order to decode the message which it represents. As alluded to earlier, listeners make great use of the context in which a word or utterance is embedded in order to reduce the processing required to deduce the message being received. In some cases the contextual cues are extremely powerful and, even with a very degraded signal, the listener could most likely decode the message. In other cases, the context is less helpful, and the listener must rely to a greater extent on the information in the speech signal.

As well as using the discourse context, listeners appear to adopt a range of listening strategies in order to facilitate the task of parsing connected speech signals and identifying the meaning of the corresponding utterance. One such strategy is that, when attempting to identify words from within a stream of connected speech, listeners tend to rely on stressed syllables which (at least in English) are particularly robust acoustically, resistant to degradation, and informative about the location of word-boundaries in connected speech (Cutler and Foss, 1977; Cutler and Norris, 1988; Cutler, 1994). This interactive, contextual versus acoustic, top-down/bottom-up strategy for speech perception has (at least) two important implications for assessment of acquired speech disorders (cf. Weismer and Martin, 1992 for a more detailed review of these issues).

First, it is possible that the active listening strategies employed by listeners may not adapt easily to the impaired segmental and prosodic patterns present. For example, in many types of dysarthric speech, the listener has to depend to a greater extent than usual on signal-dependent information (but from a signal which may be significantly degraded by virtue of the speech impairment). Indeed, as pointed out by Weismer and Martin (1992, p. 68), it is conceivable that 'speech intelligibility deficits are as much in the ear of the listener as they are in the mouth of the speaker'. Second, the fact that listeners make great use of context in speech perception means that assessments of intelligibility based on single-word recognition scores (i.e., by definition, providing no context) do not necessarily give a clear view of how intelligible the subject is in a more normal speech communication situation where speaker and listener have a shared context for their interaction.

Assessment II

Intelligibility testing is complemented by oral physical examination. Knowledge of the functioning of the component parts of the vocal tract assists the clinician when making decisions as to why the particular perceptual features prevail. Careful differential assessment of the lips, tongue, velum and so on (the point place model of Rosenbek and LaPointe, 1985) will uncover deficits which may be contributing to the picture – be it alterations of manner of articulation, loss of a place of articulation, or whatever. But, discovering spasticity, flaccidity or mistiming, or establishing a problem with tongue-tip raising is not necessarily the whole story. A discrete point perspective must take on a broader horizon from here.

A common experience is to find movement at any one point to be roughly within normal limits, or disorder appearing restricted to one anatomical component, yet intelligibility markedly impaired. If it is recalled that speech is a result of the integrated operation of the whole cognitive-linguistic and vocal tract physical systems, it becomes clear how such pictures arise. Mediocre tongue function in isolation may not stand out. However, when disordered tongue action is integrated with other articulators, it not only fails itself, but, in so doing, can interfere with the otherwise normal movement elsewhere. Thus it is important to assess not only isolates but also movement areas and couplings – e.g. mouth, velopharyngeal port, larynx, respiration, which interact to effect articulation, resonation, phonation. Rosenbek and LaPointe (1985) term the examination of speech features that depend on concerted action across articulators the *process model* of assessment. Through this the clinician observes aspects of speech which depend on the smooth running of the whole of the vocal tract.

Assessing linkages enables possible interactive breakdowns to be identified. For example, imprecise consonants may have been perceptually identified as an isolated feature contributing to unintelligibility. Point-place evaluation might have established that tongue and lips are performing within normal limits. Process assessment might disclose that the imprecise consonants are caused by poor intra-oral breath pressure due to velopharyngeal incompetency. Here work on lips and tongue would have been fruitless – the primary problem was velar dysfunction. As another example, in moderate dyspraxia, treatment priority is likely to be coordination of function between subsystems such as respiration, the larynx and tongue for voice onset/termination time, rather than sounds in isolation.

A further potentially informative component of functional speech assessment is maximum performance tests (Kent, Kent and Rosenbek, 1987), including such indicators as maximum phonation duration, maximum diadochokinetic (DDK) rate, 's/z' ratio, F_0 range, and maximum sound pressure level. The rationale for these tests may not be immediately obvious because the tasks are un-speech-like in nature. However, what these tests do is provide the therapist with information about the extremes of performance which an individual speaker is capable of. They delimit the edges of the vocal performance space available to an individual speaker. Whilst normal speakers' speech production is usually carried out well away from the margins of performance (cf. Lindblom's [1990b] account of the hyper–hypo speech continuum), as pointed out by Kent *et al.* (1987), it could be important to identify a restricted performance space.

This is because it could have implications for a speaker's ability to capitalise on the plasticity of speech motor control in order to compensate articulatorily for their impairment. Furthermore, for a speaker with a restricted space, it is possible that speech production could be particularly effortful, compared with normal speakers, with consequences for communicative efficiency. Maximum performance tests are relatively easy to carry out, and have a quantitative basis which makes them useful for monitoring changes in a speaker's overall vocal performance. However, they require careful interpretation owing to the presence of high inter-speaker variability on some of the measures, because of the inadequacies of the published normative data (see Kent *et al.*, 1987, for a detailed review of these techniques), and because of the uncertainty of their relationship with functional success of communication.

Stepping from Assessment to Therapy

After detailing all the factors contributing to the communication picture, a rank-order list of crucial variables should be drawn up. This will be derived from answers to the questions: what is causing the greatest deficit for the listener trying to understand the person's speech – and what, in turn, is causing that?

In some instances the motor deficit is not open to influence, as in motor neurone disease or progressive muscular dystrophy. In such cases therapy will have to consider how language variables (e.g. length of words and utterances; non-verbal signals for turn taking) can be accommodated to motor constraints. This introduces an important notion that should not be restricted solely to severe and progressive disorders. Rehabilitation for motor speech disorders is not just a matter of physical therapy for linguistic ends. There is a constant reciprocity. Therapy is not necessarily to restore motor function in order to make good linguistic shortcomings. Rather, at any one time, the aim will be to provide optimal language functioning within the given motor constraints. Through their interaction and interdependence, motor and linguistic strengths can be manipulated at one point to compensate for weaknesses at another. Lexicon, syntax, phonology and phonetics can be accommodated to restricted movement. A lost contrast normally signalled through sound, e.g. number or tense marking, can be signalled syntactically or lexically. For example, 'He come yesterday'; 'The girl, they like walking', are instances where the loss of plural -s is disambiguated by *they* and a poorly pronounced *came* by yesterday.

This fluidity of control and interdependence of components is in keeping with a coalitional heterarchical top-down and bottom-up view of speech-motor control. Such an attitude does not so rigidly compartmentalise into traditional categories such as phonological–phonetic, language–speech, dysphasic–dyspraxic–dysarthric, planning–execution disorder. It is in agreement with the rationale for therapy introduced by Luria (1970) of intra- and intersystemic reorganisation. *Intra-systemic therapy* tackles a problem head on – for example, improve tongue strength and speed to gain better contact with the alveolar ridge for production of /t d n/. *Intersystemic reorganisation* utilises intact skills in one system to compensate for or circumvent problems in another – for example, adjusting phrase length to breath capacity; using suprasegmental features to substitute changes in syntactic structure; using a mechanical aid to supplement or replace spoken communication.

Linguistic input is obviously but one dimension of therapy for acquired speech disorders. Communication involves the entire social and physical environment. Linguistic manipulation should be integrated into an overall plan and attitude to communication which treats not only the whole person, but their whole environment. An ideal setting in terms of listener attitude and support, background noise, lighting and so on must be created. All listeners must know the methods, attitudes and advice which most facilitate communication. This assumes even more significance in degenerative disorders where language and physical therapy cannot stem a rising tide of disability. Maximising communication, not just speech comprehensibility, must be the aim from the start. Hence with many people augmentative or alternative means of making themselves understood should partner more direct motor-speech rehabilitation, and may, in the long term, assume primacy as the communicative media. Further, people with dysarthria or dyspraxia may have other difficulties which should not be neglected – such as problems of mobility, feeding, drinking, drooling, toileting, pain, emotional lability and low self-esteem. Also, before proceeding with a more detailed discussion of treatment, it is probably worth remembering some facts about the disorders which are the subject of concern here, and which in their turn will also shape intervention.

Acquired speech disorders are not a homogeneous group. There are major divisions between speech dyspraxias, dysarthrias and other acquired speaking disorders, such as neurogenic stuttering (Deal and Cannito, 1992). Within these areas there are important sub-classifications such as ideational, ideomotor and so-called kinetic dyspraxias (Buckingham, 1986; Miller, 1986; Square-Storer, 1989; Hartman and Abbs, 1992); cerebellar, spastic, flaccid dysarthrias, and so on. Acquired speech disorders also form a heterogeneous group from the point of view of cause and course. Some conditions may expect to improve to (near) premorbid levels or to a stable plateau of impairment. Others are degenerative, irreversible over longer or shorter periods, with steady or stepwise decline which no amount of therapy, no matter how elegantly structured and applied, is going to reverse. Disorders may or may not be open to pharmacological or surgical influence. The multiple aetiologies also mean that the pronunciation disorder may be complicated by diverse associated problems – dysphasia, dysphagia, perceptual disturbances, limb deficits, visual and hearing impairment and so on.

Corresponding to this variety is an equally varied task in differential diagnosis, and in selecting appropriate therapeutic approaches. Detailed guidelines for differential diagnosis between disorders are not given here. They may be found in more general works (e.g. Wertz, LaPointe and Rosenbek, 1984; Johns, 1985; Square-Storer, 1989; Dworkin, 1991;

Vogel and Cannito, 1992). Diagnosis in terms of assigning a label of spastic dysarthria, ataxic dysarthria, or whatever, may have some worth when it comes to deciding on the appropriateness of some non-linguistic techniques (e.g. icing, brushing, drugs). As far as communication therapy is concerned, however, the prime aim of differential diagnosis is likely to be to determine which factors in sound production and perception correlate most highly with unintelligibility and which variables when manipulated produce the greatest gains for intelligibility. The concentration of this chapter is on these linguistic aspects of the task. It is taken that this does not imply neglect of all other aspects (which are covered in other works cited), including training the listener as much as training the speaker (Miller, 1989b; Vogel and Miller, 1992).

Treatment

Choice of Targets

This section looks at some direct ways in which linguistic knowledge can be applied to intervention for motor speech disorders. In teaching reacquisition of sounds, articulatory phonetics supplies the knowledge of how and where to place the articulators. Therapists may need to explain verbally, pictorially and by touch which articulators have to be placed where, and in what manner. They also need to be able to instruct the person on what he or she needs to do to produce a plosive, a fricative, an affricate, and so on, once this positioning has been achieved. This involves knowledge not just of static positions, but of movement. *What* has to move, *when* (timing, coordination) and *where to* (direction). This serves as an example of how even the most elementary lessons of phonetics are applicable in clinic.

Which sound(s) to start with will be suggested by several factors: the speech sound inventory; which sound(s) if stabilised or reintroduced are going to give the most significant improvement to intelligibility; what motor problems are present, and how much open to influence they are; which sounds are easiest for the individual and therapist to approach (visibility, manipulability, feelability, of the place and movement). In so far as speech is synonymous with movement, it is recommended to incorporate movement awareness and instruction from the start. Thus the person is taught not just static positions, but the feeling of speed, pressure, duration (of contact, etc.) and direction involved in moving on to and off articulatory configurations.

It is only in the severest cases that a person will have to start (re)constructing articulatory gestures and their corresponding sounds from scratch. For most people there will be some achievable and stable sounds already. In such cases techniques of *phonetic derivation* can be helpful. This is a technique whereby one sound is derived via progressive approximation from another. For example /ʃ/ from /s/, /s/ from /t/, /tʃ/ from /t+ʃ/. A sound might also be derived from a non-verbal gesture, such as blowing a kiss, biting the bottom lip.

For some people, attaining a particular articulatory posture may be impossible in isolation and certainly in context, even when using bursts of continuous exaggerated movement. The clinician can consider whether there is any alternative way of producing the same sound or whether another sound could stand for the unattainable segment in given situations – for instance, producing /f/ as a bilabial [ɸ]; [t d] for /θ ð/; [ŋ] for /n/; /m/ as [m̩]; /s/ as [ds] or [ts] and so on.Vowel distortions that do not create any contextual ambiguities might also be permitted. For example, collapsing the distinctions between *pier* and *pear* either to /ɪə/, /ɛə/ or a neutral /ɜ:/; or *not* and *nut* to /nat/, are unlikely to cause misunderstandings in context.

The theoretical underpinnings for these ideas are the notions of motor and perceptual equivalence. According to the former the same end result can be achieved via different motor positions/movements, i.e. in speech the same sound can be produced with quite different articulatory configurations; according to the latter, despite two sounds being produced with apparently the same articulatory setting, the perceptual end result can be two different sounds for the listener. Edwards and Miller (1989), and Hardcastle and Edwards (1992) demonstrated with electropalatography that normal-sounding speech of people with dyspraxia can be produced with what would be considered atypical articulatory activity in standard articulatory phonetics textbooks. The same has been demonstrated for normal speakers (Maurer *et al.*, 1993; Gentil, 1992).

Sometimes, however, a collapsed distinction does lead to confusions. If this is not resolvable through other methods, knowledge of articulatory and acoustic phonetics may give the clinician access to alternative solutions. A common difficulty is what is perceived by the listener as a loss of the voiced/voiceless distinction. In English, perception of this distinction does not rest solely on the vibration of the vocal folds. It is signalled in numerous ways, including the length of the preceding or following vowel, and by presence or absence of aspiration on (syllable initial) plosives. The clinician can assess which of these factors are not being used by the speaker. This is an instance where instrumental analyses can prove invaluable. The aim in therapy then would be either to tackle the deficient signal directly, (e.g. practice in producing aspiration if that cue is lacking) or by enhancing other cues to help the listener to hear a difference – for instance contrasting a long and short vowel to give the impression of voiced vs voiceless consonant. Instrumental feedback is ideal to support therapy here (see below).

A further example might be with labial and/or mandibular weakness, especially when bilateral, where problems may arise with /w/ /p/ or /b/. If mandibular support (e.g. collar) does not solve the problem, therapists can at least work at gaining sufficient variation in the acoustic phonetic cues that distinguish /p~w/. /w/ can be given a more vocalic nature, extending it to /u/, or an artificial pause inserted to simulate the closure phase of /p/. Again, instrumental back up (e.g. sound spectrography) would be ideal here. Success *vis-à-vis* listener perception can be carefully monitored by designing and carrying out labelling/discrimination tests to see if the ideal graph (e.g. Borden, Harris and Raphael, 1994) is reached. By manipulating (combinations of) variables (e.g. vowel length, aspiration) clinicians can see whether the speaker's performance comes any closer to the desired profile.

The essence of speech is not just movement. It is movements organised into a system of contrasts which, in context, take on meaning. Hence, as soon as possible, contrasts should be introduced. Again, assessment should have alerted the clinician to contrast collapses that are having a marked effect on intelligibility. Otherwise the order of contrasts introduced should reflect a balance between usefulness and ease of attainment. For one person it might be voiced–voiceless bilabials; for another oral–nasal bilabials; for another bilabials–alveolars, and so on. In some instances the problem will not be (re)establishing a sound but stabilising it. The same principles of knowing which features of place, manner and movement need to be emphasised through auditory, visual and tactile channels will apply in therapy.

Once a sound is stabilised it can be exercised in varying syllable structures – CV, VC, VCV, and CVC. As before, if the sound can be practised and contrasted in contexts which listeners are likely to confuse (e.g. *he/she/tea is in the dining room; That's my friend Ray/Roy/Ria; is that the right/white/light wine*), the aim of working towards intelligible, even if not perfect, speech is fulfilled. Some syllable structures will prove easier than others. Therapists might therefore gainfully experiment to see which is easiest for the individual and work from there. Linguistic data plus motor assessment can suggest which combinations of V + C to use, and later, when consonant clusters are introduced, which combinations.

For instance, it may be better to pair alveolar consonants with close front vowels, and velars with close back vowels, thereby lessening the degree of tongue adjustment from one to the other. Clusters like /tr ts/ may be easy for some by virtue of their sharing place of articulation. /bl/ /fl/ have the advantage that, at least in isolated syllables, the person has the opportunity to position their tongue for the second element without interfering with the first. However, large adjustments in articulator configuration are required which some people will find difficult. Similarly, if the cluster contains multiple changes in manner as well as place, this can add insuperable complexity, e.g. *sm* entails a switch not only from alveolar to bilabial and fricative to frictionless continuant, but also voiceless to voiced and oral to nasal. The lesson is, carefully match features, their totals, and the number needing change between two positions. More about syllable problems is included below.

Ease in Connected Speech

Despite carrying out some or all of the therapies mentioned so far and introducing other known facilitators for improving articulation, such as speed control (including using various types of pacer) and motor rehabilitation, the hoped-for gains may still not have been achieved and speech may continue to be poorly intelligible. In particular there may exist a large discrepancy between sounds and syllables in isolation and accurate realisation of the same in connected speech. In people with dysarthria the cause may be reduced tone, power, coordination and sensation in any or all the structures involved in speech production. In individuals with speech dyspraxia the underlying difficulty is one of effecting the fine space–time planning changes necessary to move from one target sound to another (Ziegler, 1989; Hardcastle and Edwards, 1992; but see too Katz et al., 1990).

Whichever is the case, more effective speech may be achieved through attention to the demands made in transitions which may suggest certain controlled trade-offs between permitted imperfections and intelligibility. For example, a commonly reported way to ease transitions in consonant clusters is to insert a schwa. So *green* becomes [gəɹin]; *clips* becomes [kəlɪps]; *scone* a [səkɔn]. A variation on this is to place a schwa at the start or end of the cluster sequence, in effect transferring the segment neighbouring the schwa to a separate syllable, e.g. *stay* [əs'teɪ]; *build* ['bɪldə].

The technique of altering syllable boundaries has uses beyond schwa insertion. Whole strings can be rendered more simple (articulatorily). For example 'It's like a steam roller', which has a complex VCCCVCVC-CVCCVCV(C) structure can be changed to a regular V-CV-CV-CV-CV-CV-CV-CV-CV-(C) by producing it as [tɪ zə laɪ kə sə ti mə ɹəʊ lə(ɹ)] thus accommodating it to people only able to cope with CV syllables. Those managing VC syllables best could say [ɪt ɪz əl aɪk əs ət im əɹəʊl ə(ɹ)] . The same can be applied to polysyllabic words or C_1VC_2 words where C_2 interferes with C_1 or where there are initiation difficulties. For example: *biscuit* [bɪsəkɪtə]; *a cake* [ək eɪk].

Maintaining stability of sounds in syllables across syllable boundaries can also be encouraged by controlled choice of sounds and structure of preceding and succeeding syllables, following the same principles outlined earlier. Thus the initial /k/ in *cake* could be anticipated by a context of *big cake*. If syllable final sounds tend to be the unstable ones, the same can be applied. The anticipation of /k/ in *cake* could have been used to assist the /g/ in *big*. The final /t/ in *hot* might improve in the setting *hot tea*.

Even where there are no bothersome clusters, building up to polysyllabic words using single-syllable 'bricks' proves a useful avenue. For people with dyspraxia with their greater likelihood of success with familiar real words and for those to whom the idea of splitting words into syllables is foreign, the following technique can help. *Neurology* can be worked towards via the real words: *new*, then *new row*, then *new row low*, and finally *new row low G*; *majority* via *may+jaw + re + tea*.

Splitting up into syllables can make speech sound too unusual for some, even if it improves their ability to communicate. One way of making speech sound more natural, which also has the advantage of decreasing the number and extent of necessary motor adjustments and improving fluency, is to teach chunks and words with assimilatory processes included. Thus you teach *ham + bag* rather than [hænd bæg]; [gɹiŋ kʌl(ɪ)] rather than [gɹin kʌlə(ɪ)] (green colour); and [ɪsə] not [ɪtɪzə] for *it is a*. For speech dyspraxic subjects, where disintegration of co-articulation is believed to be a significant feature, this should prove a particularly advantageous procedure. In general, though, this should remind clinicians that sounds occur in words and words in connected speech. Therapy should be geared towards this and not stick at the static decontextualised stage of isolated postures.

When syllable-level utterances are possible, therapy may need to stabilise the syllabic nucleus (Odell *et al.*, 1991; Schlenck, Bettrich and Willmes, 1993). Unpredictable or unstable nuclei are a significant factor in comprehensibility. Therapy involves developing control over laryngeal and respiratory parameters, topics covered at length in the dysarthria treatment works cited above.

Suprasegmental Aspects of Speech

Suprasegmental variation is introduced here as a useful method for increasing functional communication despite limited sound production means. If effective control over pitch and loudness (in turn resting on respiratory, laryngeal and supralaryngeal effectiveness) can be gained, then several grammatical and affective signals can be conveyed. In English as in other languages, pitch movement can provide important meaning cues (Couper-Kuhlen, 1986). Feelings of certainty, doubt and so on can also be signalled through manipulation of suprasegmental features (see also Chapter 10, this volume). Linguistic assessment will have ascertained the tones of which the person is capable. Knowledge of the tone patterns a language utilises, and the crucial articulatory-acoustic variables involved in producing them, enables the therapist to decide (a) whether the person, given their motor status, is capable of producing the necessary patterns, and (b) how to elicit and control these variables.

Contrastive stress drills may facilitate maximum use of minimum resources, though recent research indicates that this may not be so for all motor speech disordered speakers (Liss and Weismer, 1994). To capitalise on these drills it is assumed the person has access to basic phrases (subject–verb at least). By manipulating stress and intonation different implications of a statement can be conveyed. For example 'you're coming' can be said as a statement, question or command. According to how it is spoken it can also contrast *you* with a supposed alternative (she, we, etc.), *coming* with *going*, *are* with *are not*. 'The old man won some money' can be given different nuances in response to different questions such as: 'Which man won some money? Did the bald man win some money? Did he lose some money? Did he win some whisky?' (See also Chapter 10, this volume.) Minimal pair work can be incorporated here at any level (compare the *he–she–tea* example above).

Other types of stress and intonation drill borrow from real-life situations where these linguistic features occur in a predictable and limited range of variations: for example, reading football results, the shipping forecast, station/airport announcements, recipes and the like. Words can be chosen to reflect the sounds, syllable structure and stress patterns being currently worked on, e.g. *Tottenham 2 – Totterdown 10*, for practising /t/; *Celtic 6 – Selkirk 7*, for /s/. Hargrove and McGarr (1994) detail integrated programmes for managing different aspects of prosody.

Such drills are especially useful for those with limited syntax or lexicon. It permits them to produce different meanings with the same basic syntactic structure. In these cases another productive drill is using a carrier word or phrase (*I wanna; I'm gonna; it's a...*) with contrastive stress to give different meanings with different filler words. For example, *I'm gonna come* with interrogative intonation to ask 'am I coming, can I come' contrasts with the use of imperative intonation to mean 'I will come' or 'I insist on coming'.

Paradoxically, teaching abnormal stress and intonation, as a temporary or permanent strategy, may benefit some patients. Such patients typically have weak breath support, very slow articulator movements, or rapid fatigue leading to decreased movement range even though they might have attained the target position initially. Some people with dyspraxia may have particular difficulty moving from stressed to unstressed syllables, or vice versa, losing or severely distorting the unstressed element. In cases like these giving each syllable full and equal stress may assist. Thus, 'early becomes ['ɜ(ɪ)'li]; *undo* becomes ['ʌn'du]; *po'tato* becomes ['pʌ'teɪ'təu]. Intelligibility may be helped even more by inserting a pause or extra small inspiration between syllables to forestall deletion or contamination across syllables (Yorkston *et al.*, 1990). Speakers often adopt their own compensatory strategies along these lines (e.g. Hunter, Pring and Martin, 1991; the case report by Vance, 1994).

The technique also helps when incorporating a sound into a multisyllable word. If it can be arranged on to the stressed one, or stress altered to accommodate this, success is more likely. Thus, it might be easier to introduce /d/ into 'Deeside before in de'cide or alter decide temporarily to 'de'cide or ' decide.

The Broader Context

Throughout the progression from single sound or simple syllable to connected phrase level output, or as speech has to be gradually scaled down in degenerative conditions, linguistics provides a framework and guidelines for principled change. The choice of syllable structure and sound patterns within it and the controlled introduction and manipulation of some suprasegmental features have been mentioned. Useful gains may also be made by attending to syntactic and lexical variables. This will be specially pertinent where the speech disorder presents with a concomitant dysphasia.

In people with dyspraxia of speech the precise relationship between syntactic loading/complexity and articulatory breakdown remains unresolved, but there are cases where syntax clearly does influence performance. Care must be taken, when (re)introducing or stabilising a sound, not to undermine success by stretching syntactic and morphological complexity too soon.

In most people with dysarthria, when there is no accompanying language or cognitive deficit, it will be the length rather than the syntactic complexity of utterances which requires control. Limited breath capacity, movement range and speed may demand that utterances be made in a series of short phrases, and ways need to be found of producing grammatical variety within the same length of utterance. If longer utterances are used, therapy may attend to identifying natural boundaries for insertion of breath intakes without loss of intelligibility.

For some individuals with speech dyspraxia the greater the propositional weight on an utterance – i.e. the more conscious deliberate planning has to go into it – the more speech is influenced negatively. Less familiar words tend to be more in error than ones used daily. At certain stages in remediation this might become a crucial variable to control. It can help people with dyspraxia and/or dysarthria if syntactically and propositionally undemanding structures are used which enable them to concentrate on the sound/movement in question. Hence it should be easier to concentrate on /k/ realisation in cup of coffee than in composer Kodály. Some aspects of speech–language interaction in intelligibility are broached by Miller (1989b), Hammen, Yorkston and Dowden (1991), and Vogel and Cannito (1992).

Dysphasia, severe dyspraxia or severe dysarthria may restrict some people to reliance on a limited number of words with limited syllable structure. In such instances the choice of sounds, syllable structures and content must be chosen wisely to permit maximum communication with minimum words. The stress and intonation exercises outlined above may expand possibilities somewhat, but in such severe cases augmentative or alternative means of communicating may be indicated.

Instrumental Support for Therapy

Up to now little mention has been made of the possibilities afforded by articulatory and acoustic instrumentation which, as well as providing very useful assessment information, can also have a role as a provider of biofeedback during a therapy programme. Many instrumental techniques permit real-time visualisation of relevant speech production parameters, enhancing the speaker's awareness of those parameters, and thereby potentially leading the speaker to greater control over them.

Instrumental techniques which have been used in this way include spectrography (Maki *et al.*, 1981), electromyography (Carman and Ryan, 1989), and electropalatography (Morgan Barry, 1989; Goldstein *et al.*, 1994). Whilst these techniques can be very useful, it is important to emphasise the potential nature of the learning which can be achieved in this way. Merely exposing a speaker to a visual representation of his or her own speech performance does not automatically lead to the speaker learning how to control the relevant parameters, any more than seating the speaker in front of a mirror gave the instant cure to placement problems without the therapist teaching the person what to observe and how to control movements. Application of such techniques requires some understanding of the complex factors which underlie learning of complex motor skills.

This is not the place for a review of such factors (see Schimdt, 1991). However, as an example of the type of issue that is relevant to the use of biofeedback techniques, it is interesting to point to the increasing evidence in the motor-learning literature which suggests that learning is enhanced by the provision of more restricted feedback (Wulf and Schmidt, 1989; Wulf, Schmidt and Deubel, 1993). This finding runs contrary to the prevailing view that more frequent and more informative feedback will enhance learning. A further difficulty with many of the available real-time visual displays of speech production is that the image which is produced is extremely complex, and innaccessible without specialist knowledge. With this in mind, attempts have been made to convert the raw instrumental images into a more user-friendly form for the purposes of application in therapy; eg. the Speechviewer system for monitoring of acoustic parameters (LeDorze *et al.*, 1992; Barry, 1994).

Evaluating Other Intervention Through Linguistics

Knowledge of linguistic correlates of communication breakdown can also contribute to decisions regarding other means of intervention, such as medical or surgical. To know whether these are going to have a beneficial effect on speech it is necessary to know: (a) what features of linguistic impairment are linked with loss of intelligibility, (b) what underlying impairment (tone, power, coordination, sensation; site of impairment...) is bringing about the linguistic picture, both points which have been discussed in the assessment sections earlier, and (c) whether the proposed intervention will effect the desired change in the variables of (a) and (b).

A case in point could be prosthetic or surgical management of velopharyngeal function. Speech and language assessment must identify whether or not soft palate dysfunction is a major contributing factor to poor communication. If it is, prostheses or surgery may help. If it is not, then time, effort and morale are being squandered. The same applies to other treatments.

Drug therapy may ameliorate some features in Parkinsonian speech, but not necessarily all. In upper motor neuron lesions anti-spastic drugs might appear to be indicated. However, the speech clinician must establish whether it is the alleged hypertonus influencing speech, or variables beyond this. Abbs, Hunker and Barlow (1983) provide a prime example of where a drug regime would have been contra-indicated in their case of spastic dysarthria. It could be that instead of expensive and possibly harmful drugs a straightforward alveolar plate (with roughened surface to increase sensory awareness) would suffice. Again, linguistically informed speech evaluation should predict this.

Amplifiers may suit some people with quiet voices. However, the clinician must ask: is it merely the quietness that is impairing speech, or would providing an amplifier simply enable the person to project a dysarthrophonic voice further and highlight even more their poor articulation? In such cases tackling articulation and voice quality would have to precede (artificial) amplification. This process of cause–effect establishment applies to similar cases: for example, use of a bite block to stabilise the mandible, cervical collar to support the mandible; or abdominal girdle for supporting the stomach wall and diaphragm.

New products are forever appearing on the market. Clinicians need to be able to weigh up their worth. Careful consideration of which linguistic variables may and may not be helped will enable an evaluation of the makers' claims, general usefulness and specific applicability.

Conclusion

The direction here has been to outline a framework and rationale for relating (linguistic) assessment and therapy, and in so doing give a flavour of some of the ways in which linguistic training can apply to therapy for motor speech disorders. Though not exhaustive, the intention was to provide some practical examples within a broader disciplined setting.

The essential messages are that, first, linguistics provides a principled framework and descriptive method for analysing and measuring communicative performance. It provides the background theory and knowledge for (a) what is normal speech, (b) what variables interact to produce normal intelligible speech and therefore, in turn, (c) what features might be targets for therapy and be manipulated to regain effective communication. The detailed analyses possible within a linguistic framework enable the clinician to target precise loci of breakdown, thereby making therapy at once directly relevant and parsimonious. Time and effort are not wasted on coincidental or irrelevant features that would not effect improvement, even if they could be rehabilitated. Linguistics also makes possible the careful charting of progress (or deterioration) on several levels and breaking down of therapy into graded subgoals. This is vital if therapy efficacy is to be measured.

There are two important lines of influence on linguistic elements within the domain of motor speech disorders. Sound is produced by movement, and this is dependent on motor planning and execution. Speech and, in turn, speech therapy, is for social ends and not merely an academic exercise in phonetic and phonological analysis. Thus, intervention must relate the linguistic to the motor and social contexts. It has been stressed that the relationship between linguistic variables and either of these is not a direct one-to-one affair. Although this makes the search for solutions (theoretical and practical) more complex, it nevertheless permits a flexible approach to disorders. Each element (motor, linguistic, social) is interdependent on the others, as are variables within these elements (planning, execution; voice onset time, formant transition time, release burst; listener familiarisation etc.). This opens the door to therapy which reorganises and redistributes which variables are given prominence in gaining intelligibility within and across the motor–linguistic–social triad.

It is further stressed that, whilst linguistics enables an exhaustive assessment of communication parameters from macrosocial down to microphonetic, it is not necessary to apply this in a wholesale manner. Clinicians need not encumber themselves with endless data, nor speech-impaired individuals with endless tests. Linguistic knowledge should also permit a clinician to select judiciously those assessments and therapy resources that will lead to selective and effective application of that knowledge. Finally, one may note that a broad linguistic approach is compatible with, and supportive of, a whole-person, whole-context attitude to communication.

References

Abbs, J. (1988). Neurophysiologic process of speech movement control. In: N. Lass *et al.* (Eds), *Handbook of Speech Language Pathology and Audiology*. Toronto: Decker.

Abbs, J., Hunker, C. and Barlow, S. (1983). Differential speech motor subsystem impairments with suprabulbar lesions: neurophysiological framework and supporting data. In: W. Berry (Ed.), *Clinical Dysarthria*. San Diego: College Hill Press.

Ackerman, H. and Ziegler, W. (1991). Articulatory deficits in Parkinsonian dysarthria: an acoustic analysis. *Journal of Neurology, Neurosurgery & Psychiatry* 54, 1093–1098.

Ansel, B.M. and Kent, R. (1992). Acoustic phonetic contrasts and intelligibility in dysarthria associated with mixed cerebral palsy. *Journal of Speech & Hearing Research* 35, 296–308.

Barry, S. (1994). Review of Speechviewer 2. *Child Language Teaching and Therapy* 2, 206–213.

Borden, G., Harris, K. and Raphael, L. (1994). *Speech Science Primer*, 3rd edn. Baltimore, MD: Williams & Wilkins.

Browman, C. and Goldstein, L. (1990). Tiers in articulatory phonology: with some implications for casual speech. In: J. Kingston *et al.* (Eds), *Papers in Laboratory Phonology 1*. Cambridge: Cambridge University Press.

Buckingham, H. (1986). Scan copier mechanism and the positional level of language production. *Cognitive Science* 10, 195–217.

Caramazza, A. and Hillis, A. (1990). Where do semantic errors come from? *Cortex* 26, 95–122.

Caramazza, A. and Miceli, G. (1990). Structure of the lexicon. In: J.-L. Nespoulous *et al.* (Eds), *Morphology, Phonology and Aphasia*. Berlin: Springer-Verlag.

Carman, B. and Ryan, G. (1989). Electromyographic biofeedback and the treatment of communication disorders. In: J.V. Bakmajian (Ed.), *Biofeedback: Principles and Practice for Clinicians*. Baltimore, MD: Williams & Wilkins.

Connolly, J. (1989). Functional linguistic analysis and the planning of remediation. In: P. Grunwell *et al.* (Eds), *The Functional Evaluation of Language Disorders*. London: Croom Helm.

Couper-Kuhlen, E. (1986). *Introduction to English Prosody*. London: Edward Arnold.

Crary, M. (1993). *Developmental Motor Speech Disorders*. London: Whurr Publishers.

Cutler, A. (1994). Segmentation problems, rhythmic solutions. *Lingua* 92, 81–104.

Cutler, A. and Foss, D.J. (1977). On the role of sentence-processing in speech perception. *Language Speech* 20, 1–10.

Cutler, A. and Norris, D. (1988). The role of strong syllables in segmentation for lexical access. *Journal of Experimental Psychology: Human Perception and Performance* 14, 113–121.

Deal, J. and Cannito, M. (1992). Acquired neurogenic dysfluency. In: D. Vogel and M. Cannito (Eds), *Treating Disordered Speech Motor Control*. Austin, TX: Pro-ed.

Docherty, G. and Ladd, D. (Eds) (1992). *Papers in Laboratory Phonology II*. Cambridge: Cambridge University Press.

Docherty, G. and Miller, N. (in preparation). The phonetics–phonology issue in speech disorders.

Dworkin, J. (1991). *Motor Speech Disorders: a Treatment Guide*. St Louis, MO: Mosby.

Dworkin, J. and Aronson, A. (1986). Tongue strength and alternate motion rates in normal and dysarthric subjects. *Journal of Communication Disorders* 19, 115–132.

Edwards, S. and Miller, N. (1989). Electropalatographic sudy of dyspraxic misarticulation. *Clinical Linguistics & Phonetics* 3, 111–126.

Folkins, J. and Bleile, K. (1990). Taxonomies in biology, phonetics, phonology and speech motor control. *Journal of Speech & Hearing Disorders* 55, 596–611.

Forrest, K., Adams, S., McNeil, M. and Southwood, H. (1991). Kinematic, electromyographic, and perceptual evaluation of speech apraxia, conduction aphasia, ataxic dysarthria and normal speech production. In: C. Moore *et al.* (Eds), *Dysarthria and Apraxia of Speech*. Baltimore, MD: Brookes.

Forrest, K., Weismer, G. and Turner, G.S. (1989), Kinematic, acoustic, and perceptual analyses of connected speech produced by Parkinsonian and normal geriatric adults. *Journal of the Acoustical Society of America* 85, 2608–2622.

Fowler, C. (1985). Current perspectives on language and speech production – a critical review. In: R. Daniloff (Ed.), *Speech Science*. London: Taylor & Francis.

Fowler, C. (1986). *An event Approach to the study of speech perception from a direct realist perspective.* Journal of Phonetics 14, 3–28.

Gentil, M. (1992). Variability of motor strategies. *Brain & Language* 42, 30–37.

Goldstein, P., Ziegler, W., Vogel, M. and Hoole, P. (1994). Combined palatal-lift and EPG-feedback therapy in dysarthria: a case study. *Clinical Linguistics & Phonetics* 8, 201–218.

Hammen, V., Yorkston, K. and Dowden, P. (1991). Index of contextual intelligibility. In: C. Moore *et al.* (Eds), *Dysarthria and Apraxia of Speech*. Baltimore, MD: Brookes.

Hardcastle, W. and Edwards, S. (1992). EPG-based description of apraxic speech disorders. In: R. Kent (Ed.), *Intelligibility in Speech Disorders*. Amsterdam: Benjamins.

Hardcastle, W. and Marchal, A. (1990). *Speech Production and Speech Modelling*. Amsterdam: Kluwer.

Hargrove, P. and McGarr, N. (1994). *Prosody Management of Communication Disorders*. London: Whurr Publishers.

Hartman, D. and Abbs, J. (1992). Dysarthria associated with unilateral upper motor neuron lesion. *European Journal of Disorders of Communication* 27, 187–196.

Hawkins, S. (1992). Introduction to task dynamics. In: G. Docherty *et al.* (Eds), *Papers in Laboratory Phonology II*. Cambridge: Cambridge University Press.

Hertrich, I. and Ackermann, H. (1993). Acoustic analysis of speech prosody in Huntington's and Parkinson's disease – a preliminary report. *Clinical Linguistics & Phonetics* 7, 285–297.

Hunker, C.J., Abbs, J. and Barlow, S.M. (1982). The relationship between Parkinsonian rigidity and hypokinesia in the orofacial system: a quantitative analysis. *Neurology* 32, 749–754.

Hunter, L., Pring, T. and Martin, S. (1991). Use of strategies to improve speech intelligibility in cerebral palsy. *British Journal of Disorders of Communication* 26, 163–174.

Jackson, H. (1878). On affections of speech from disease of the brain. *Brain* 1, 304–330.

Johns, D. (Ed.) (1985). *Clinical Management of Neurogenic Conmunication Disorders*, 2nd edn. Boston: Little, Brown.

Katz, R., Machetanz, J., Orth, U. and Schönle, P. (1990). Kinematic analysis of anticipatory coarticulation in the speech of anterior aphasics using electromagnetic articulography. *Brain & Language* 38, 555–575.

Kent, R. (Ed.) (1992). *Intelligibility in Speech Disorders*. Amsterdam: Benjamins.

Kent, R., Kent, J.F. and Rosenbek, J.C. (1987). Maximum performance tests of speech production. *Journal of Speech & Hearing Disorders* 52, 367–387.

Kent, J., Kent, R., Rosenbek, J.C., Weismer, G., Martin, R., Sufit, R. and Brooks, B.R. (1992). Quantitative description of dysarthria in women with amyotrophic lateral sclerosis. *Journal of Speech & Hearing Research* 35, 723–733.

Kent, R. and Rosenbek, J.C. (1983). Acoustic patterns of apraxia of speech. *Journal of Speech & Hearing Research* 26, 231–249.

Ladefoged, P. and Fromkin, V. (1969). Electromyography in speech research. *Phonetica* 15, 219–242.

Le Dorze, G., Dionne, L., Ryalls, J., Julien, M. and Oullet, L.(1992). The effects of speech and language therapy for a case of dysarthria associated with Parkinsons disease. *European Journal of Disorders of Communication* 27, 313–324.

Leinonen-Davies, E. (1988). Assessing the functonal adequacy of children's phonological systems. *Clinical Linguistics & Phonetics* 2, 257–270.

Leuschel, A. and Docherty, G.J. (1995). Prosodic assessment of dysarthria: effects of sampling task and issues of variability. In: Robin, D., Yorkston, K. and Beukelman, D. (Eds), *Disorders of Motor Speech: Assessment, Treatment and Clinical Characterization*, pp. 155–178. Baltimore, MD: Paul H. Brookes.

Lindblom, B. (1990a). On the notion of possible speech sound. *Journal of Phonetics* 18, 135–152.

Lindblom, B. (1990b). Explaining phonetic variation. In: W. Hardcastle *et al.* (Eds), *Speech Production and Speech Modelling*. Amsterdam: Kluwer.

Liss, J. and Weismer, G. (1994). Selected acoustic characteristics of contrastive stress production in control geriatric, apraxic, and ataxic dysarthric speakers. *Clinical Linguistics & Phonetics* 8, 45–66.

Ludlow, C. and Bassich, C. (1983). Results of acoustic and perceptual assessments of two types of dysarthria. In: W. Berry (Ed.), *Clinical Dysarthria*. San Diego, College Hill Press.

Luria, A. (1970). *Traumatic Aphasia*. The Hague: Mouton.

Maki, J., Gustafson, M.S., Conklin, J.M. and Humphrey-Whitehead, B.K. (1981). The speech spectrographic display: interpretation of visual patterns by hearing-impaired adults. *Journal of Speech & Hearing Disorders* 46, 379–387.

Maurer, D., Gröne, B., Landis, T., Hoch, G. and Schönle, P. (1993). Re-examination of the relation between the vocal tract and the vowel sound with electromagnetic articulography in vocalisations. *Clinical Linguistics & Phonetics* 7, 129–143.

McNeil, M., Liss, J., Tseng, C. and Kent, R. (1990). Effects of speech rate on the absolute and relative timing of apraxic and conduction aphasic sentence production. *Brain & Language* 38, 135–158.

Miller, N. (1986). *Dyspraxia and its Management*. Beckenham: Croom Helm

Miller, N. (1989a). Apraxia of speech. In: C. Code (Ed.), *Characteristics of Aphasia*. London Taylor & Francis.

Miller, N. (1989b). Using the functional approach in the rehabilitation of acquired dysphasia. In: P. Grunwell and A. James (Eds.), *Communicative Perspectives in Clinical Linguistics*. Beckenham: Croom Helm.

Morgan Barry, R. (1989). EPG from square one: an overview of electropalatography as an aid to therapy. *Clinical Linguistics and Phonetics* 3, 81–91.

Netsell, R. (1969). Evaluation of velopharyngeal function in dysarthria. *Journal of Speech and Hearing Disorders* 34, 113.

Odell, K., McNeil, M., Rosenbek, J. and Hunter, L. (1990). Perceptual characteristics of vowel and prosody production in apraxic, aphasic and dysarthric speakers. *Journal of Speech & Hearing Research* 34, 67–80.

Ohala, J. (1990). There is no interface between phonology and phonetics. *Journal of Phonetics* 18, 153–171.

Olson Ramig, L. (1992). The role of phonation in speech intelligibility: a review and preliminary data from patients with Parkinson's disease. In: R. Kent (Ed.), *Intelligibility in Speech Disorders*. Amsterdam: Benjamins.

Rosenbek, J. and LaPointe, L. (1985). The dysarthrias. In: D. Johns (Ed.), *Clinical Management of Neurogenic Communication Disorders*, 2nd end. Boston: Little, Brown.

Saltzman, E. and Munhall, K. (1989). A dynamical approach to gestural patterning in speech production. *Ecological Psychology* 1, 333–382.

Schlenck, K.-J., Bettrich, R. and Willmes, K. (1993). Aspects of disturbed prosody in dysarthria. *Clinical Linguistics & Phonetics* 7, 119–128.

Schmidt, R. (1991). *Motor Learning and Performance: From Principles to Practice*. Champaign, IL: Human Kinematics Books.

Seikel, J.A., Wilcox, K. and Davis, J. (1991). Dysarthria of motor neuron disease. *Journal of Communication Disorders* 23, 417–431.

Schönle, P.W., Grabe, K., Wenig, P., Hohne, J., Schrader, J. and Conrad, B. (1987). Electromagnetic articulography: use of alternating magnetic fields for tracking; movements of multiple points inside and outside the vocal tract. *Brain & Language* 31, 26–35.

Solomon, N.P. and Hixon, T. (1993). Speech breathing in Parkinson's disease. *Journal of Speech & Hearing Research* 36, 294–310.

Square-Storer, P. (Ed.) (1989). *Acquired Apraxia of Speech in Aphasic Adults*. London: Taylor & Francis.

Square-Storer, P. and Apeldoorn, S. (1991). An acoustic study of apraxia of speech in patients with different lesion loci. In: C. Moore et al. (Eds), *Dysarthria and Apraxia of Speech*. Baltimore, MD: Brookes.

Stevens, K. (1989). On the quantal nature of speech. *Journal of Phonetics* 17, 3–45.

Svensson, P., Henningson, C. and Karlsson, S. (1993). Speech motor control in Parkinson's disease: a comparison between a clinical assessment protocol and a quantitative analysis of mandibular movements. *Folia Phoniatrica* 45, 157–164.

Till, J. and Alp, L. (1991). Aerodynamic and temporal measures of continuous speech in dysarthric subjects. In: C. Moore et al. (Eds), *Dysarthria and Apraxia of Speech*. Baltimore, MD: Brookes.

Vance, J. (1994). Prosodic deviation in dysarthria: a case study. *European Journal of Disorders of Communication* 29, 61-76.

Vogel, D. and Cannito, M. (Eds) (1992). *Treating Disordered Speech Motor Control*. Austin, TX: Pro-ed.

Vogel, D. and Miller, L. (1992). Top down approach to treatment of dysarthric speech. In: D. Vogel and M. Cannito (eds) *Treating Disordered Speech Motor Control*. Austin, TX: Pro-ed.

Weismer, G., Kent, R., Hodge, M. and Martin, R. (1988). The acoustic signature for intelligibility test words. *Journal of the Acoustical Society of America* 84, 1281–1289.

Weismer, G. and Liss, J. (1991). Acoustic/perceptual taxonomies of speech production deficits in motor speech disorders. In: C. Moore et al. (Eds), *Dysarthria and Apraxia of Speech*. Baltimore, MD: Brookes.

Weismer, G. and Martin R. (1992). Acoustic and perceptual approaches to the study of intelligibility. In: R. Kent (Ed.), *Intelligibility in Speech Disorders*. Amsterdam: Benjamins.

Weismer, G., Martin, R., Kent, R. and Kent, J. (1992). Formant trajectory characteristics of males with amyotrophic lateral sclerosis. *Journal of the Acoustical Society of America* 91, 1085–1098.

Wertz, R., LaPointe, L. and Rosenbek, J. (1984). *Apraxia of Speech and its Management*. New York: Grune & Stratton.

Wilson, W. and Morton, K. (1990). Reconsideration of the action theory perspective on speech motor control. *Clinical Linguistics & Phonetics* 4, 341–362

Wulf, G. and Schmidt, R. (1989). The learning of generalized motor programs: reducing the relative frequency of knowledge of results enhances memory. *Journal of Experimental Psychology: Learning, Memory, Cognition* 15, 748–757.

Wulf, G., Schmidt, R. and Deubel, H. (1993). Reduced feedback frequency enhances generalized motor program learning but not parameterization learning. *Journal of Experimental Psychology: Learning, Memory, Cognition* 19, 1134–1150.

Yorkston, K., Hammen, V.L., Beukelman, D.R. and Traynor, C.D. (1990). The effect of rate control on the intelligibility and naturalness of dysarthric speech. *Journal of Speech & Hearing Disorders* 55, 550–560.

Ziegler, W. (1989). Anticipatory articulation in aphasia: more methodology. A reply to Sussman *et al.* and Katz. *Brain & Language* 37, 172–176.

Ziegler, W., Hartmann, E. and Hoole, P. (1993). Syllabic timing in dysarthria. *Journal of Speech & Hearing Research* 36, 683–693.

Index

385